Anaesthesiology and Resuscitation
Anaesthesiologie und Wiederbelebung
Anesthésiologie et Réanimation

40

Editores

Prof. Dr. R. Frey, Mainz · Dr. F. Kern, St. Gallen
Prof. Dr. O. Mayrhofer, Wien

Ketamine

Bericht über das internationale Symposion
am 23. und 24. Februar 1968 in Mainz

Herausgegeben von

H. Kreuscher

Mit 94 Abbildungen

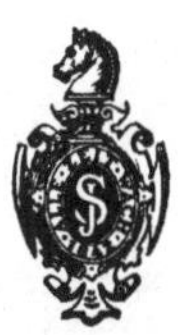

Springer-Verlag Berlin Heidelberg New York 1969

ISBN-13: 978-3-540-04412-3   e-ISBN-13: 978-3-642-99958-1

DOI: 10.1007/978-3-642-99958-1

Titel-Nr. 7396

Vorwort

Der vorliegende Band der Schriftenreihe befaßt sich mit einem neuen parenteralen Narkosemittel. Er ist ein vollständiger Bericht über das internationale Symposion, das am 23. und 24. Februar 1968 in Mainz veranstaltet wurde.

Wissenschaftler aus Belgien, Deutschland, Frankreich, Jugoslawien, den Niederlanden, Österreich, Schweden, der Schweiz und den USA berichteten und diskutierten über ihre Erfahrungen mit dem neuen injizierbaren Narkosemittel Ketamine.

Dieses Symposion sollte dazu beitragen, einerseits den derzeitigen Stand unseres Wissens und unserer Erfahrungen mit Ketamine, andererseits Lücken in der Erforschung der klinischen Anwendbarkeit dieses Mittels zu erkennen.

Damit wurde zum zweiten Male in Deutschland die Eignung eines neuen Narkosemittels vor seiner Einführung in den Arzneimittelhandel im Rahmen eines Symposions zwischen erfahrenen Fachleuten öffentlich diskutiert. Das rege Interesse wurde durch die Teilnahme von über 200 Anaesthesisten, Pharmakologen und Toxikologen aus 9 Ländern offenbar.

Allen Teilnehmern, insbesondere den Referenten und Korreferenten sowie Diskussionsrednern, sei auch an dieser Stelle für ihren Beitrag zum Gelingen des Symposions gedankt.

Mainz, im Februar 1969   R. FREY und H. KREUSCHER

Inhaltsverzeichnis

I. Die pharmakologischen Grundlagen von Ketamine

(Vorsitz: G. KUSCHINSKY, Mainz)

II. Klinische Untersuchungen

(Vorsitz: G. CORSSEN, Birmingham, Alabama und M. ZINDLER, Düsseldorf)

III. Klinische Erfahrungen

(Vorsitz: R. Frey, Mainz, M. Gemperle, Genf und J. Lassner, Paris)

Verzeichnis der Referenten

Beaumanoir, A., Dr. Hôpital Cantonal, Dép. d'Anesthésiologie, Genf

Benke, A., Dr., Facharzt f. Anaesthesie, Wien, Klosterneuburgerstraße

Böhmert, F., OMR., Dr., Anaesthesie-Abt., Städt. Krankenhaus Bremen

Bornemann, F., cand., med. Institut für Anaesthesiologie d. Universität Mainz

Brunckhorst, B., Dr., Anaesth.-Abt., Univ.-Krh. Hamburg-Eppendorf

Chen, G., Dr., Fa. Parke, Davis & Co., Ann Arbor, Michigan (USA)

Corssen, G., M. D., Medical Center, University of Michigan, Ann Arbor (USA)

Dangel, P., Dr., Anaesthesieabteilung, Kinderspital Zürich

Dillon, J. B., M. D., Prof., UCLA Med. School, Los Angeles, Californien (USA)

Doenicke, A., Priv.-Doz., Dr. Chirurg. Poliklinik München

Dudeck, J., Dr., Inst. f. Med. Statistik u. Dokument

Eckart, I., Dr., Anaesth.-Abt., Städt. Rud.-Virchow-Krankenhaus, Berlin

Emmert, K., Dr., Chirurgische Poliklinik München

Fuchs, S., Dr., Inst. f. Anaesthesiologie der Universität Mainz

Gauch, H., cand. med., Inst. f. Anaesthesiologie der Universität Mainz

Gemperle, G., Dr., Hôpital Cantonal, Dép. d' Anesthésiologie, Genf

Gemperle, M., Priv.-Doz., Dr., Hôpital Cantonal, Dép. d'Anesthésiologie, Genf

Henschel, W. F., OMR., Dr., Allg. Anaesthesieabt., Städt. Krankenanst. Bremen

Kassel, H., Dr., Landeskrankenhaus Sanderbusch/Oldenburg

Kaump, D. H., M. D., Fa. Parke, Davis & Co., Ann Arbor Michigan (USA)

König, G., Dr., Anaesth.-Abt., Chirurg. Klinik Hamburg-Eppendorf

Kreuscher, H., Priv.-Doz., Dr., Inst. f. Anaesthesiologie der Universität Mainz

Kugler, J., Priv.-Doz., Dr., Nervenklinik der Universität München

Kurka, P., Dr., Leitender Facharzt für Anaesthesiologie der II. Chirurg. Abteilung, Wilhelminenspital, Wien

Kuschinsky, G., Prof. Dr., Pharmakol. Institut der Universität Mainz

Langrehr, D., OMR, Dr., Anaesthesieabt., Zentralkrankenhaus Bremen-Nord

Lassner, J., Prof. Dr., 130, Rue de la Pompe, Paris 16

Laub, M., Dr., Anaesthesieabteilung der Chir. Poliklinik München

LEASE, G. O., M. D., Fa. Parke, Davis & Co., Ann Arbor, Michigan (USA)

LECRON, L., Dr., 12, Rue Saint Fiacre, Epinois, Belgien

MORET, P., Dr., Hôpital Cantonal, Dép. d'Anesthésiologie, Genf

NAGEL, F., Dr., HNO-Klinik der Universität Mainz

MISONNE, P., 52, Rue Antoine, Brüssel 6, Belgien

MÜNCHHOFF, W., Dr., Inst. f. Anaesthesiologie, Zweckverband-Krh.,
    Minden

NOLTE, H., Priv.-Doz., Inst. f. Anaesthesiol., Zweckverb.-Krankenh.,
    Minden

PODLESCH, I., Dr., Abt. f. Anaesth,. Universität Düsseldorf

ROLLY, G., Dr., Univers. of Ghent, Akademisch-Ziekenhuis, Gent, Belgien

RUMPF, K., Dr. Dipl.-Psych., Psychiatrische Universitätsklinik Mainz

SOETENS, A., Dr., Hazelarenstraat 16, Antwerpen-Anvers, Belgien

STÖCKER, L., Dr., Anaesthesieabteilung, Städt. Krankenhaus Essen

STOLP, W., Dr., Anaesthesieabt., Zentralkrankenhaus Bremen-Nord

SZAPPANYOS, G. G., Dr., Hôpital Cantonal, Dép. d'Anesthésiologie, Genf

TEUTEBERG, H., Dr., Institut f. Anaesthesiologie der Universität Mainz

UNGER, W., Facharzt f. Anaesthesie, II. Chir. Abt., Kr.-Anst. Rudolfstift,
    Wien

WESTHUES, G., Dr., Anaesth.-Abteil. d. Universitäts-Kinderklinik München

ZEGVELD, C., Dr., Alkmaar, Niederlande, Irenelaan 8

ZINDLER, M., Prof. Dr., Abt. f. Anaesthesie, Universität Düsseldorf

The Pharmacology of Ketamine

By **G. Chen**

Fa. Parke, Davis & Co., Ann Arbor, Michigan, USA

2-(O-chlorophenyl)-2-methylaminocyclohexanone · HCl (Ketamine, CI-581) is a member of the arylcycloalkylamines (Fig. 1). They are a distinct class of centrally-acting drugs, the neuropharmacologic properties of which were uncovered ten years ago. 1-Phenyl(-1-cyclohexyl)piperidine (phencyclidine, Sernylan) was the first compound investigated in laboratory animals and subsequently studied in man as a general anesthetic agent [4, 8, 9, 12].

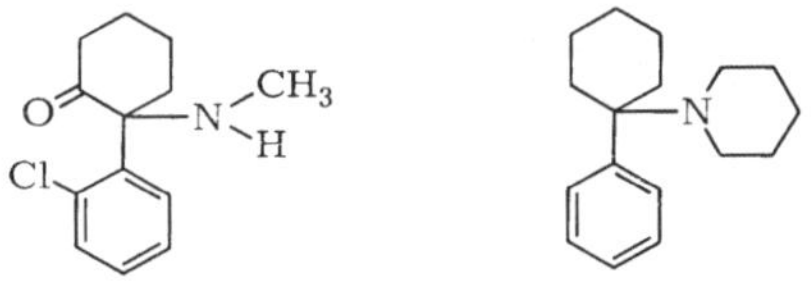

Ketamine
(Cl-581)

Phencyclidine
(Cl-395)

Fig. 1. Arylcycloalkylamines

By way of introduction I would like to discuss briefly certain differences in their overt effects in laboratory animals and in man between the arylcycloalkylamines and the barbiturates. The signs induced in animals by the two classes of drugs given in Table 1 are shown at increasing dose levels. The effects will be in a reversed order during recovery from anesthesia. The arylcycloalkylamines differ from the barbiturates in producing a state of catalepsy without hypnosis at non-anesthetic doses. Only a transitory cataleptic effect was seen in animals with the barbiturates during emergence from anesthesia. This difference in neuropharmacologic properties might account for some of the differences in their central effects during the post-anesthetic period. Another difference from the barbiturate anesthetics was the occurrence of convulsions in some animal species with doses of the arylcycloalkylamines above the anesthetic levels. Electroencephalographically, the barbiturates produced in the cat the characteristic slow-high amplitude spindles (Fig. 2). Under the influence of the arylcycloalkylamines, on the other hand, the EEG consisted of slow and high amplitude continuous synchronous waves [1]. Whereas cumulative effect and tolerance would result from the repeated administration of the barbiturates, this was not to be the case with the arylclycoalkylamines (Figs. 3, 4, Table 2) [13].

Table 1. *The Central Effects of Arylcycloalkylamines and Barbiturates on the Central Nervous System*

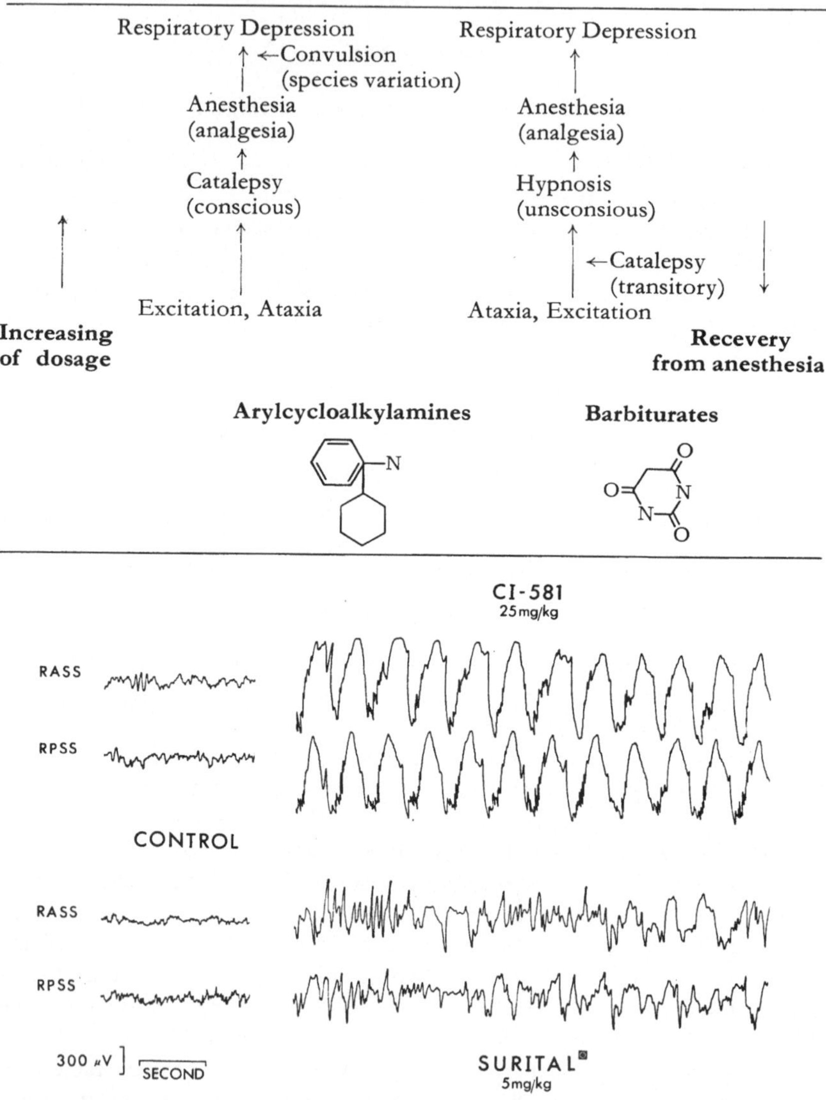

Fig. 2. The EEG of cats, immobilized with decamethonium (2 mg/kg i. v.) given CI-581 or Thiamyl sodium. RASS = right anterior suprasylvian gyrus, RPSS = right posterior suprasylvian gyrus

Table 2. *Some Differences in Neuropharmacologic Properties between Arylcycloalkylamines and Barbiturates*

	Catalepsy	Hypnosis	Convulsions at large doses	Species Variation	Cumulative effect	Tolerance
Aryl-cyclo-alkyl-amines	+	−	+, −	+	−	−
Bar-bitur-ates	−	+	−	−	+	+

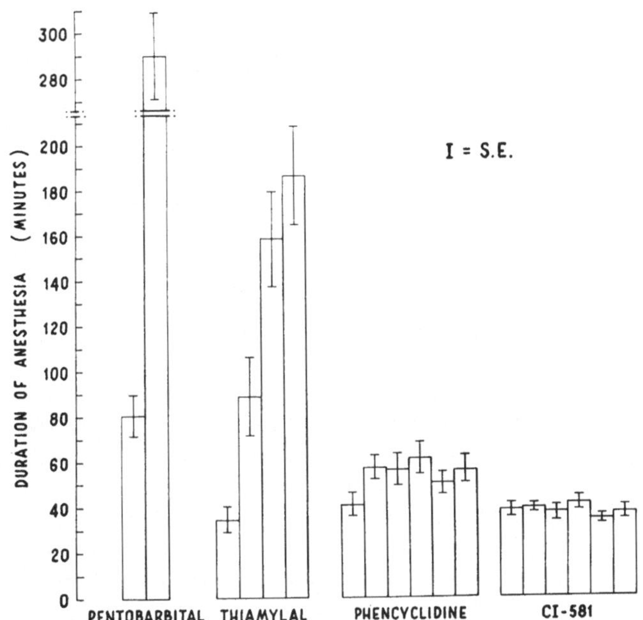

Fig. 3. Effect of successive anesthetization on the duration of anesthesia in monkeys with barbiturates and arylcycloalkylamines (cumulative effect). The duration of anesthesia was taken from the time of completing intravenous injection of the anesthetic to the time of emergence from anesthesia when the monkey was just capable of raising its head and fore-limbs. The successive injections of a fixed dose of the anesthetic were made as soon as the monkey recovered from anesthesia. The doses and the number of monkeys used were: pentobarbital-17 mg/kg, 4; thiamylal-14 mg/kg, 6; phencyclidine-1 mg/kg, 11; and CI-581-20 mg/kg, 6 monkeys. The bar grams from the left to right indicate the average durations of anesthesia and standard errors upon successive injections

1*

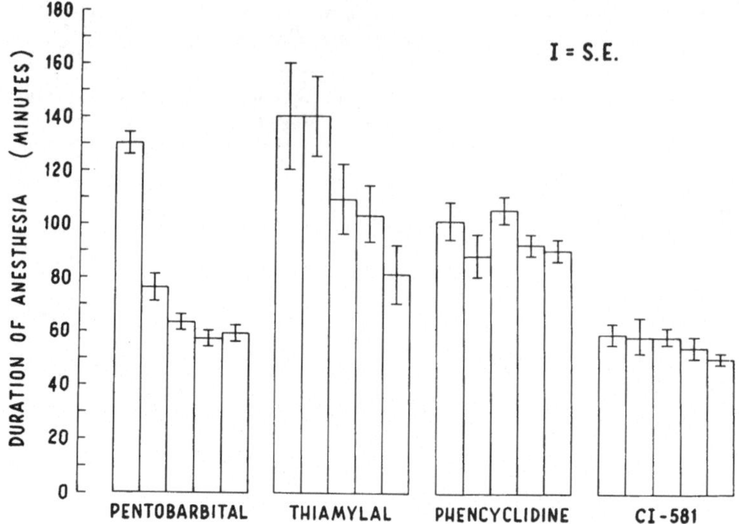

Fig. 4. Effect of daily anesthetization on the duration of anesthesia in monkeys with barbiturates and arylcycloalkylamines (tolerance development)

The same experimental procedure was followed as that for Fig. 3 except that a fixed dose of the anesthetic was given once a day. The doses and the number of animals used were: pentobarbital-22 mg/kg, 14; thiamylal-28 mg/kg, 8; phency-clidine-3 mg/kg, 8; and CI-581-30 mg/kg, 8 monkeys

The marked catalepsy produced by the arylcycloalkylamines without being accompanied by hypnosis may account for certain of the post-anesthetic reactions which have occurred in a few human subjects. The catalepsy is a characteristic akinetic state with the loss of the body righting reflex. The reflex movement of the neck and head to external stimulus is not affected and there is no impairment of consciousness [3]. The extremities appear to be paralyzed by motor deprivation, perhaps with sensory deprivation as well. It resembles the condition of "sleeping-paralysis" in man. The catalepsy is more prolonged in lower animal species than in primates. Fig. 5 shows the typical cataleptic conditions in a mouse and in a monkey. The mouse whose body was immobilized was capable of stretching its neck and vocalizing. The rhesus monkey was incapacitated, but alert, and could turn its head without difficulty. The onset and the extent of catalepsy proceeded in an ascending order. The lower parts of the body were affected before the upper regions. The order was reversed during recovery. Those regions of the body which were affected first, lasted longer also. Thus, the different parts of the body appeared to be dissociated or disconnected. Most likely, it is at the cataleptic phase during emergence from surgical anesthesia that sensory and motor disturbances might appear in human subjects; such as the alteration in the perception of body size, weight, position and time, feeling of numbness and separation of the body from the extremities. Had the arylcycloalkylamines a hypnotic action, these sensory and motor disturbances would not have been perceived during emergence from anesthesia. Indeed, the post-anesthetic reactions in human subjects could be prevented by hypnosis. To differentiate the anesthetic state induced by the conventional anesthetics, the term "dissociative anesthesia" has been suggested for that by the arylcycloalkylamines [10]. Insofar as the mode and the site of action of the arylcycloalkylamines on the central nervous system are not understood, exept that general anesthesia could also be produced by phencyclidine in decorticated monkeys [5], the word "dissociative" is more appropriate to describe the post-anesthetic effects rather than to imply the nature and cause of anesthesia.

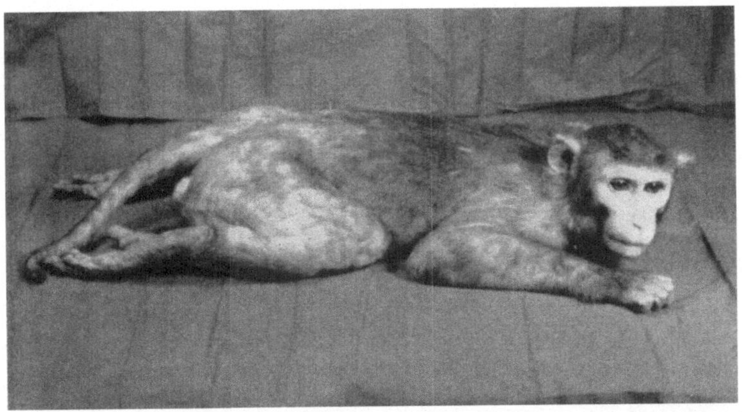

a

b

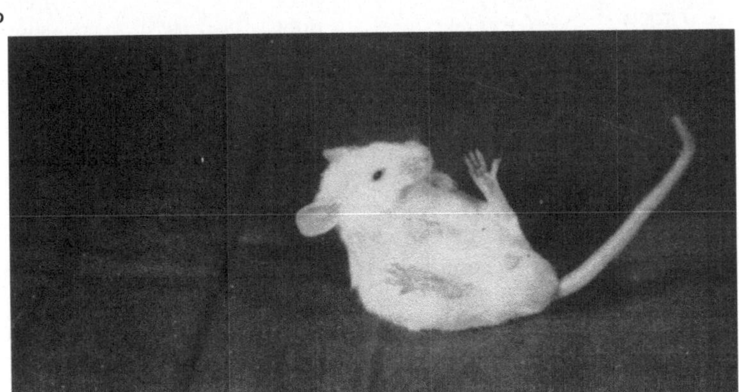

Fig. 5. Catalepsy during recovery from general anesthesia. Monkey, given 15 mg/kg CI-581 I. V., Mouse, given 200 mg/kg CI-581 I. P.

A distinction for their modes of action in producing these two different states of depression is shown by the fact that in certain animal species, such as the rabbit, catalepsy only, but not general anesthesia, may be induced by the arylcycloalkylamines. There is evidence also that a brief period of general anesthesia may be produced in pigeons, mice and monkeys by a few arylcycloalkylamines without marked catalepsy during recovery.

Because of the prolonged post-anesthetic reactions produced by some of the arylcycloalkylamines, notably phencyclidine, a search was then made to find a compound that would provide adequate surgical anesthesia and rapid recovery. CI-581 was found to meet these requirements in laboratory animals [6, 13] and subsequently was investigated as an intravenous and intramuscular anesthetic in humans [10, 14]. CI-581 is much shorter acting than phencyclidine. Table 3 gives a comparison of the effects

Table 3. *The Overt Effects of Phencyclidine (P) and CI-581*

Species	Compound	Ex-citation	Dys-ergia	Cata-lepsy	Anesthesia	Convulsion	Duration
Pigeon	P	—	+	+	—	+	long
	CI-581	—	+	+	+	—	short
Mouse	P	+	+	+	—	+	long
Rat	CI-581	+	+	+	+	—	short
Guinea	P	—	+	+	—	+	long
pig	CI-581	—	+	+	—	—	short
Rabbit	P	—	+	+	—	—	long
	CI-581	—	+	+	—	—	short
Cat	P	—	+	+	+	rare	long
	CI-581	—	+	+	+	rare	short
Dog	P	—(+ ?)	+	+	poor	+	long
	CI-581	—(+ ?)	+	+	poor	+	short
Monkey	P	—	+	+	+	+	long
	CI-581	—	+	+	+	very rare	short
Man	P	—	+	+	+	?	long
	CI-581	—	+	+	+	?	short

of the two drugs in laboratory animals and in man. The data reveal also the species variation in response to the central action of these drugs. A very marked difference is indicated by the ability of CI-581 to produce general anesthesia in pigeons and in mice. Anesthesia could not be induced in these animals with phencyclidine. Mydriasis and lacrimation occurred in mice with CI-581 at the stage of general anesthesia and the degree of mydriasis is proportional to the depth of anesthesia. These ocular manifestations did not consistently appear in other species with CI-581; miosis was not a cardinal sign for surgical anesthesia with this drug. In some human subjects receiving intravenous CI-581, the eyes began to open widely with profuse lacrimation on approaching the stage of general anesthesia. Therefore, the eye signs commonly used in judging the stage of anesthesia for the conventional anesthetics are not applicable to that for CI-581. Respiration was not markedly affected by CI-581 at the stage of surgical anesthesia. In some animals, a transitory apnea might occur right after intravenous injection or following intramuscular administration of a large dose of CI-581. In pigeons, mice and monkeys, the injection of a lethal dose of CI-581 resulted in respiratory failure without being preceded by frank convulsions. Phencyclidine, in contrast, caused convulsions in these animals at doses above the anesthetic levels.

CI-581 was absorbed rapidly following oral or parenteral administration. Surgical anesthesia could readily be induced in monkeys and in other species by intramuscular injection of CI-581. GLAZKO and co-workers have shown that the uptake of CI-581 by the central nervous system and distribution into other tissues also occured rapidly [2, 7]. Apparently, the rapid redistribution of CI-581 from the brain into other tissues may principally account for the short acting anesthetic property of this drug. CI-581 is metabolized very rapidly in the body of most animal species with the appearance of several metabolites in the urine. Three metabolites have been isolated and identified from the urine of rats, dogs, monkeys, and humans. Their structures and the possible metabolic pathways are shown in Fig. 6. Demethylation appears to occur first to the free amino compound; hydroxylation of the cyclohexanone ring then follows and finally results in the form of the cyclohexene derivative. The three metabolites are excreted in different proportions in the urine of rats, dogs, monkeys and humans. The metabolite III is mainly in the form of conjugate with glycuronic acid. The metabolite II appeared to be predominant in the urine from man, monkey and dog. Metabolites I and III predominated in the rat urine. The liver contains the highest level of CI-581 and appears to be the principal site for the metabolic disposition of the drug.

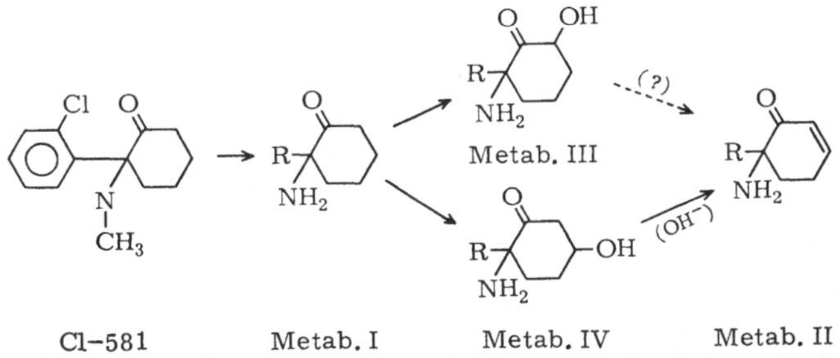

Fig. 6. The metabolites of CI-581 and the possible metabolic processes

The transfer of CI-581 across the placental barrier was found to be rapid in dogs and monkeys. Both the unchanged drug and the metabolites have been identified in the fetal tissues.

The cataleptic and anesthetic activities of metabolites I and II were very weak about 0.1 and 0.01 those of CI-581 respectively. They did not show any striking neuropharmacologic properties different from those of CI-581. In view of the rapid induction and the brevity of surgical anesthesia, CI-581 per se appears to be responsible for the general anesthesia, although the metabolites may contribute an additive effect during the period of recovery from anesthesia.

In regard to the cardiovascular effect of CI-581, the intravenous administration of CI-581 in rats, dogs and humans gave rise to a slight rise in systolic and diastolic pressure and an increase in heart rate [7]. VIRTUE and associates observed in man an increase in cardiac output with hypertension and tachycardia but without any apparent change in peripheral resistance [14]. The hypertension was seen also in adrenalectomized rats with CI-581. Only at extremely large doses, transitory hypotension and bradycardia occurred. The CI-581-induced hypertension in dogs was partially, and sometimes completely, suppressed by the preadministration of chlorpromazine and some other α-adrenergic blocking drugs, by pronethalol, and by hexamethonium. CI-581 did not markedly potentiate the pressor response to norepinephrine or suppress that of phenethylamine indicating the lack of an indirect sympathomimetic action on the vascular system [7].

The arrhythmia induced by epinephrine in dogs under methoxyflurane anesthesia was not aggrevated but was attenuated by the preadministration of CI-581 [7]. A weak antiarrhythmic effect of CI-581 was observed in dogs

Table 4. *Some Observations in Animals with CI-581*

Preparation	Testing	Observation
Dog, Apomorphine	Emesis	—
Hydrated Rat	Diuresis	Slight
Mouse, electroshock (Extensor-seizure)	Sympathomimetic (Indirect)	—
Rabbit Cornea	Local anesthesia (5 % solution)	—
Dog, B. P. (Arterenol, isopropylarterenol)	Adrenergic blockade ($x + \beta$)	
Dog, B. P. (DMPP)	Ganglionic blockade	—
Dog, B. P. (Acetylcholine)	Anticholinergic	—
Dog, B. P. (Histamine)	Antihistaminic	—
Cat, Tibialis muscle	Neuromuscular blocking	—

with ventricular tachycardia following ligation of the anterior descending coronary artery [7]. In dog heart-lung preparation and in isolated rabbit and guinea-pig hearts, only negative chronotropic and inotropic effects of CI-581 were obtained. No significant difference was found in norepine-ephrine contents of the heart in untreated rats and in rats given CI-581. The uptake or release of tritiated norepinephrine in the rat heart was not affected by CI-581 [7]. These results on the cardiovascular system appeared to indicate that the hypertension and tachycardia produced by CI-581 were principally either due to a direct or an indirect stimulating action on the cardio-stimulating center of the brain [7, 11]. That CI-581 may cause an acute intravascular release of epinephrine resulting in combined alpha and beta adrenergic receptor stimulation has also been suggested for the hypertensive effect and tachycardia [14].

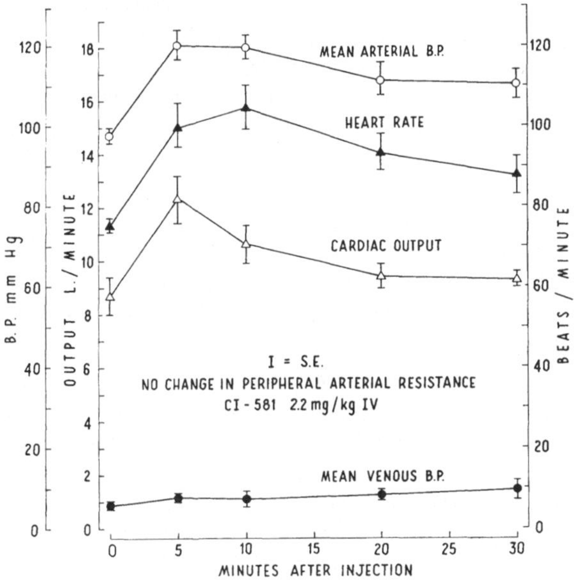

Fig. 7. The cardiovascular effects of CI-581 in humans. The graphs were made with the experimental data from the paper of VIRTUE ET AL. (20)

Certain other pharmacologic properties of CI-581 that have been investigated are shown in Table 4. CI-581 was without effect on apomorphine-induced emesis in dogs. In hydrated rats, CI-581 caused a slight diuresis at small doses. It did not potentiate the effect of dopa on electrically-induced extensor-seizure threshold in mice indicating the lack of an indirect sympathomimetic action on the central nervous system. No local anesthetic action was evident when a 5% solution of CI-581 was applied to rabbit's cornea. CI-581 was devoid of an alpha and beta blocking, ganglionic blocking, anticholinergic, antihistaminic, or a neuromuscular blocking activity. To summarize, it may be stated that CI-581 acts principally on the central nervous system.

Zusammenfassung

2-(O-chlorophenyl)-2-(methylamino)cyclohexanon-HCl (Ketamine, CI-581) ist eine kataleptisch, analgetisch und anaesthetisch wirkende Verbindung ohne hypnotische Eigenschaften und darum unterschiedlich von den herkömmlichen Barbituraten. Die Katalepsie ist ein charakteristischer, akinetischer Zustand mit Verlust des Körperaufrichtereflexes beim Versuchstier und ohne Beeinträchtigung des Bewußtseins. Die Extremitäten scheinen durch motorischen und sensorischen Ausfall paralysiert zu sein. Die Tiefe der Analgesie und allgemeinen Anaesthesie durch Ketamine variiert mit der Spezies: sie ist ausgeprägter bei Menschen, Affen, Katzen, Ratten und Mäusen als bei Tauben, Meerschweinchen, Hunden und Kaninchen. Im Gegensatz zu Barbituraten tritt nach der wiederholten Applikation von Ketaminen kein kumulativer Effekt oder erhöhte Toleranz auf.

Ketamine hat für die Erzeugung einer Allgemeinanaesthesie eine breite Dosierungsspanne ohne Erzeugung einer erkennbaren respiratorischen Depression. Unter dem Einfluß von Ketamine ist ein leichter Anstieg des Blutdruckes und der Herzfrequenz zu beobachten. Der Effekt auf das cardio-vasculäre System erfolgt vorwiegend über die zentralen regulatorischen Mechanismen. Ketamine wird nach oraler oder parenteraler Applikation schnell resorbiert; die Aufnahme von Ketamine durch das zentrale Nervensystem und die Verteilung in andere Gewebe erfolgt ebenfalls rasch. Die schnelle Weiterverteilung von Ketamine vom Hirn in andere Gewebe kann grundsätzlich für die kurzwirkenden anaesthetischen Eigenschaften dieses Pharmakons verantwortlich gemacht werden. Die Verbindung wird sehr schnell im Körper der meisten Versuchstiere metabolisiert. Verschiedene Metaboliten sind im Urin nachweisbar. Die Hauptmetaboliten wurden als N-alkylierte Amine indentifiziert: zwei Verbindungen mit Hydroxylierung des Cyclohexanon-Ringes und des korrespondierenden Cyclohexenamins.

References

1. Bond, H. W.: A Comparative Study of the Effect of CI-581 and Thiamylal (Surital[R]) on the Electrocorticograms in the Cat. Unpublished observations. (1967).

2. CHANG, T., W. A. DILL, and A. J. GLAZKO: Metabolic Disposition of 2-(0-chlorophenyl)-2-methylaminocyclohexanone (CI-581) in Laboratory Animals and Man. Fed. Proc. **24**, 268 (1965).
3. CHEN, G.: Evaluation of Phencyclidine-type Cataleptic Activity. Arch. int. Pharmacodyn. **157**, 193–201 (1965).
4. —, C. R. ENSOR, D. RUSSELL, and B. BOHNER: The Pharmacology of 1-(1-phenylcyclohexyl)piperidine · HCl. J. Pharmacol. **127**, 241–250 (1959).
5. — —, and B. BOHNER: An Investigation on the Sympathomimetic Properties of Phencyclidine by Comparison with Cocaine and Desoxyephedrine. J. Pharmacol. **149**, 71–78 (1965).
6. — — — The Neuropharmacology of 2-(0-chlorophenyl)-2-methylaminocyclohexanone hydrochloride. J. Pharmacol. **152**, 332–339 (1966).
7. —, A. J. GLAZKO, and D. H. KAUMP: Laboratory Summary on CI-581, June, 1967. Exper. Therap. Dept., Research Division, Parke, Davis & Co.
8. CHEN, G. M., and J. K. WESTON: The Analgesic and Anesthetic Effect of 1-(1-phenylcyclohexyl)piperidine · HCl. Anesth. Analg. **39**, 132–137, (1960).
9. DOMINO, E. F.: Neurobiology on Phencyclidine (Sernyl). Int. Rev. Neurobiol. **6**, 303–347 (1964).
10. —, P. CHODOFF, and G. CORSSEN: Pharmacologic Effects of CI-581, A New Dissociative Anesthetic in Man. Clin. Pharmacol. Ther. **6**, 279–291 (1965).
11. DOWDY, E. G., and K. KAYA: Studies in the Circulatory Effects of CI-581. Presented at the Annual Meeting of the American Society of Anesthesiologists, October 1, 1967.
12. GREIFENSTEIN, F. E., M. DEVAULT, J. YOSHITAKE, and J. E. GAJEWSKI: A Study of a 1-acrylcyclohexylamine for Anesthesia. Anesth. Analg. **37**, 283–294 (1958).
13. MCCARTHY, D. A., G. CHEN, D. H. KAUMP, and C. R. ENSOR: General Anesthetic and other Pharmacological properties of 2-(0-chlorophenyl)-2-methylaminocyclohexanone · HCl (CI-581). J. New Drugs **5**, 21–33 (1965).
14. VIRTUE, R. W., J. M. ALANIS, M. MORI, R. T. LAFARGUE, J. H. K. VOGEL, and D. R. METCALF: An Anesthetic Agent: 2-orthochlorophenyl, 2-methylaminocyclohexanone · HCl (CI-581). Anesth. **28**, 823–833 (1967).

Toxicology of Ketamine

By **D. H. Kaump, S. M. Kurtz, R. A. Fisken, J. L. Schardein, D. E. Roll**
and **T. F. Reutner**

Fa. Parke, Davis & Co., Ann Arbor, Michigan, USA

Ketamine (CI-581, 2-(0-chlorophenyl)-2-(methylamino)-cyclohexanone hydrochloryde, is a parenteral anesthetic agent with unique pharmacologic and physiologic properties [1, 2]. In addition to the routine acute and chronic toxicity studies accorded most new pharmacologic agents, the anesthetic nature and numerous potential variations in the clinical application of Ketamine dictated that specialized studies be carried out under circumstances approximating the projected clinical uses. Therefore, experiments were designed to study how such variables as the age of the animals, various patterns of repeated drug administration, and the prior administration of an agent known to stimulate microsomal enzymes affected its toxicity. These experiments, and minor variations in the routine toxicity studies, are described in this report.

Materials and Methods

Ketamine is supplied as the hydrochloride salt, of which 86.7% constitutes the base component. All drug doses in these experiments are expressed in terms of the base component. Ketamine is a white crystalline solid with a m. p. of 259° C. It is soluble in water to form a 20% clear, colorless solution. A 10% aqueous solution has a pH of 3.5.

Experimental design and Methods of Study

Acute Toxicity Determinations. LD_{50} determinations have been done in rodents and in rhesus monkeys. Each animal was given a single dose of Ketamine at several dose levels, by various routes, following which all grossly evident effects were observed and recorded. The number of surviving animals at each dose level was noted at the end of the observation period, and the LD_{50} value was calculated by the MILLER-TAINTER [3] method. Local toleration to intramuscular, intravenous, and intra-arterial injection was evaluated during the course of repeated injection studies.

Repeated Dose Studies. Preliminary studies in dogs were conducted after intramuscular injection of Ketamine either on several successive days or after repeated injections on the same day.

In further studies, pairs of dogs and monkeys were given Ketamine in daily increasing dosage levels until the animals either died or were sacrificed in moribund condition.

Based upon information obtained in these preliminary trials, intermediate term tolerance studies were done in which groups of rats, dogs, and monkeys were administered Ketamine daily. Rats and monkeys were treated intravenously, and dogs were treated intramuscularly. In addition to the observation and recording of grossly evident reactions and weight changes, extensive clinical and laboratory studies were performed.

Laboratory studies included evaluation by standard methods of the peripheral blood, bone marrow, and serum chemistry. Hemoglobin, hematocrit, sedimentation rate (dogs and monkeys), and total and differential leukocyte counts were determined on the peripheral blood before drug treatment, and at varying intervals throughout the study. Study of all bone marrow biopsy and autopsy specimens from dogs and monkeys included total nucleated cell counts, total erythrocyte counts, and nucleated cell differential counts. In addition, GIEMSA stained sections from a thrombin clot in the monkey and decalcified rib in the dog were examined for drug-related changes. Portions of the femur were removed from the rat at autopsy, decalcified, embedded in paraffin, sectioned, and stained by the GIEMSA method for further hematologic evaluation.

Microchemical determinations of serum chloride, calcium, sodium, potassium, phosphate, alkaline phosphatase, CO_2, glucose, urea nitrogen, cholesterol, total protein, albumin, globulin, bilirubin, and SGO- and SGP-transaminase were done initially, and at various intervals during the study on all animals.

Prior to initiation of drug treatment, open surgical biopsy was performed on all dogs and monkeys. Specimens of the liver, kidney, and bone marrow were prepared for histological evaluation. These tissues were again biopsied at interim and/or termination of the study.

Complete autopsies on all sacrificed animals were done after perfusion with saline, followed by perfusion with 10% formalin. The following organs and tissues from all autopsies were procured for microscopic examination: lung, heart, liver, gallbladder (rats excluded), kidney, spleen, pancreas, salivary glands, esophagus, stomach, duodenum, jejunum, ileum, cecum, colon, brain, spinal cord (monkeys), thyroid, parathyroid, pituitary, adrenal, bone, bone marrow, lymph nodes, thymus, striated muscle, eye (dogs and monkeys), urinary bladder, breast (rats and monkeys), and genital organs. Paraffin sections were stained routinely with hematoxylin and eosin. In addition, sections of liver, kidney, and adrenal of all animals were stained for fat with Oil Red 0, and biopsy specimens of the liver and kidney of all dogs and monkeys were stained with PAS. Bone marrow was stained with GIEMSA. Pituitary was stained with the trichrome-PAS method, and brain and spinal cord with thionin.

Results

Acute Toxicity Studies. The acute toxicity studies were done in three different classes of rodents. These comprised studies in young males, studies in newborn and 14-day-old animals, and studies in animal pretreated with either Ketamine or phenobarbital sodium. In the first experiment, groups of 10 or more young adult (6-to 10-weeks-old) mice or rats were given single doses of Ketamine by one of several routes of administration. The LD_{50} values are summarized in Table 1.

Table 1. *Ketamine : Acute Toxicity (LD_{50}) values expressed as mg/kg active Moiety*

Route	Mouse	Rat	Monkey
Oral	616.6 ± 33.6	446.7 ± 10.6	—
I. P.	223.9 ± 3.91	223.9 ± 3.7	—
I. V.	—	58.88 ± 1.22	60*

* Value Supplied by Dr. D. A. MC CARTHY.

Ketamine is somewhat more toxic in rats than in mice when it is given orally. However, after intraperitoneal injection, the LD_{50} values correspond closely. The induced clinical signs were common to both mice and rats regardless of route of administration. There was initial excitement and irritability, rapidly followed by depression, severe incoordination, and prostration. Recovery followed in a reverse sequence. Most of the deaths occurred within 2 hours of drug administration. Complete autopsy examination of a number of rats surviving treatment at, or greater than, the LD_{50} values revealed no evidence of organ damage.

In the second acute toxicity study, LD_{50} values were determined after intraperitoneal injection of Ketamine in rodents of 3 age groups. These animals were either in the neonatal period (under 24 hours), the preweaning period (14 days), or young adult period (42 to 49 days). The LD_{50} values are summarized in Table 2.

Table 2. *Ketamine : Acute Toxicity (LD_{50}) after intraperitoneal Injection (values expressed as mg/kg active Moiety)*

Age Group	Mice	Rats
Neonatal	275.4 ± 7	146.2 ± 4.8
Preweaning	208.9 ± 4.6	169.8 ± 6.4
Young Adult	229 ± 4.7	248 ± 4.5

Most deaths occurred within 1 hour after dosing in the preweaning and young adult animals. The animals in the neonatal age had reduced respiration, cyanosis, and death was delayed up to 6 hours. The LD_{50} values were very similar in mice in the 3 age groups, but in rats there was some slight lessening of acute toxicity with increasing age. In general, however, the values were not sufficiently different to suggest undue toxitity in the very young.

The final acute toxicity study with Ketamine was done in male albino rats as an attempt to determine whether the LD_{50} values were altered by pre-administration of a known microsomal enzyme stimulator, or by previous treatment with Ketamine itself. For this study we injected the animals intraperitoneally for 3 consecutive days with 20 mg/kg of either phenobarbital sodium or Ketamine. After several periods of time, we determined the LD_{50} values after intraperitoneal injection of Ketamine. These values are summarized in Table 3.

Table 3. *Ketamine : Acute Toxicity after intraperitoneal Injection (values expressed as mg/kg active Moiety)*

Day	Pretreated with		Not pretreated
	Ketamine	PB Na	Control
3	224 ± 7.0	218.8 ± 9.6	173.8 ± 11.8
7	252 ± 8.0	252 ± 8.0	224.0 ± 11.0
14	252 ± 2.3	263 ± 9.2	240.0 ± 8.2
28	252 ± 5.9	252 ± 7.0	240.0 ± 10.0

There were no significant differences in the LD_{50} values between either of the pretreated groups or the untreated control animals.

Local Toleration Studies. Local toleration to injections of Ketamine was determined in rabbits, rats, and dogs. Rabbits were injected intra- muscularly with 0.5 cc of either a 1% or 5% solution. Both solutions induced local pressure necrosis which underwent rapid resolution. Intraarterial injections were given using 1% and 5% solutions in both rats (aorta) and dogs (femoral). The only injury produced in these animals was arterial mural damage incident to the trauma of injection, and was similar to the damage produced by injection of saline in control animals. Subsequent trials were done in rats and monkeys which will be described. There was no evidence of vascular damage beyond that which would be expected from repeated venipuncture.

Intermediate Term Repeated Dose Studies. Groups of male and female rats were given daily intravenous injections of Ketamine for 6 weeks, at dosage levels of 2.5, 5, and 10 mg/kg. There was a dose level related brief period of anesthesia of similar depth and duration in males and females at each dose level. There was an associated slight food intake and moderate weight gain depression which was dose level related in males, but not in females. While minor aberrations in clinical laboratory values did occur at autopsy, neither gross nor microscopic organ damage was seen that suggested a drug-related effect.

Dogs were given Ketamine intramuscularly. In the initial experiment, pairs of dogs were either given doses of 40 mg/kg on each of 4 successive days, or 5 injections at 30-minute intervals on the same day. The dogs given single daily injections had incoordination, followed in 1 or 2 minutes by prostration. In these animals, there was a return of the righting reflex within 33 to 54 minutes. In those given repeated doses on the same day, there was a prolonged state of anesthesia. Both treatment schedules were well tolerated, and there were no significant changes in the multiple peripheral hematologic, urine, or bone marrow values. Except for a moderate elevation of transaminase levels, serum chemistry values remained within normal limits. The elevated transaminase values may have resulted from local muscle damage which was more prominent than in the saline injected control animals. Similar gross and microscopic findings were present both in the animals treated with Ketamine, and in the control animals handled similarly but injected with saline. An additional pair of dogs was given increasing daily injections over a 29-day period, starting with doses of 1 mg/kg, and reaching a final level of 160 mg/kg. At this time the dogs were sacrificed in good clinical condition. Clinical signs were related strictly to the pharmacologic activity of the drug, and included excitement with slight tremors, followed by incoordination, and, finally, prostration. At the time of deepest anesthesia, there was an increased pulse rate, depressed respiratory rate, and depressed rectal temperature. During recovery, there was increased activity and vocalizing. In both dogs, there was a slight increase in blood alkaline phosphatase, and a moderate increase in transaminase values, both perhaps associated with weight loss and local tissue damage. There was no significant evidence of organ damage either by gross or microscopic examination.

The final study in dogs was done with daily intramuscular injections for 6 weeks. Three groups of 4 animals each were given doses of 4, 20, or 40 mg/kg of Ketamine. Two animals from each group were sacrificed after 6 weeks, while the remaining dogs were maintained for an additional 28 days without further treatment. The treated dogs had elevated values for blood cholesterol, urea, alkaline phosphatase, and transaminase which were most prominent in the animals given doses of 40 mg/kg. The values returned to normal levels after cessation of treatment. In view of the anorexia, weight loss, local muscle damage, and minor histologic changes, these aberrant laboratory values cannot be definitely ascribed to the primary activity of the drug.

In rhesus monkeys, anesthesia was induced by an intravenous injection of 20 mg/kg at the rate of 0.1 cc (5 mg) every 15 seconds. Thereafter, anesthesia was maintained by supplemental injections through an intra-venous catheter at 12 mg/kg every 15 minutes. Groups of 4 animals each were maintained under anesthesia for either 1 hour, 3 hours, or 6 hours at twice weekly intervals. The dosage schedule is summarized in Table 4.

Table 4. *Ketamine : Dosage Schedule in Monkeys*

Duration of Anesthesia (in hours)	Av. total Dose mg/kg	Treatment Period in Days	No. of Doses	Recovery Period in Days
6	296	28	8	21
3	152	41	12	7
1	56	41	12	7

Induction of anesthesia in monkeys was rapid, smooth, and began after the introduction of about 10 mg/kg. The anesthetic state was accompanied by a blank stare, ptosis, myoclonic jerking, and initial relaxation. Later there was variable mydriasis, tremors, and salivation. The respiratory rate was generally somewhat depressed, and there was a slight hypothermia with return to pre-anesthetic body temperature near the end of the treatment period. The heart rate was somewhat diminished, and there was a fall in blood pressure which was variable in degree and in time of appearance. Hematologic changes consisted of occasional instances of leukocytosis, neutrocytosis, and sedimentation rate increase. There was a non-dose related variable elevation in transaminase values. There was an increase in blood glucose values in those animals held under longer periods of anesthesia. Electrocardiograms were made prior to treatment, during treatment, and at the end of the last period of anesthesia. There was a slight slowing of the heart rate in all animals, but no significant changes in the configuration of the complexes. There were no distinct drug-related lesions either by gross or microscopic examination.

During the course of these experiments, the pattern of recovery and time of recovery after treatment were observed in order to determine whether evidence for development of tolerance might occur in the several species. In rats, there was no evidence of either a diminution or an increase in the responses to 2.5, 5.0, or 10.0 mg/kg over the 42-day dosing period. The time of recovery from the anesthetic effect of Ketamine was measured from the time of injection using the righting and standing reflexes as evidence of recovery in dogs. There was no apparent shortening of the time required for righting or standing over the 6-week period after doses

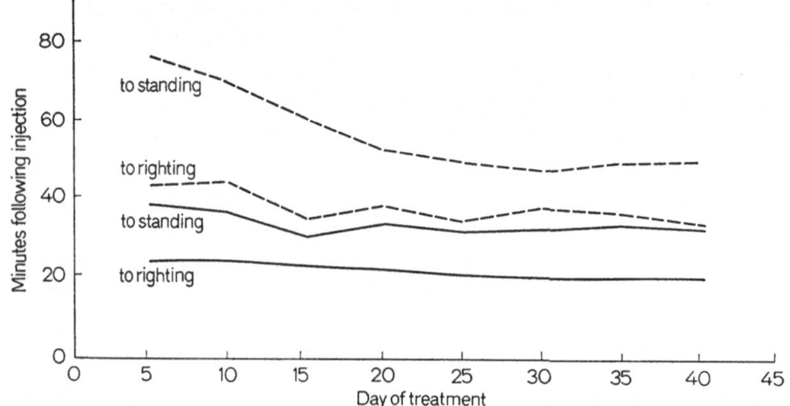

Fig. 1. CI-581: Recovery after intramuscular injection in dogs (average of 4 dogs per dose group). – – – – – – 40 mg/kg, —————— 20 mg/kg

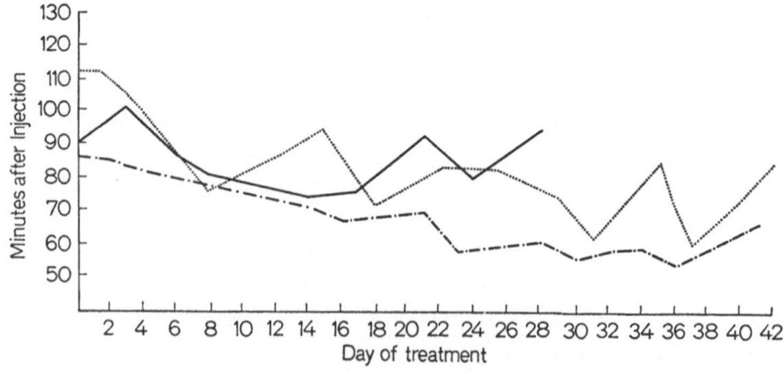

Fig. 2. CI-581: Recovery after last injection in monkeys (average time to walking). Anesthetic periods of: –·–·–·– 1 hour, – – – – – – – 3 hour, —————— 6 hour

of 20 mg/kg/day of Ketamine. After daily doses of 40 mg/kg, there was an anticipated longer time to recovery, with no shortening of the time required for righting, but perhaps some shortening of the time required to stand (Fig. 1).

As evidence of recovery in monkeys, the times to righting, to lifting of shoulders, and to walking were used. In general, these 3 recovery times were quite parallel. Fig. 2 plots only the time to walking.

These recovery times possibly suggest slight tachyphylaxis in the animals anesthetized for periods of 1 or 3 hours, but not in those anesthetized for periods of 6 hours.

Zusammenfassung

Die intravenöse Injektion von Ketamine bei Affen oder Ratten und die intramuskuläre Applikation bei Hunden erzeugt sehr schnell eine Anaesthesie ohne Muskelentspannung. Die Aufwachperiode war bei Ratten und Hunden, jedoch nicht bei Affen, durch Hyperaktivität charakterisiert. Unter den extremen Bedingungen der durchgeführten Untersuchungen konnten gelegentlich Zeichen einer leichten Tachyphylaxie beobachtet werden. Die wiederholte Anwendung von Ketamine zeigte bei den ausgiebigen autoptischen Untersuchungen der Versuchstiere nur geringe Toxicität. Die Verbindung wurde nach intravenöser Injektion bei Ratten und Affen, nach intraarterieller Injektion bei Ratten und Hunden sowie nach intramuskulärer Injektion bei Kaninchen und Hunden gut vertragen.

References

1. CHEN, G.: Presented at International Symposium on Ketamine (CI-581), University of Mainz, 23 and 24 February 1968. This book pp. 1—11.
2. McCARTHY, D. A., G. CHEN, D. H. KAUMP, and C. ENSOR: J. New Drug 5, 21–33 (1953).
3. MILLER, L. C., and M. L. TAINTER: Proc. Soc. exp. Biol. (N. Y.) 57, 261 (1944).

Ketamine-Scope of Clinical Program

By **G. O. Lease**

Parke, Davis & Co., Ann Arbor, Michigan, (USA)

The development of Ketamine, like most pharmaceutical agents, involved synthesizing and screening a large number of compounds that wer passed through pharmacology, toxicology, and clinical investigation. Most of these chemicals are eliminated during the evaluations. Finally, one compounds, in this case Ketamine, survives critical evaluation and is ready for wide clinical use.

A stepwise development is accurate chronologically for the initiation of each step or phase. Sufficient data must be collected and evaluated in one phase before a decision can be reached to proceed to the next phase. Eventually, with the addition of potential uses, evaluation is occurring in all phases simultaneously.

You have already heard from Dr. CHEN regarding the pharmacological evaluation of Ketamine and from Dr. KAUMP regarding the toxicological studies of Ketamine. We divided the clinical evaluation into three phases. Briefly, Phase I involves the clinical pharmacological evaluation. Elaborate monitoring of all major systems is done to detect the first evidence of toxicity. Dose range employed is generally very wide, beginning with a low dose and proceeding cautiously to a level that may very well exceed the final recommended therapeutic range.

Phase II involves early therapeutic trials and whenever practical, low doses are used initially in relatively healthy people. Indepth laboratory evaluations are carried out at frequent intervals. The early dose response studies, including metabolic disposition, are done in Phase II.

Phase III involves trials where, by virtue of experience, less extensive controls are necessary. Significant laboratory parameters have been defined in Phases I and II and only these are done routinely in Phase III. A full battery of laboratory tests are used to check any system function as necessary.

The first clinical trial involving a compound related to Ketamine was initiated in mid 1957. However, the first injection of Ketamine was not given until seven years later on August 3, 1964. This was carried out by Drs. CORSSEN and DOMINO. The Phase I evaluation, as described in four protocols, was continued in 50 normal volunteers. The subjects were carefully screened by means of physical examination and laboratory testing prior to entry into the program. Before administering Ketamine, each subject was connected to a polygraph so that EEG, EKG, respiration, and arterial blood pressure could be monitored continuously. These early trials in humans confirmed previous animal data indicating no significant depression of the cardiovascular and respiratory systems. In addition, these trials established a dose required to induce anesthesia with profound, peripheral analgesia.

With the above information in hand, Dr. Corssen began the first clinical Phase II trial on November 17, 1964. The patient was a 19-year-old female, admitted to the hospital for cystoscopic examination. The study was continued and evidence accumulated that Ketamine could be a valuable drug.

Further Phase II trials followed and additional information justified a decision to proceed with Phase III trials. As you can see from the earlier definitions, separation of Phases II and III for Ketamine is difficult. Many trials begin as Phase II studies and become Phase III at some point in time. These phases can be recognized by the cautious approach adopted early in a trial as compared with the somewhat more confident approach later in the trial after experience has developed.

At this point in time Ketamine has been evaluated in 32 countries. Of the 9,670 case records received in the U.S. by December 31, 1967, 2,552 came from Europe. Inasmuch as we are evaluating many studies in Munich, the total number of case records provided by the investigators is larger than indicated and, as a result, the per cent from Western Europe is larger. A total of 169 protocols, including the clinical pharmacology trials, were negotiated during the period 1964 through 1967. Of the 154 trials actually initiated, 54 were in Europe, 46 were in the U.S.A., and 55 were in the rest of the world. The difference between 169 and 154 is the 15 cancelled studies, 13 of which were in the U.S.A., one in Canada, and only one in Europe. The high initiation rate for trials in Europe reflects the responsibl enthusiasm of the investigators here.

Diskussion

Corssen: Herr CHEN hat in seinem Vortrag erwähnt, daß wir seit Beginn unserer Untersuchungen immer wieder auf den Begriff „dissoziative Anaesthesie" hingewiesen haben. Wir haben inzwischen eine Reihe von Untersuchungen an Katzen angestellt, um zu beweisen, daß der Ausdruck „dissoziative Anaesthesie" tatsächlich seine Begründung hat. Wir haben in Zusammenarbeit mit dem Department für Pharmakologie an unserer Universität in Michigan (Dr. MIASAKA und Dr. BLUMENHOFF) Elektroden in verschiedene Teile des Katzengehirns gelegt und an 5 Katzen den Effekt von Ketamine studiert:

5 min nach der intravenösen Gabe von 4 mg/kg Ketamine sehen wir wenig Aktivität im Thalamus und geringe Aktivität im Hippokampus. Nach 15 min läßt die Delta-Aktivität im corticalen Bereich nach, während im Hippokampus noch immer starke Aktivität vorherrscht. Nach 30 min kommen die corticalen Anteile zur Ruhe; während die Katze sich jetzt aufrichtet und sehr irritiert erscheint, kommt es zu einer starken Aktivierung des Hippokampus. Wir sehen auch, daß die thalamische Komponente nicht aktiviert ist. Wir glauben, damit beweisen zu können, daß es sich bei Ketamine tatsächlich um einen dissoziativen Effekt handelt, Außerdem haben wir den Effekt von Ketamine auf somatosensorische „avoke potentials" studiert. Ich kann leider nicht auf Einzelheiten eingehen, ich will nur sagen, daß wiederum im corticalen Bereich eine starke depressorische Komponente vorherrscht, während z. B. im Mittelhirn, der formatio reticularis, praktisch überhaupt kein Effekt erzielt werden konnte. Wir sehen also wieder eine Dissoziation zwischen corticalem und subcorticalem Effect. Den besten Beweis für eine Dissoziation sehen wir in dem Effekt von Ketamine auf neocorticale Anteile des Gehirns im Vergleich zu subcorticalen Bereichen. Nach Ketamine typische Delta-Aktivität, d. h. Depression der corticalen Zentren und praktisch kein Effekt auf subcorticale Bezirke. Nach 15 min sehen wir, daß die typischen „burst suppression"-Symptome auftreten. Wir sehen Phasen, wo noch immer Delta-Aktivität vorherrscht und dann eine „low voltage"-Aktivität einsetzt. Wir sehen aber außerdem, daß nach 15 min noch immer eine deutliche Dissoziation zwischen corticalem und subcorticalem Bereich vorhanden ist. Nach 30 min kehrt das EEG schließlich zur Ausgangslage zurück.

Im EEG eines zehnjährigen Kindes sahen wir 20 sec nach der Injektion von 2 mg/kg Ketamine eine rasch eintretende Veränderung des Ausgangs-EEG in seiner Theta-Aktivität; aber der Angriff ist schneller im frontalen

Cortex, als es z. B. im Vertex oder im okzipitalen Bereich der Fall ist. Außerdem sehen wir, daß die Theta-Aktivität noch nach 2 min anhält, aber viel stärker im frontalen als im okzipitalen Bereich. Diese Erscheinung haben Domino und ich interpretiert als einen typischen Beweis für die Prädominanz der Ketamine-Wirkung im Assoziationsareal des Cortex. Generell gesagt: Es handelt sich um eine Dissoziation des Effektes zwischen frontalen, corticalen und okzipitalen Zentren.

Ich wollte das hier nur zur Sprache bringen, weil ich weiß, daß Dr. Chen noch immer den Begriff „Dissoziation" nicht gerne mag. Aber wenn wir noch eine Weile darüber sprechen, werden wir eines Tages sicher auch ihn dazu bekehrt haben, so daß er sich uns anschließt und auch von „dissoziativer Anaesthesie" spricht.

NN: I would like to ask Dr. Chen: Is there any catecholamine effect of CI-581?

Chen: So far we know, we cannot detect these catecholamines, I am sorry. Well, I would like to ask Dr. Corssen, I wonder, can you use the term selected so right as dissociative? You are complicating if you say, a selective effect is rather a dissociative one.

Corssen: I would still like to work a little longer on this matter, but when the cat comes out the emergency phase, the cat sits up because the errective reflexes are complete and then we stimulate the cat. The cat is very irritable and then we measure from our electrodes and we see, that the cortex is practically back to normal, while the hippokampus is greatly activated. To our knowledge there is not one anaesthetic yet available neither chloroform nor ether which has shown this phase of dissociation. They all either depress or they don't depress.

Netter: I would like to ask Dr. Kaump one question: I understand from your slides that the stimulation of the metabolic system does not change the LD 50 and therefore probably not the duration of anaesthesia. Now, what determines the duration, the excretion by the kidney or the metabolition? It seems to be rather the excretion by kidney.

Kaump: I think, that Dr. Netter meant the table of metabolism. I think probably the duration of anaesthesia then will be determined by the rate of metabolism of the compound and not so much by the excretion.

Netter: This would mean, that the duration can be shortened by pretreatment with phenobarbital?

Kaump: No, it was not shortened by pretreatment, because phenobarbital did not hasten that known metabolism of Ketamine.

Netter: Well, so we can say, that you cannot stimulate the metabolism and this does not change the duration of anaesthesia. Well, the determination of the action will rather be the excretion in urine. So it seems to be not quite clear yet.

Zindler: Dr. KAUMP, didn't you say, this is mainly a case of redistribution which is the case in barbiturates and other compounds?

Kaump: They are weak but they do retain some of the pharmacologic activities of compared compounds. The injected compound is very rapidly distributed throughout the tissues. As Dr. CHEN indicated, there is a very high concentration in liver earlier as the rapidly distributed compound will be metabolized.

Zindler: This wouldn't mean, that this is a termination of anaesthesia, not a distribution -but do you think the excretion?

Kaump: I think probably excretion.

Chen: I think, that this anaesthesia is entirely terminated by distribution.

Zindler: One more question to Dr. CHEN: Did you ever try to give it in the carotid artery with any objective?

Chen: Yes, we did so with the same dosage.

Der Einfluß von Ketamine
auf verschiedene Vitalfunktionen des Menschen
(Experimentelle Untersuchungen
und klinische Erfahrungen bei 1300 Fällen)*

Von **D. Langrehr** und **W. Stolp**

Aus der Anaesthesieabteilung des Zentralkrankenhauses Bremen-Nord,
Städt. Krankenanstalten, Bremen (Direktor: O.-Med.-Rat Dr. D. Langrehr)

Das von G. Chen u. Mitarb. (1959–1967) inaugurierte und von
G. Corssen u. Mitarb. (1964–1968) in die Klinik eingeführte Phencyclidin-
Derivat Ketamine (CI-581; 2-(o-chlorophenyl)-2-methylamino-cyclohexa-
non-HCl) hat uns wegen seiner besonderen Eigenschaften veranlaßt, durch
experimentelle und klinische Untersuchungen zur Klärung des Wirkungs-
spektrums beizutragen. An Hand unserer Erfahrung in mehr als 1300 Fällen
möchten wir darlegen, welchen Einfluß Ketamine auf verschiedene Vitalfunktionen des Menschen hat und welche Indikationen zur klinischen Anwendung sich für uns ergeben haben.

Methodik

Die Mehrzahl der Angaben zur Methodik sind bereits früher dargelegt
(Langrehr u. Mitarb. 1967), worauf hier verwiesen wird. Bislang nicht mit-
geteilte methodische Details sind hier angefügt.

a) Die Substanz CI-581 lag als Hydrochlorid in wasserklarer Lösung 50 mg/ml
(5 %), 25 mg/ml (2,5 %) und 10 mg/ml (1 %) mit einem pH von 4,2 vor und wurde
i.v. oder i.m. (letztere Applikationsform nur mit 5 %-Lösung) als Einzel- oder
Repetitionsdosis von 0,5–10,0 mg/kg Körpergewicht injiziert.

b) Bei insgesamt mehr als 1300 dissoziativen Anaesthesien mit Ketamine
beziehen sich Prozent-Angaben und Zahlen (Nebenwirkungen u. a.) auf die
ersten 1000 Fälle.

In 252 Fällen wurde keine Prämedikation verabfolgt. Bei Bronchoskopien
wurde 15–45 min vor CI-581 eine Prämedikation von 0,5 mg Bellafolin und
7,5 mg Dicodid gegeben. In den übrigen Fällen erhielten die Patienten 15–45 min
vor CI-581 50–100 mg Dolantin und 0,5 mg Bellafolin oder 1–2 ml Thalamonal
und 0,5 mg Bellafolin i.m. Die Mehrzahl der geburtshilflichen Fälle erhielt
0,25–0,5 mg Bellafolin i.v. oder i.m.

---

* Mit Unterstützung der Deutschen Forschungsgemeinschaft.

Soweit Kinder zu den Fällen mit Prämedikation zählen, wurde die Dolantin-Bellafolin-Vorgabe nach Maßgabe einer von uns benutzten Tabelle je nach Körpergewicht (Langrehr u. L'Allemand, 1962) vorgenommen; die Bellafolinmengen bewegen sich dabei zwischen 0,15–1,0 mg, die Dolantinmengen zwischen 5–90 mg.

Bei Bronchoskopien, Bronchographien sowie Appendektomien wurde in insgesamt 303 Fällen neben CI-581 noch Succinylcholin 50–200 mg i.v. verabfolgt und mit O_2 beatment. In 116 Fällen von Narkoseeinleitung mit CI-581 wurden 1–2 mg/kg Ketamine injiziert und die Anaesthesie mit einer Kombinationsnarkose ($N_2O:O_2$; Fluothane; Relaxation) fortgeführt. In den übrigen 581 Fällen wurde Ketamin, eventuell neben der Prämedikation, als alleiniges Anaesthetikum verabreicht. In 52 Fällen wurden wiederholte Anaesthesien mit Ketamin bei dem gleichen Patienten (bis maximal 11 mal) durchgeführt. 109 von 1000 Fällen waren vom anaesthesiologischen Standpunkt als Risikofälle aufzufassen (siehe auch Tab. 2).

c) Im Rahmen einer noch nicht abgeschlossenen spinal-motorischen Analyse wurde an laminektomierten Katzen in oberflächlicher intraperitonealer Nembutal-Anaesthesie der monosynaptische Massenreflex (MMR) eines Extensor-Motoneuronen-Verbandes nach submaximaler elektrischer afferenter Einzelschockreizung des peripheren N. gastrocnemius aus einem entsprechenden Vorderwurzel-Filament abgeleitet. Die dosisabhängige Veränderung der MMR-Amplitude nach Ketamine gibt Aufschluß über die Veränderung der Entladungsbereitschaft lumbaler Motoneurone. Einzelfilamentableitungen afferenter Muskelspindel-entladungen (Hinterwurzelfilamente) vor und nach Durchtrennung entsprechender Vorderwurzeln gaben Auskunft über direkte Ketamine-Wirkungen auf deefferentierte Proprioceptoren sowie über Änderungen der retikulären Antriebe der γ-Muskelspindelschleife (efferent innervierte Muskelspindeln als Indikator der γ-Motoneuronaktivität). Einzelheiten der Ableitmethodik für die spinalmotorische Analyse siehe bei Henatsch, Langrehr, Schulte u. Kaese (1962).

d) Nach Beobachtung der Häufigkeit von initialen, sprunghaften, seitensynchronen Pupillenerweiterungen (Hippus) innerhalb der ersten 2–3 min nach Ketamine wurde in 100 Fällen die endgültige Pupillenweite registriert.

e) Zur Beurteilung der Wirkung von Ketamine auf atmungszentrale Substrate wurden bei 6 Patienten Atemantriebe im Rückatmungsversuch mit dem Almara-4-Glocken-Spirographen (Wassner, 1961) durchgeführt. Die CO_2-Antwortkurven des wachen Patienten wurden mit denen nach 1,5 oder 3 mg/kg Ketamine am gleichen Patienten in Beziehung gesetzt.

f) Zum Vergleich mit dem früher mitgeteilten Verhalten des Blutzuckerspiegels nach Ketamine (Langrehr u. Mitarb., 1967) wurden die Blutzuckerwerte von 5 Diabetikern bis zu 3 Std nach 4 mg/kg CI-581 bestimmt. Die Patienten, die sich kleineren chirurgischen Eingriffen zu unterziehen hatten, wurden etwa 2–3 Std nach morgendlichem Frühstück und Insulingabe der dissoziativen Anaesthesie unterworfen.

g) In Zusammenarbeit mit dem Zoologischen Garten Wuppertal wurden 50 Narkosen mit Ketamine an verschiedenen Tierspezies und -individuen durchgeführt, wobei nach i.m.-Applikation der 5%igen Lösung (5–25 mg/kg) jeweils die Zeit der chirurgischen Toleranz und die Zeit bis zum Ende der ersten Erholungsphase, d. h. bis das Tier sich aus eigener Kraft auf die Beine stellen konnte oder zu laufen und klettern begann, registriert. Diese Untersuchungen dienten der Klärung von Dosis-Wirkungsdauerbeziehungen und der veterinär-anaesthesiologischen Indikation für die Anwendung von Ketamine (Langrehr u. Mueller, 1967).

Tabelle 1. *Arithmetische Blutdruck- und Herzfrequenzmittelwerte nach Ketamine unter verschiedenen Ausgangsbedingungen*

RR mmHg vor Puls/min	nach 1 min	3 min	5 min	7 min	10 min	Maximale Steigerung mmHg Freq./min	%	Bedingung
1. 138/81 110	160/91 128	166/93 127	156/88 126	149/84 119	143/82 114	28/12 18	20/14 16	100 × 1–2 mg/kg Normotonie
2. 210/109 101	239/125 109	261/139 115	256/129 113	236/115 109	217/111 112	51/30 14	24/28 14	14 × 1–1,5 mg/kg Hypertonie
3. 130/82 99	145/87 114	155/93 121	153/90 124	145/86 108	139/84 109	25/11 25	19/13 25	15 × 1–2 mg/kg ohne Prämedikation
4. 93/69 114	119/81 123	119/79 123	122/79 123	120/79 116	123/79 112	30/12 9	30/18 8	58 × 1–5 mg/kg Hypotonie, Risikofälle
5. 144/80 110	151/94 112	166/98 121	169/99 125	168/100 119	152/89 115	25/20 15	18/25 14	15 × 1,5 mg/kg 2-min-Injektion
6. 142/77 107	165/92 125	169/99 123	169/94 124	163/90 117	152/88 115	27/22 18	19/28 16	15 × 1,5 mg/kg 5-sec-Injektion
7. 125/75 110	144/80 138	158/90 130	150/92 127	140/86 115	130/82 108	33/15 28	25/20 25	10 × 1 mg/kg Einleitung kombinieter Narkose
8. 132/81 96	149/87 114	157/95 115	153/92 119	149/93 111	144/88 107	25/14 23	19/17 24	81 × 1–5 mg/kg Risikofälle
vor	nach 4 min	8 min	12 min	16 min	20 min			
9. 127/79 94	153/94 99	150/93 111	141/90 110	135/86 107	130/84 107	26/15 17	20/19 18	10 × 3 mg/kg ohne Prämedikation Eröffnungsperiode Kreißender

h) Die Aufzeichnung der Uteruskontraktionen bei Kreissenden während der Eröffnungsperiode nach Ketamine (3 mg/kg) wurde mittels externer Tokometrie (Frankfurter Tokograph nach Siener der Firma Hartmann & Braun, Frankfurt/M. und Atlas-Recorder 8001) gewonnen. Die Beurteilung der Neugeborenen nach geburtshilflichen Eingriffen in dissoziativer Anaesthesie erfolgte 60 sec nach der Geburt, unabhängig vom Abnabelungstermin, nach dem von V. Apgar angegebenen Schema.

i) Die Bestimmung relativer Herzzeitvolumenwerte und des thorakalen Blutvolumens nach Ketamine wurde mit Hilfe von Farbverdünnungskurven durchgeführt, die über eine Ohreinheit mit zugehörigem Atlas-Doppeloxymeter synchron auf Direktschreiber und Fotoschreiber (Atlas Combicard, 15 cm Papierbreite) registriert werden konnten.

Ergebnisse

1. Blutkreislauf und Myokard

Nach der i.v.-Applikation von CI-581 kommt es ohne initiale Schwankungen zu einem kontinuierlichen Blutdruckanstieg, der sein Maximum bei rascher Injektion (5 sec) etwa um die dritte Minute p. i. erreicht, bei langsamer Injektion (2 min) um die 4.–5. min. Die allmähliche Rückkehr des Systemblutdruckes zum Ausgangsniveau dauert meist länger als 10 min und ist in der 20. min fast immer erreicht. Die Höhe der Initialdosis (0,5–6 mg/kg i.v.) spielt für den Grad der Druckerhöhung keine wesentliche Rolle (siehe auch Domino, Chodoff und Corssen, 1965). Repetierte Einzeldosen bewirken dementsprechend nur dann eine erneute Blutdrucksteigerung, wenn die Druckerhöhung schon wieder deutlich rückläufig war. Der langsame Anstieg des systolischen und diastolischen Druckes ohne größere Amplitudenänderung zusammen mit einer synchronen Pulsfrequenzsteigerung betrifft normotone, hypotone und hypertone Patienten gleichermaßen. Während die prozentuale Veränderung keine ausgeprägte Abhängigkeit von den verwendeten Dosierungen, dem Ausgangsniveau und der Prämedikation zeigt, findet sich eine solche jedoch bei extrem unterschiedlichen Ausgangslagen, z. B.: i.m.-Injektion, bei Kindern mit gesundem Gefäßsystem gegenüber i.v.-Injektionen bei ausgeprägtem stabilem Hypertonus. Die Tabelle 1 faßt unsere Befunde über das Blutdruckverhalten unter verschiedenen Bedingungen zusammen. Wir weisen insonderheit auf zwei Punkte hin:

a) Auch bei hypotoner Ausgangslage und im Schock findet sich nach Ketamine fast immer diese Blutdruckerhöhung.

b) Wegen der möglicherweise unerwünschten weiteren Blutdrucksteigerung bei malignen Hypertonien sehen wir im Vorliegen eines Hypertonus von mehr als 200 mmHg systolischem Blutdruck eine Kontraindikation gegen die Anwendung von Ketamine.

Wir fanden bei der peripheren Durchblutungsmessung im Tierexperiment (Katze; Hund und Affe verhalten sich in bezug auf Blutdrucksteigerung und peripheren Widerstand offenbar nicht einheitlich, CHEN u. Mitarb. 1967; SZAPPANYOS u. GEMPERLE 1968; TRABER u. Mitarb. 1968) eine Vasokonstriktion der Extremitätenstrombahn (LANGREHR u. Mitarb. 1967). Zusammen mit den Befunden am Menschen (Herzzeitvolumen, peripherer Widerstand; ähnliche Ergebnisse auch bei VIRTUE u. Mitarb. 1967 sowie KREUSCHER u. Mitarb. 1967), dem langsam und kontinuierlich verlaufendenden Blutdruck- und Pulsfrequenzanstieg, den Befunden über das initiale Pupillenspiel und die spinale Motorik (siehe weiter unten) halten wir diesen Kreislaufeffekt für nervös bedingt und sehen in ihm den Ausdruck für eine substanzbedingte Zunahme des Sympathikotonus. Während ILETT u. Mitarb. (1966) für andere Phencyclidinderivate auch eine direkte Wirkung auf adrenergische α-Rezeptoren diskutieren, halten CHEN u. Mitarb. (1967) die Herz-Kreislaufeffekte für den Ausdruck einer Stimulierung kardio-vasomotorischer rhombencephaler Substrate. Sie fanden keinen Anhalt für Änderungen des Catecholaminspiegels im Blut von Rattenherzen.

Die Abb. 1 zeigt das Verhalten von Blutdruck, Herzfrequenz, Herzzeitvolumen und thorakalem Blutvolumen bei 4 Patienten nach jeweils 2 mg/kg CI-581 i.v. Mit steigendem Blutdruck und Herzfrequenz finden sich mehr oder weniger ausgeprägte Anstiege des Herzzeitvolumens, in unseren Fällen bis maximal 28% über den Ausgangswert, bei gleichzeitiger Abnahme des thorakalen Blutvolumens in 3 Fällen. Nur in einem Fall (Abb. 1, links oben 14 ♂, 48 kg) findet sich eine Zunahme des thorakalen Blutvolumens. In allen 4 Fällen findet sich eine mäßige Zunahme des errechneten peripheren Gesamtwiderstandes, die nur in einem Fall (links unten, 32 ♂, 62 kg) größer ist und maximal 30% vom Ausgangswert erreicht (LANGREHR 1969).

Die Steigerung der Herzauswurfleistung mit synchron steigendem Blutdruck und steigendem Venendruck sowie nicht vermindertem, eher erhöhtem peripheren Gesamtwiderstand steht im Einklang mit der Vorstellung über die Stimulierung kreislaufzentraler Substrate.

Beim Zustandekommen dieses Effektes von Ketamine spielen mechanosensible Herz- und Gefäßrezeptoren im Sinne einer Verminderung ihrer afferenten Impulse zu den rhombencephalen Zentren wohl keine Rolle. Wegen der nur geringen lokalanaesthetischen Nebenwirkung von Ketamine werden Vorhofs- und Aortenrezeptoren im Tierexperiment erst durch Maximaldosierungen in ihren Entladungen gehemmt, deren Rezeptor-Kontaktkonzentrationen bei klinischen Dosierungen kaum erreicht werden dürften (LANGREHR u. Mitarb. 1967; DOWDY u. KAYA 1968). In Übereinstimmung mit MC CARTHY und CHEN (1966, 1967) sowie WHEELOCK fanden auch wir im Tierexperiment keinen Hinweis auf wesentliche myokarddepressorische Wirkungen von Ketamine, erst bei sehr hohen Konzentrationen (0,2 mg/ml Ketamine in der Badflüssigkeit) am Herz-Lungenpräparat (TRABER u. Mitarb. 1968; 1969) und bei zusätzlicher Basisnarkose (DOWDY u. Mitarb. 1968) wurde über negativ inotrope Effekte berichtet.

Entsprechend konnten wir auch beim Menschen, selbst in Riskofällen und Schocksituationen keinen deutlichen Blutdruckabfall oder Herzrhythmusstörungen beobachten, worauf wir unsere Empfehlung der dissoziativen Anaesthesie für Risikofälle stützen (siehe auch KASSEL 1968; STANLEY u. Mitarb. 1968 und Zeile 4. u. 8. der Tabelle 1).

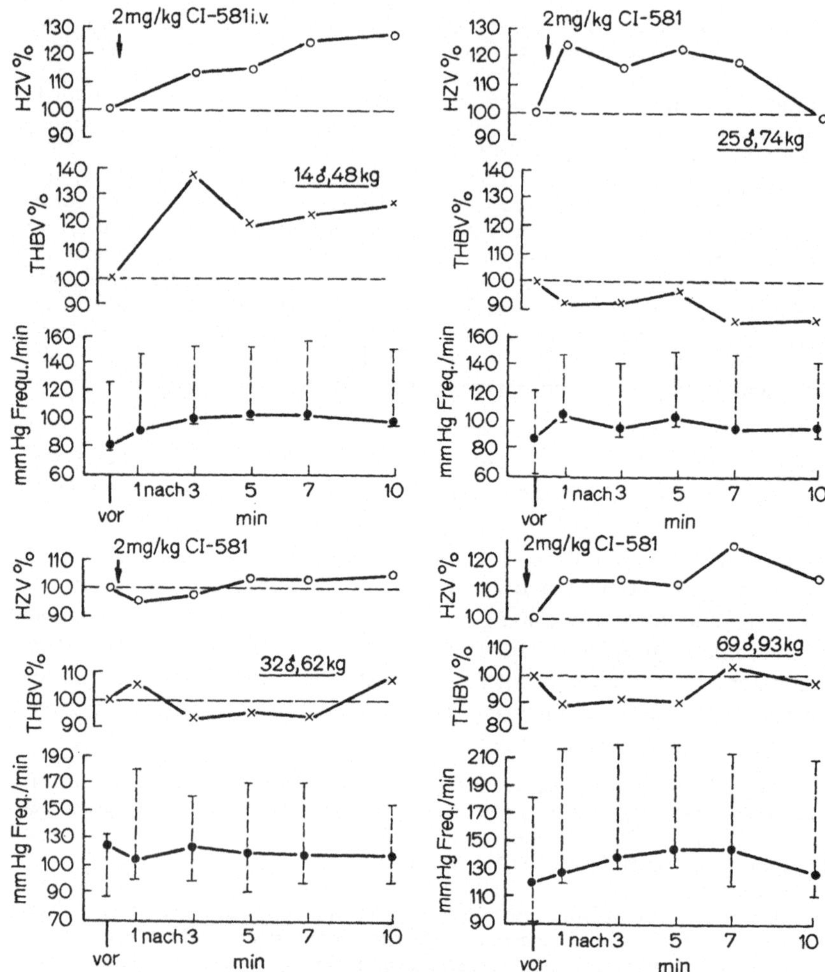

Abb. 1. Verhalten von Blutdruck, Pulsfrequenz, Herzzeitvolumen, thorakalem Blutvolumen nach 2 mg/kg Ketamine bei 4 Patienten. Jeweils von oben nach unten: relatives Herzminutenvolumen in %, thorakales Blutvolumen in %, Blutdruck und Pulsfrequenz

Die Abb. 2 zeigt den Vergleich des Verhaltens von Systolendauer, Austreibungszeit, Anspannungszeit, Herzfrequenz, des Quotienten Austreibungszeit/Anspannungszeit und des Quotienten Austreibungszeit/Herzfrequenz unter der Wirkung von 2 mg/kg Ketamine i.v. und 2 Vol.-% Fluothane. Diese Meßgrößen bieten nach den Angaben von Holldack, Blumberger u. Meiners (Kreuscher, 1966) die Möglichkeit einer Beurteilung der Myokardkontraktionskraft.

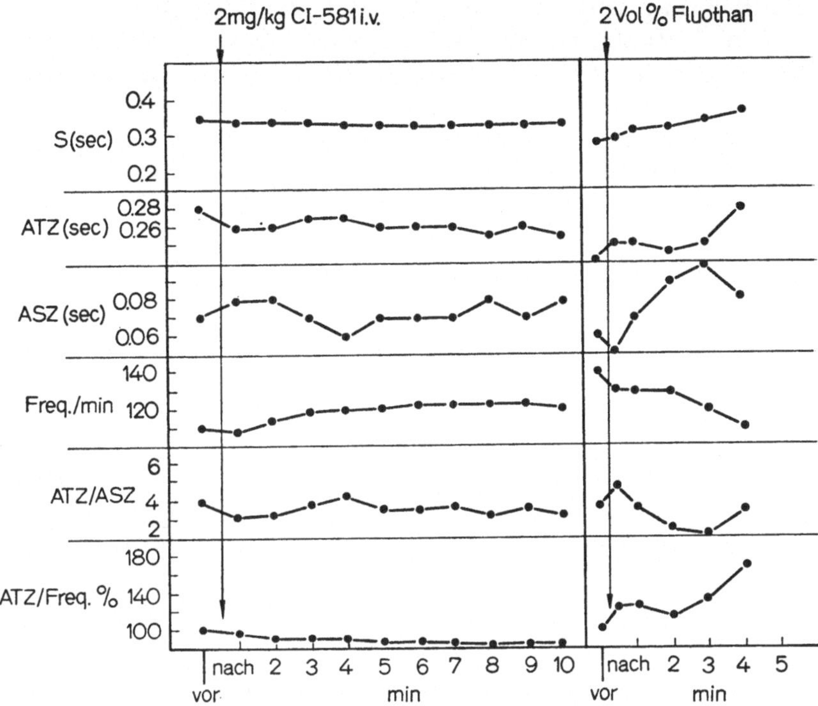

Abb. 2. Vergleich der direkten Myokardwirkung von 2 mg/kg Ketamine i.v. und 2 Vol.-% Fluothane. S = Systolendauer, ATZ = Austreibungszeit, ASZ = Anspannungszeit, ATZ = Hinweis auf die Kontraktionskraft nach Blumberger, ATZ/Freq. = relative Austreibungszeit nach Meiners. Jeder Punkt arithmetisches Mittel von 10 aufeinanderfolgenden Herzrevolutionen (± 1,0 %). Werte aus der Registrierung von Herzschall, EKG, Druck A. axillaris

Während schon wenige Minuten nach 2 Vol.-%-Fluothane-Applikation bei fallender Herzfrequenz die Anspannungszeit (ASZ) deutlich verlängert ist und die relative Austreibungszeit (ATZ/Freq.) weit über die zulässige Grenze von 110% ansteigt (deutliche Myokarddepression), findet sich nach Ketamine keine signifikante Abweichung von den Ausgangswerten.

2. Atmung

Nach der i.v.-Applikation von Ketamine bis zu Dosen von 6 mg/kg i.v. bleiben der Tonus der Zungengrund- und Rachenmuskulatur erhalten, ebenso die Rachenreflexe, d. h. die Atemwege frei. Als Beleg für die im allgemeinen suffiziente Spontanatmung dienten uns Blutgasanalysen bei alten Patienten in reduziertem Allgemeinzustand und bei Frauen während geburtshilflicher Eingriffe (Langrehr u. Mitarb. 1967; Stolp u. Mitarb. 1968). In Übereinstimmung mit Befunden von Virtue (1967), Podlesch u. Zindler (1967), Corssen u. Mitarb. (1965 bis 1967) fanden sich keine signifikanten Abweichungen der Blutgaswerte vom Normbereich. Darüber hinaus zeigt die Abb. 3 den Vergleich der CO_2-Antwortkurven bei 4 Patienten im Wachzustand und während dissoziativer Anaesthesie mit 1,5 oder

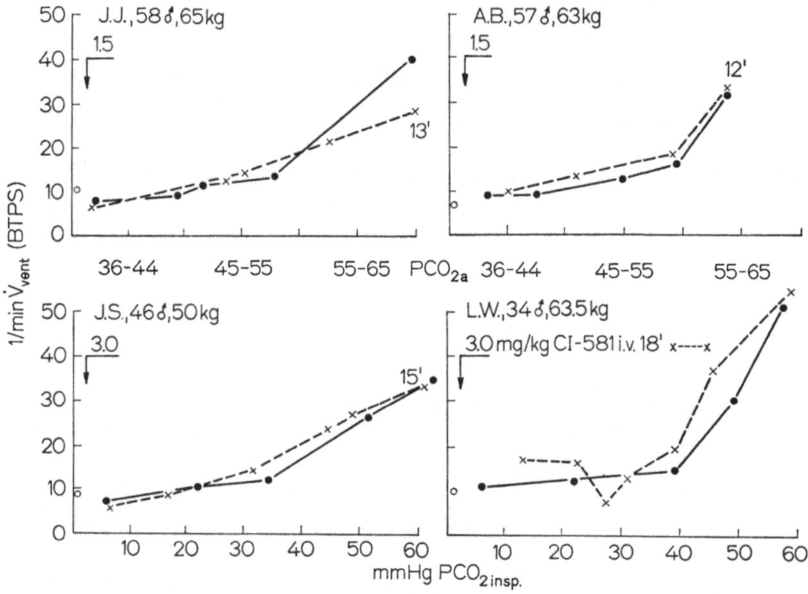

Abb. 3. CO_2-Antwortkurven von 4 Patienten, oben nach 1,5, unten nach 3,0 mg/kg Ketamine i.v. Rückatmung, Almara-4-Glocken-Spirograph. Atemminutenvolumen ($\dot{V}$ vent) jeweils im steady state des inspiratorischen P_{CO_2}-Wertes. Zwischen den oberen und unteren Kurven Näherungswerte des P_{CO_2} im arteriellen Blut nach den Erfahrungen einer anderen Versuchsreihe unter den Bedingungen des Rückatmungsversuches. (·————· Atemantrieb wacher Patienten, × - - - × nach Ketamine)

3 mg/kg Ketamine. Im Gegensatz zu der bekannten Verminderung der Ansprechbarkeit atmungszentraler Substrate auf CO_2-Erhöhung nach nahezu allen bekannten Narkosemitteln finden wir nach Ketamine in diesen Fällen keine signifikante Depression des Atemantriebes. Die gleichzeitige Bestimmung des globalen O_2-Verbrauchs zeigt während der Ketamine-Anaesthesie keinen Abfall desselben, sondern eher eine Tendenz zum Anstieg, was wohl in erster Linie mit der Tonuszunahme der Skelettmuskulatur in Zusammenhang gebracht werden kann.

Wenn auch im allgemeinen die Spontanatmung suffizient und die Atemwege frei bleiben, müssen wir VIRTUE u. Mitarb. (1966) sowie PODLESCH u. ZINDLER (1967) beipflichten, daß auch bei der Ketamine-Anaesthesie eine Beatmungsmöglichkeit immer vorhanden sein muß. Wir waren bei 1000 Fällen 12mal gezwungen, wegen apnoischer Phasen oder Glottiskrampf manuell zu beatmen. Bei meist suffizienter äußerer Atmung finden sich doch regelmäßig charakteristische Rhythmusstörungen:

1. Steigerung der Atmungstiefe bei verlangsamter Frequenz.

2. Serien frequenter kleinvolumiger Atemzüge.

3. Apnoische Phasen bis zu maximal 40 sec Dauer, gefolgt von

4. tiefen seufzerartigen Inspirationen bis zu 2000 ccm Zugvolumen mit endinspiratorischem Plateau.

Eine Tendenz zur Verschiebung der Atemmittellage nach der Inspirationsseite, d. h. zur Vergrößerung des exspiratorischen Reservevolumens hin, ist während der Ketaminewirkung nicht selten zu beobachten. Sie wird zum Ende der Narkose beim Übergang in den Nachschlaf wieder ausgeglichen und ist nach unserer Meinung der Grund für die Anhebung der Basislinie bei der externen Tokometrie (siehe weiter unten). Wir konnten sie bei unseren Zootiernarkosen, vor allem bei Huftieren, regelmäßig beobachten, wobei sie leicht eine Tympanie des Bauchraumes vortäuschen kann.

Die Rhythmusänderungen der Spontanatmung, insbesondere die tiefen Atemzüge und die endinspiratorischen Plateaus, haben gewisse Ähnlichkeit mit der Atmung nach Vagusdurchgrennung im Tierexperiment. Inwieweit für das Zustandekommen solcher Atmungsformen ein zentraler Effekt ursächlich in Frage kommt, muß zunächst offen bleiben. Eine periphere pharmokologische Deafferentierung durch Beeinträchtigung der pulmonalen Dehnungsrezeptoren ist hierfür wohl auch verantwortlich zu machen. Wir fanden endoanaesthetische Nebeneffekte (ZIPF, 1953) von Ketamine auf Lungendehnungsrezeptoren im Tierexperiment (LANGREHR, 1967).
Andererseits werden die nociceptiven Afferenzen der oberen Luftwege (rasch adaptierende Rezeptoren, Afferenzen des Hustenreflexes) wesentlich weniger beeinflußt als die pulmonalen Dehnungsrezeptoren (langsam adaptierend, Inspirationshemmung). Das steht im Einklang mit dem unbeeinträchtigten Hustenreflex auf der einen Seite und den inspiratorischen Plateauphasen nach Ketamine auf der anderen.

3. Intraokularer Druck, Sehstörungen, Pupillenspiel

Ganz ähnlich wie bei anderen Narkoseformen (LANGREHR, ADELSTEIN u. L'ALLEMAND, 1966) folgt der intraokulare Druck während der Ketaminewirkung dem Systemblutdruck (LANGREHR, 1967). Die intraokularen Druckanstiege von 2–8 cm H_2O gestatten die Anwendung von

Ketamine z. B. auch bei Glaukompatienten. Nach initialem Vertikal- oder Horizontalnystagmus (vor allem bei Kindern) sind in der Aufwachphase der dissoziativen Anaesthesie bis zur völligen Orientierung und noch darüber hinaus Sehstörungen im Sinne von Konvergenzschwäche, Doppelbildersehen und Flimmern als Nebenwirkung typisch und können möglicherweise für das Auftreten von Schwindegefühl, Übelkeit und Erbrechen (s. Tab. 2) verantwortlich gemacht werden. Die Bedeutung solcher Sehstörungen für die Beurteilung der Straßenfähigkeit liegt auf der Hand. Im Rahmen der Beurteilung der Adaptationsschwierigkeiten in der Aufwachphase (Psychomimetik s. weiter unten) spielen diese Störungen ebenfalls eine wesentliche Rolle.

Auf das Phänomen von sprunghaften seitensynchronen Pupillenerweiterungen in den ersten Minuten nach Ketamineapplikation (Hippus) hat Mundeleer hingewiesen. Wir fanden dieses Phänomen bei 100 daraufhin untersuchten Patienten in jedem Fall. Danach stellte sich die Pupillenweite in der Mehrzahl der Fälle (90%) auf eine mittlere Weite (2–4 mm Durchmesser) ein. Eine Dosisabhängigkeit der endgültigen Pupillenweite fanden wir nicht. Zur Erklärung der unregelmäßigen Innervationssteigerung des M. dilatator pupillae können 2 Möglichkeiten herangezogen werden:

1. Eine vermehrte Aktivität im Grenzstrang des Sympathicus,

2. eine vermehrte neuronale Aktivität im Nucleus nervi oculomotorii, die ihrerseits über Kollateralen der zentralen Sehbahn (N. interstitialis reticularis Cajal) induziert sein kann.

Neben der Störung der Akkomodations- und Fusionskonvergenz sind offenbar unter dem Einfluß von Ketamine verschiedene Hilfsmechanismen des Auges betroffen.

Im Zusammenhang mit der diskutierten Wirkungsweise von Ketamine auf die Atmungs- und Kreislaufregulation gehen wir wohl bei der Betrachtung der zusätzlichen okularen Phänomene nicht fehl in der Annahme, daß es sich um eine an der Retikulärformation aktive, zumindest nicht depressiv wirkende Substanz handelt. Dafür sprechen auch die Befunde der spinalmotorischen Analyse und die EEG-Ableitungen (Kugler u. Doenicke, Szappanyos u. Gemperle, Corssen u. Domino).

4. Spinale Motorik

Im Gegensatz zu der bei anderen Anaesthesieformen üblichen Dämpfung spinalmotorischer Substrate finden sich nach Ketamine einige Besonderheiten: Erhaltener Skelettmuskeltonus, erhaltene oder gesteigerte Eigenreflexe, suffiziente Atemmotorik, faszikuläre Muskelzuckungen vorwiegend der oberen Rumpf- und Armmuskulatur, langsame koordinierte Kopf- und Extremitätenbewegungen nach Art athetotischer Bewegungsabläufe, stärkere motorische Exzitationen insbesondere bei niedrigen Dosierungen. Der gemeinsame Nenner dieser Effekte ist in einer gesteigerten Entladungsbereitschaft bestimmter Motoneuronenverbände zu suchen, ein Phänomen, welches z. B. auch die Phenoxyessigsäurederivate auslösen. Bei diesen Stoffen konnte eine Wirkung im Bereich der Stammhirn-Retikulärformation wahrscheinlich gemacht werden (BRINLING, SHOPIRO u. SIGG 1962; LANGREHR u. L'ALLEMAND 1963, 1964; WIRTH u. HOFFMEISTER 1964). Zur Detailanalyse der spinalmotorischen Effekte von Ketamine, die noch nicht abgeschlossen ist, können wir bislang folgendes beitragen: An deefferentierten Muskelspindeln ließ sich kein Direkteffekt von Ketamine nachweisen. Auf der anderen Seite zeigten efferent innervierte Spindeln sowohl eine Verminderung ihrer durch Ohrmuschelreiz (Pinna) induzierten Hemmung wie auch eine Vermehrung der Pinna-Förderung nach Ketamine. Die Abb. 4 zeigt die dosisabhängige Vergrößerung

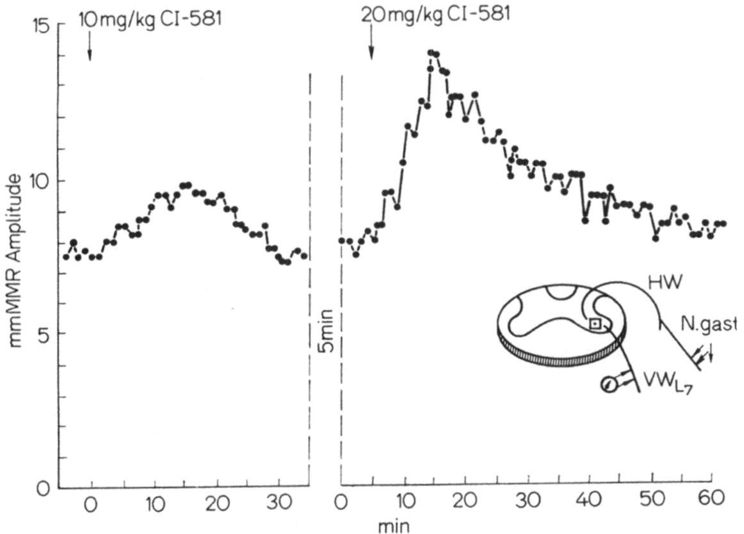

Abb. 4. Dosisabhängige Steigerung der Entladungsbereitschaft lumbaler Motoneurone nach Ketamine i.v. Katze, intraperitoneale Nembutal-Narkose, laminektomiert. MMR = monosynaptischer Massenreflex eines Extensor-Motoneuronenverbandes, Reizung des peripheren N. gastrocnemius mit submaximalen Einzelschocks, Ableitung des MMR aus VW L7-Filament

der Amplitude der durch submaximale Einzelschockreize des N. gastrocnemius induzierten monosynaptischen Massenentladung (MMR) eines Extensor-Motoneuronenverbandes und belegt die Verstärkung der Entladungsbereitschaft solcher Motoneuronenverbände durch Ketamine.

3*

Als vorläufiges Resultat dieser Untersuchungen kann festgehalten werden, daß

1. eine gesteigerte Entladungsbereitschaft spinaler Motoneuronenverbände vorliegt, und daß diese

2. mit einer Vermehrung zentrifugaler Antriebe (Retikulärformation) auf die γ-Muskelspindelschleife einhergeht. Diese Befunde stehen in Übereinstimmung mit der Tatsache, daß dem Ketamine, im Gegensatz zu anderen anaesthetischen Pharmaka, eine ausgesprochen antikonvulsive Eigenschaft fehlt (Chen u. Mitarb. 1967). Auf der anderen Seite besitzt es aber selbst in höheren Dosierungen im Tierexperiment auch keine krampfauslösende Wirkung (Chen u. Mitarb. 1967). Unsere Befunde bei zwei Raubkatzen (siehe weiter unten), bei denen es zu tonisch-klonischen Krampfanfällen kam, sind mit großer Wahrscheinlichkeit auf einen artspezifischen Metabolismus (starke Abbauverzögerung, Überdosierung) zurückzuführen. Die vereinzelten Fälle von „Krämpfen" nach Ketamine beim Menschen (Helrich; Dowdy; Corssen; Sbarounis [4 Fälle]) betreffen cerebral vorgeschädigte Individuen. Drei von uns einer dissoziativen Anaesthesie unterzogene Patienten mit genuiner Epilepsie zeigten keine Besonderheiten, auch konnten wir unter 1300 Fällen keine tonisch-klonischen Krämpfe beobachten. Im Einklang mit den mitgeteilten EEG-Befunden kann demnach die Gefahr für das Auftreten von epileptiformen Krampfanfällen nach Ketamine wohl nicht als gravierend betrachtet werden (siehe auch Corssen u. Mitarb. 1968).

5. Laborbefunde, Blutzuckerspiegel

In Übereinstimmung mit Befunden von Domino u. Mitarb. (1965, 1966) sowie McCarthy u. Mitarb. (1965) konnten wir bei einem ganzen Spektrum von Laborwerten nach Ketamine keine signifikante Änderung irgendeines Wertes feststellen, die uns veranlaßt hätte, weitere Untersuchungen dieses Wertes vorzunehmen. Es wurden untersucht: Hämoglobin, Erythrocytenzahl, Leukocytenzahl, BSG, Urinstatus, Differentialblutbild, Rest-N, SGOT, SGPT, LDH (Langrehr u. Mitarb. 1967). Nur weil von einer Substanz mit sympaticomimetischer Wirkung ein Effekt auf den Blutzuckerspiegel erwartet werden kann, haben wir diesen bei 20 Patienten bis zu 4 Std nach 4 mg/kg CI-581 i.v. kontrolliert.

Die Abb. 5 zeigt oben die Einzelbestimmungswerte bei 20 normoglukämischen Patienten bezogen auf den Ausgangswert = 100%. Es findet sich ein leichter Anstieg der arithmetischen Mittelwerte bei diesen Patienten, die während der 1. Std nach CI-581 gleichzeitig einem chirurgischen Eingriff unterzogen wurden. Unten zeigt die Abb. 5 das Verhalten des Blutzuckerspiegels bei 5 Diabetikern nach der gleichen Dosis Ketamine, die ebenfalls während der 1. Std kleineren chirurgischen Eingriffen unterzogen wurden. Die nach dem Frühstück und morgendlicher Insulingabe normalerweise leicht fallende Tendenz der Blutzuckerwerte wird durch eine dissoziative Anaesthesie ca. 2–3 Std nach dem Frühstück nicht verändert.

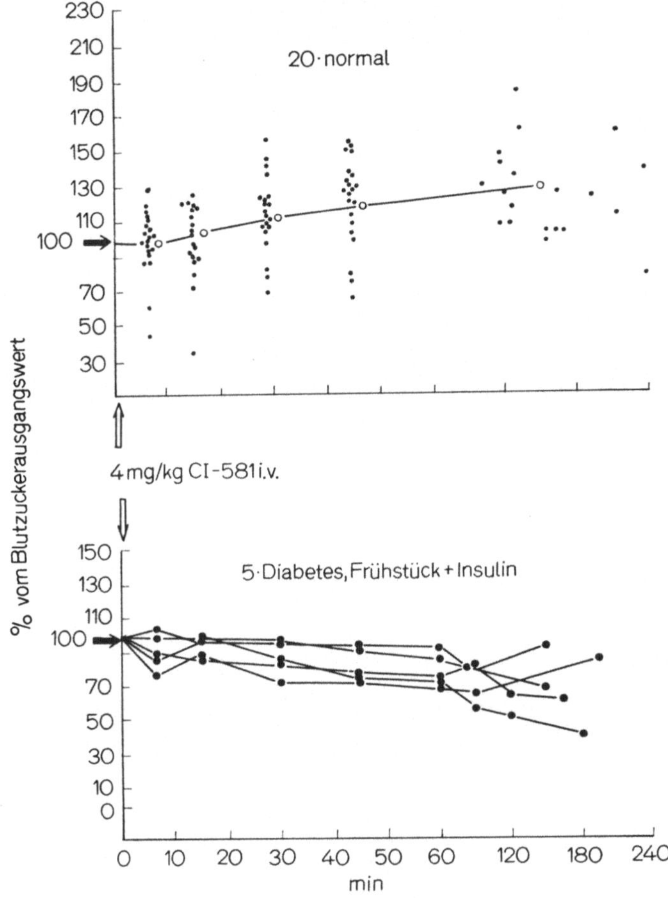

Abb. 5. Verhalten des Blutzuckerspiegels bei 20 normoglucämischen Patienten nach 4 mg/kg Ketamine i.v. (oben) und bei 5 Diabetikern nach 4 mg/kg Ketamine i.v. (unten). Umrechnung aller bis zu 4 Std p.i. gefundenen Werte auf Prozent vom Ausgangswert = 100 % (Punkte); arithmetische Mittelwerte jeder Zeitgruppe oben (Kreise)

Dieser Befund steht im Einklang mit der Erfahrung bei einer ganzen Reihe von kleineren chirurgischen Eingriffen an Diabetikern, die wir bevorzugt in dissoziativer Anaesthesie durchgeführt haben und bei denen die Blutzuckerwerte erst wieder mittags und abends bestimmt wurden.

6. Dosis-Wirkungsdauer, Stoffwechsel, Toxizität, diaplacentarae Passage, Uteruswirkung

Die Abb. 6 zeigt die von uns gefundene Dosis-Wirkungsdauerbeziehung für Ketamine bis zu 6 mg/kg i.v. als Mittelwerte bei 500 Erwachsenen teils mit, teils ohne Prämedikation und von 6–10 mg/kg i.m. als Mittelwerte bei 60 Kindern bis zu 6 Jahren. Sofern nicht mehr als 0,5 bis maximal 1,0 ml der 5%igen Lösung in ein Injektionsdepot der gut durchbluteten Oberschenkelstreckmuskulatur bei Kindern injiziert wird (bei benötigten größeren Mengen also mehrere Depots) schließen sich die Wirkungszeiten nach i.m.-Applikationen direkt an den Kurvenverlauf derjenigen nach i.v.-Applikation an. Lediglich die Latenz zwischen Injektion und Wirkungs-eintritt verlängert sich von 20–40 sec i.v. auf 2–4 min i.m. Sobald punktier-bare Venen vorhanden sind, würden wir auf die i.m.-Injektion, so wertvoll ihre Möglichkeit für Kleinkinder und Säuglinge ist, verzichten. Unter die-sen Voraussetzungen können wir die Angabe: i.m. = 3–5fach höhere Dosierung zur Erzielung gleicher Wirkungszeiten wie i.v., nicht bestätigen.

Werden größere Mengen Ketamine (5–10 mg/kg) bei größeren Kindern als Depot an einen einzigen Ort i.m. injiziert, so kommt es allerdings wegen der protrahierten Resorption zu einer von den Toleranzzeiten der Abb. 6

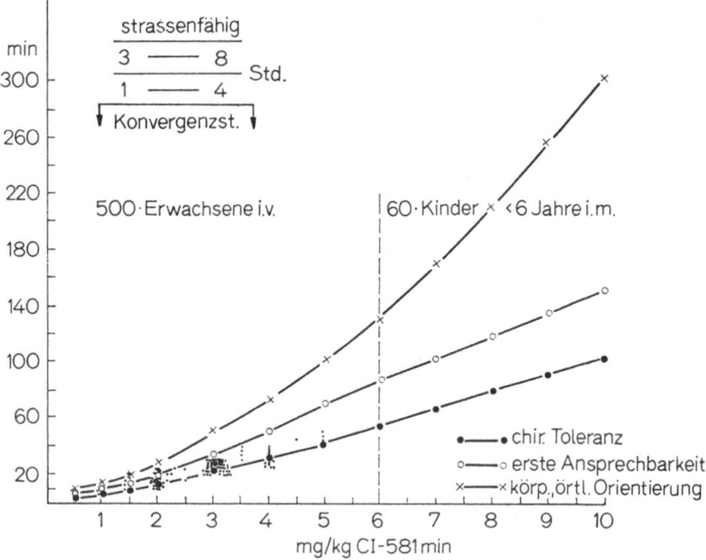

Abb. 6. Dosis-Wirkungsdauerbeziehung von Ketamine nach i.v.-Applikation (0,5–6,0 mg/kg; Mittelwerte von 500 Erwachsenen, teils mit, teils ohne Prä-medikation) und i.m.-Applikation (6,0—10,0 mg/kg; Mittelwerte von 60 Kindern bis zu 6 Jahren). Einzelheiten siehe Text. Punkte = Toleranzzeiten bei 100 geburts-hilflichen Eingriffen

abweichenden Verkürzung der für chirurgische Eingriffe nutzbaren Zeit, während die Erholungsphasen ungefähr gleich ausgedehnt bleiben. Dieselben Zusammenhänge sind auch bei unseren Zootier-Narkosen mit i.m.-Applikation in Ansatz zu bringen (siehe weiter unten). Kalkuliert man Resorptionsverzögerungen mit ein, so kommt bei Beachtung des oben Gesagten nach unserer Erfahrung für die i.m.-Applikation höchstens eine $1\frac{1}{2}$–2fache Menge der i.v.-Dosierung in Ansatz.

Wir haben, wie die Abb. 6 zeigt, die Wirkungsdauer vierteilig erfaßt:

1. Dauer der Toleranz gegenüber chirurgischen Eingriffen.

2. Dauer bis zum ersten verbalen Kontakt. In dieser Zeit besteht noch eine erhebliche Analgesie und eine komplette Amnesie, obwohl evtl. schon Lautäußerungen und Extremitätenbewegungen zu beobachten sind. Diese Phase könnte der chirurgischen Toleranz noch zugeschlagen werden, jedoch sollten wegen der weiter unten zu erläuternden Vermeidung von starkem Afferenzeinstrom in der Aufwachphase (Psychomimetik) jetzt alle Manipulationen am Patienten beendet sein.

3. Der Zeitraum von der ersten Ansprechbarkeit bis zur völligen zeitlichen, örtlichen und körperlichen Orientiertheit kommt für eine chirurgische Intervention nicht mehr in Frage. In dieser zweiten Aufwachphase spielen sich die Adaptationsvorgänge ab, die weiter unten unter „Psychomimetik" noch näher erläutert sind.

4. Daran anschließend findet sich noch ein individuell stärker in bezug auf die Dauer schwankender Zeitraum, in dem neben langsam abklingenden Konvergenzstörungen (1–4 mg/kg CI-581 i.v. = 1–4 Std) ein Gefühl der Abgeschlagenheit und ein Ruhe- oder Schlafbedürfnis die Erlangung der sogenannten Straßenfähigkeit weiter verzögert (1–4 mg/kg CI-581 i.v. = 3–8 Std) (LANGREHR u. Mitarb. 1967).

Diese von uns beobachteten Wirkungszeiten stehen in guter Übereinstimmung mit den Befunden anderer Untersucher (STEPHEN u. Mitarb. 1966; ROBERTS 1967 u. a.) sowie mit den EEG-Schlaftiefekurven und Leistungsprüfungen von DOENICKE u. Mitarb. (1967. 1968) und den Gewebe-Halbwertzeiten (McCARTHY u. Mitarb. 1966; DILL u. Mitarb. 1963). Sie charakterisieren Ketamine als einen Stoff mit länger dauernden Nachwirkungen, der nach unseren rechtlichen Gegebenheiten für die ambulante Narkose Erwachsener kaum in Frage kommt. Bei der Verwendung für ambulante Kleinkindernarkosen kann von Fall zu Fall anders entschieden werden, wir haben die Ketamine-Anwendung für ambulante Anaesthesien allerdings nur selten in Betracht gezogen.

Die Abb. 7 zeigt die Dosiswirkungsdauerbeziehungen, die bei 50 Narkosen an Zootieren verschiedener Spezies mit Ketamine im. gewonnen wurden (LANGREHR u. MUELLER 1967).

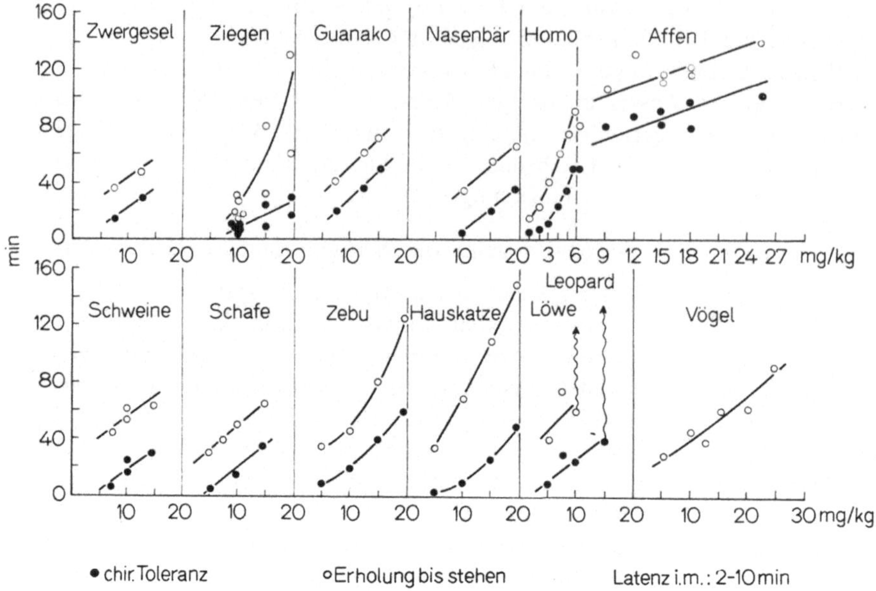

Abb. 7. Dosis-Wirkungsdauerbeziehung bei 50 Ketamine-Anaesthesien an verschiedenen Zootier-Spezies. 5–30 mg/kg Ketamine i.m. Einzelheiten siehe Text

Mit Ausnahme von Affen, die eine ähnliche Empfindlichkeit gegenüber Ketamine wie der Mensch zeigen, benötigen Nicht-Labortiere verschiedener Spezies etwa 3–4fach höhere Dosierungen zur Erzielung gleicher chirurgischer Toleranzzeiten im Vergleich zum Menschen. Dabei muß jedoch die entsprechend dem Körpergewicht notwendige großvolumige Dosis i.m. mit berücksichtigt werden, die zwar häufig auf zwei Injektionsstellen verteilt wurde, jedoch immer noch zu einer erheblichen Resorptionsverlangsamung gegenüber der i.v.-Gabe führt. Versager haben wir, ebenso wie beim Menschen, nicht beobachtet. Die Bedeutung von Ketamine für die Veterinäranaesthesie ist an anderer Stelle dargestellt (LANGREHR u. MUELLER 1967). Zwei Leoparden entwickelten nach 10 und 15 mg/kg CI-581 i.m. langdauernde tonisch-klonische Krämpfe, die nach ausgedehntem Nachschlaf ohne Folgen überstanden wurden. Dieser Befund ist insofern von Bedeutung, als Ketamine unter den üblichen Prüfbedingungen (CHEN u. Mitarb. 1967) keinen Anhaltspunkt für krampfauslösende Wirkungen zeigte. Besondere Stoffwechselverhältnisse bei großen Raubkatzen mit stark verlangsamter Metabolisierung sind wohl für den Effekt von Bedeutung (CHEN, SOERING, pers. Mitteilung). Bei zwei jungen Löwen fanden wir einen solchen Effekt bei niedrigerer Dosierung (5 und 7,5 mg/kg i.m.) nicht.

Von dem bei Versuchstieren parenteral wie oral aufgenommenen CI-581 sind nach Dill u. Mitarb. (1963), McCarthy u. Mitarb. (1966) und Chen u. Mitarb. (1967) nach aufeinanderfolgender Demethylierung und Oxydation 4 Metaboliten bekannt, die ihrerseits eine geringe kataleptische Effektivität zeigen. Somit sind die länger anhaltenden Nachwirkungen letzten Endes von der Gewebsverteilung und der Ausscheidung (Niere) abhängig.

Auf der anderen Seite zeigt Ketamine eine bemerkenswert geringe Toxizität und eine große therapeutische Breite sowohl im akuten und chronischen Tierversuch (McCarthy 1965; Bree u. Corssen 1967; Chen u. Mitarb. 1967) wie auch nach Maximaldosierungen beim Menschen (25–50 mg/kg i.v.; Stephen u. King 1966; Corssen 1968; Dangel 1968).

Die diaplacentare Passage erfolgt rasch (Dill u. Mitarb. 1963, Affen). Das intrauterine Kind am Ende der Gravidität zeigt nach mütterlichen Dosierungen von 2–5 mg/kg CI-581 i.v. jedoch keine signifikanten Herzfrequenzänderungen. Nach erfolgter Geburt findet sich bei unseren mehr als 200 geburtshilflichen dissoziativen Anaesthesien kein Anhalt für eine Verschlechterung des zu erwartenden Apgarwertes durch Ketamine, wenn man etwa die nach unserer Erfahrung heute günstige Kombinationsnarkose (Propanidid, N$_2$O; O$_2$; 0,5 Vol.-% Fluothane) zum Vergleich heranzieht.

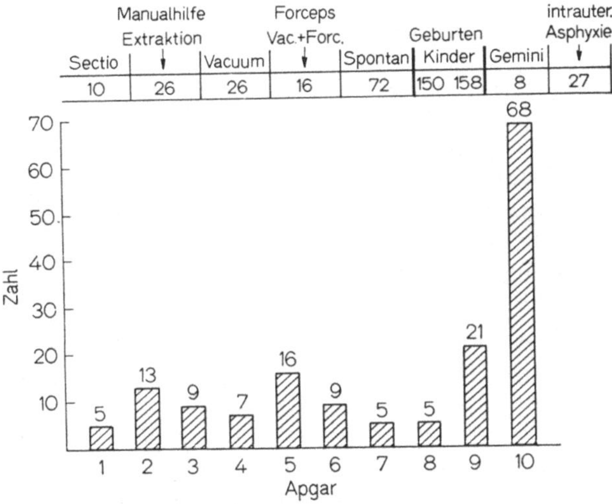

Abb. 8. Statistik der geburtshilflichen Eingriffe und der postpartal gefundenen Apgarwerte bei 150 Ketamine-Anaesthesien

Die Abb. 8 zeigt die Statistik der geburtshilflichen Eingriffe unter Ketamine-Anaesthesie und die gefundenen Abgarwerte bei den Neugeborenen. Wir halten unter diesen Umständen die dissoziative Anaesthesie für empfehlenswert bei geburtshilflichen Eingriffen (Chodoff u. Stella 1966; Stolp, Langrehr u. Sokol 1968). Die Wehentätigkeit des Uterus unter der Geburt wird nicht beeinträchtigt, wie wir durch externe Tokometrie bei zehn Frauen während der Eröffnungs- oder Austreibungsphase registrieren konnten. Die Abb. 9 zeigt eine Wehenregistrierung unter 3 mg/kg CI-581 i.v. Auch die postpartale Kontraktionsbereitschaft des entleerten Uterus sowie seine Ansprechbarkeit auf Wehenmittel blieb ungestört (Stolp u. Mitarb. 1968).

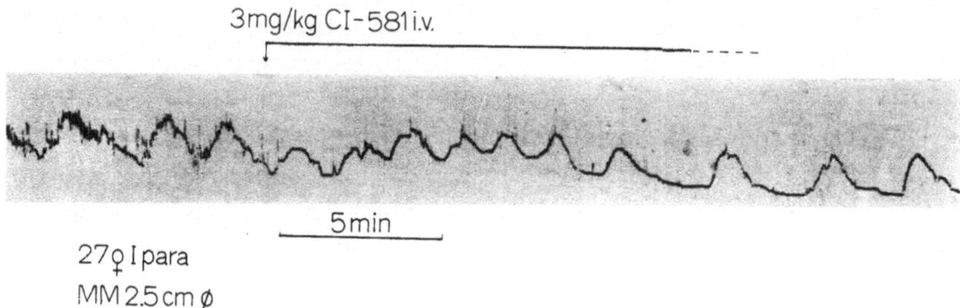

Abb. 9. Ungestörte Wehentätigkeit nach 3 mg/kg Ketamine i.v. 27jährige I para, Eröffnungswehen, MM 2,5 cm Durchmesser, externe Tokometrie

7. Allgemeine Symptomatik, Nebenwirkungen, Psychomimetik

Nach der i.v. Injektion von Ketamine wird mit einer von der Kreislaufzeit abhängigen Latenz von 20–40 sec (i.m. 2–4 min) schlagartig das Toleranzstadium erreicht. Der Patient hat jeden Kontakt zur Zeit, Umwelt und seinem eigenen Körper verloren, chirurgische Maßnahmen sind ohne Schmerzäußerungen und ohne schmerzbedingte Kreislauf- und Atmungseffekte sofort möglich. Die Rachenreflexe (Husten, Würgen) sind intakt, der Tonus der Zungen- und Schlundmuskulatur erhalten, so daß die Atemwege im allgemeinen ohne weitere Hilfestellung, auch in Seiten- oder Bauchlage, frei bleiben. Die tieferen Luftwege sind trocken, wir sahen keine Bronchokonstriktion, auch nicht bei Emphysembronchitis und Asthma bronchiale. Eine vermehrte orale Salivation in 3,8% der Fälle (s. Tab. 2) betrifft nur solche Patienten ohne Atropinprämedikation. Obwohl der mäßig vermehrte Speichelfluß nach unserer Erfahrung keine Aspirationsgefahr darstellt und Ketamine wegen seines sympathicomimetischen Effektes keine Bradykardie hervorruft, bevorzugen wir in letzter Zeit die i.v. Zugabe kleiner Atropinmengen, um auch die mögliche Salivation zu vermeiden. Die Augen sind häufig weit geöffnet, die Lidreflexe manchmal abgeschwächt, die Pupillen reagieren nach Abklingen des initialen Hippus prompt auf Licht. Die Bauchdeckenreflexe sind auslösbar, die Muskeleigenreflexe gesteigert, pathologische Reflexe kamen nicht zur Beobachtung.

In 2,4% der Fälle (s. Tab. 2) sahen wir in den ersten Minuten des Toleranz-stadiums blitzartige faszikuläre Muskelzuckungen vorwiegend der Hals- und Extremitätenmuskulatur. Eine stärkere motorische Unruhe in 1,3% der Fälle, die den Eingriff jedoch meist nicht wesentlich störte und als Bewegungen der oberen Extremitäten und des Kopfes manchmal mit athetotischen Bewegungsabläufen imponierte, wird nach unserer Er-fahrung am besten sofort durch $N_2O:O_2$ Fluothane-Zugabe oder auch Barbituratinjektion unterbunden, da sie häufig solche Patienten betrifft, die ohne Zusatznarkose dann später besonders ausgeprägte Adaptations-schwierigkeiten in der Aufwachphase zeigen. In 2,2% der Fälle sahen wir Schwitzen im Gesicht und am Rumpf, in 4,6% fiel eine passagere Gesichts- oder Gesichts-Rumpfrötung der Haut auf, die nach einigen Minuten abgeklungen war.

Tabelle 2. *Tabelle der Nebenwirkungen und Drogen-Kombinationen bei den ersten 1000 Ketamine-Anaesthesien (Einzelheiten siehe Text)*

1000 × CI-581	
Nebenwirkungen	
Salivation	38
Nystagmus	16
Muskelzuckungen	24
motorische Exzitation	13
Schwitzen	22
Gesichts-Rumpfrötung	46
> 20 sec Apnoe, Zunge, Glottis	12
Schwindel	6
Übelkeit	9
Erbrechen	6
Lautäußerungen	23
Unruhe, postoperative Überwachung – 60 min	16
Spontanbericht, Träume	60
möchte Narkose nicht wieder	7
Kombinationen	
ohne Prämedikation	252
CI-581 + SCh	303
CI-581 + Kombinierte Narkose	116
CI-581 Mono- vetl. Prämedikation	581
Mehrfachnarkosen (bis 11 ×)	52
Risikofälle	109
Todesfälle	2

Das Erwachen geschieht langsam und ist zwischen Ende der Toleranz-phase und dem Erreichen der völligen Orientierung durch eine relativ lange Erholungsphase mit mehreren Wiedereinschlafintervallen gekennzeichnet.

Gewährleistet die Gesamtdosierung eine Beendigung des chirurgischen Eingriffs innerhalb des Toleranzstadiums, so daß die Erholungsphase in ruhiger Umgebung mit einem Minimum an exteroceptivem Afferenzeinstrom vor sich gehen kann, so bestehen für den Patienten nur geringe Adaptationsschwierigkeiten, er schließt auf Aufforderung bereitwillig eine Nachschlafperiode an (Selbstversuche). In 2,1% der Fälle registrierten wir postnarkotischen Schwindel, Übelkeit oder Erbrechen (0,6%); diese Nebenwirkungen müssen wir eher den Konvergenzstörungen oder auch einer Dolantin-Prämedikation zur Last legen, als einer direkten Ketamine-Wirkung. Ketamine hat keinen emetischen Effekt, sondern einen geringen antiemetischen (Chen u. Mitarb. 1967). Die dissoziative Anaesthesie gehört zu den Verfahren mit sehr geringer Häufigkeit von postnarkotischem Erbrechen, was im Einklang mit der Erfahrung bei einer größeren Zahl nicht sicher nüchterner Patienten bei dringlichen Anaesthesien steht.

Versager im engeren Sinne, d. h. die Analgesie blieb aus und die Dekonnektion des Patienten kam nicht zustande, sahen wir bei Dosierungen von 1 mg/kg i.v. an aufwärts nicht. Die Gefäßverträglichkeit der Substanz ist als gut zu bezeichnen, wir sahen keine Venenreaktion. Selbst die intraarterielle Injektion im Tierexperiment blieb ohne Folgen (Kaump u. Mitarb. 1967; Langrehr u. Mitarb. 1967).

Nicht nur hinsichtlich der beschriebenen Nebenwirkungen stellt Ketamine einen deutlichen Fortschritt gegenüber früher klinisch erprobten Phencyclidinderivaten dar (Rosenbaum u. Mitarb. 1959; Scholler u. Mitarb. 1960; Johnstone 1960; Greifenstein u. Mitarb. 1958; Gött 1960; Lear u. Mitarb. 1959; Langrehr u. Mitarb. 1967). Auch hinsichtlich der psychomimetischen Nebenwirkungen liegt im Ketamine ein Stoff vor, dessen Adaptationsvorgänge in der Aufwachphase durchaus zu handhaben sind. Wir haben, nicht zuletzt auf Grund von Selbstversuchen, die in Übereinstimmung mit den Erfahrungen von Stöcker und Lassner stehen, die psychomimetischen Adaptationsvorgänge zum größten Teil auf Konvergenzstörungen, analgetische Mißempfindung und Schwierigkeiten bei der Bewältigung des erinnerungsfähigen Erlebnisses vom „dissoziativen Traum" zurückgeführt (Langrehr u. Mitarb. 1967). Echte Halluzinationen (Kloos 1951) sahen wir nicht. Die mit diesem Terminus in Einzelfällen belegten Adaptationsstörungen (Bjarnesen u. Corssen 1967), die nach unserer Erfahrung immer mit dem Erreichen der völligen Orientierung sistieren, möchten wir am ehesten einer Fehleinschätzung der Wirkungsdauer von Ketamine zur Last legen.

Beachtet man in der Aufwachphase die möglichst weitgehende Verminderung des exteroceptiven Afferenzeinstromes (Cohen u. Mitarb. 1960), fordert man den unruhigen Patienten auf, die Augen zu schließen und weiter zu schlafen, da er noch nicht ganz aufgewacht sei, begegnet man den wenigen Fällen von größerer motorischer Unruhe und Lautäußerungen

(2,3%) noch vor dem Erreichen der ersten Ansprechbarkeit mit einer Zusatznarkose und kurzfristiger Schlafverlängerung und erklärt man einer kleinen Zahl von Patienten später den Aufwachvorgang auf ihre Frage hin, so erfährt die dissoziative Anaesthesie nur von seiten ganz weniger Patienten (0,7%, Tab. 2) eine endgültige Ablehnung. Dabei handelte es sich in unseren 7 Fällen 5mal um Patienten, die nahezu alles im Zusammenhang mit ihrer Behandlung ablehnten.

Über das erinnerungsfähige Erlebnis des dissoziativen Traumes berichteten 6% der Patienten spontan, in mehr als 50% der Fälle wird es auf Befragen mehr oder weniger konkret bestätigt. Der Inhalt solcher „Träume", von LASSNER mit den Ketamine-Effekten auf die Retikulärformation und andere Stammhirnzonen in Zusammenhang gebracht, ist dargelegt worden (LANGREHR u. Mitarb. 1967). Ketamine gehört mit den früher getesteten Phencyclidinderivaten, mit α-Chloralose, GHB und Initialwirkungen des Äthers in eine Gruppe von Anaesthetica, durch welche gleichartige zentralnervöse Effekte ausgelöst werden, die etwa bei Barbituraten, Fluothane, Lachgas, Trichlorethylen u. a. nicht zur Beobachtung kommen (WINTERS u. Mitarb. 1967). Daher sind für den Anaesthesisten zunächst ungewohnte Reaktionen auffällig, deren Zustandekommen aufgeklärt und deren Auswirkungen bei der Beurteilung der klinischen Verwendbarkeit eines neuen Stoffes zusammen mit anderen vorteilhaften Effekten abgewogen werden müssen. Die für Ketamine und ähnliche Stoffe bislang gefundenen zentralnervösen Wirkungen (Wirkungsdissoziation zwischen Neocortex-Thalamus und Limbisch-reticulär-System, CORSSEN u. Mitarb. 1968) unterscheiden sich in einer Reihe von Einzelheiten jedoch deutlich von denen der bekannten Halluzinogene (β-Phenethylamine = Mescalin und α-Lysergsäurediethylamid = LSD) (LONGO 1967; HOFFER und OSMOND 1967).

8. Eingriffsarten, Kombination mit anderen Anaesthesieverfahren, Altersverteilung

Die Tab. 3 zeigt die Eingriffsarten, bei denen in unseren ersten 1000 Fällen Ketamine zur Anwendung kam. Die hier aufgeführten Eingriffe stimmen nicht in allen Punkten mit den heute für uns geltenden Indikationen für die dissoziative Anaesthesie überein (siehe weiter unten).

Die Tab. 2 zeigt oben die Häufigkeit der früher schon besprochenen Nebenwirkungen, unten die von uns verwendeten Kombinationen mit anderen Drogen. Von 1000 Fällen wurde 252mal Ketamine ohne Prämedikation verwendet. In 52 Fällen wurde die dissoziative Anaesthesie wiederholt (bis zu 11mal, septische Chirurgie, Verbrennungen), 109 Patienten müssen als Risikofälle gewertet werden. Die 2 Todesfälle innerhalb von 12 Stunden nach der Anaesthesie können, in Übereinstimmung mit anderen ähnlich gelagerten Fällen, die inzwischen mitgeteilt wurden (Report 1967), nicht dem Ketamine zur Last gelegt werden. Es handelt sich um Patienten in schlechtestem Allgemeinzustand mit mehreren konkomitierenden Grundkrankheiten, die diesen letzten Endes trotz operativer Bemühungen zum Opfer fielen. Wir hatten, wie bei den übrigen Risikopatienten, den Eindruck, daß die dissoziative Anaesthesie mit O_2- oder $N_2O:O_2$-Beatmung eine relativ optimale Narkoseform darstellte. Von 1000 Anaesthesien wurde bei 303 Patienten zusätzlich Succinylcholin und O_2-Beatmung angewandt, bei 116 eine Kombinationsbeatmungsnarkose ($N_2O:O_2$:Fluothane:Relaxation) der initialen Ketamineapplikation angeschlossen, während bei 581 Patienten Ketamine als Monoanaesthetikum, teils mit, teils ohne Prämedikation, verwendet wurde. Veränderungen der Relaxationsdauer bei der Kombination von Imbretil, Succinylcholin und Ketamine fanden wir nicht, die neuromuskuläre Erregungsübertragung wird durch Ketamine nicht verändert (Telivuo 1968), das Wiederingangkommen der Spontanatmung nach Bronchoskopien unter Ketamine-Succinylcholin-O_2-Beatmungsnarkose war gegenüber dem Barbiturat-Succinylcholin-O_2-Verfahren deutlich besser.

Tabelle 3. *Tabelle der Eingriffsarten, bei denen Ketamine in den ersten 1000 Fällen zur Anwendung kam*

CI-581-Eingriffsarten	
V. sectio, Punktion, Incision, Wundversorgung, sekund. Naht, Drainage-, Verbandwechsel, Nagelextr., Anus-praeter-Abtr., P.E., Lymphkn.-Exstirp., Fraktur-Rep. + Gips, Phimosen-Op., Semicastratio, Pylorotomie, Tonsillektomie, Zahnextraktion	267
Bronchoskopie, Bronchographie, Cystoskopie, Oesophagoskopie, Starck-Sonde, Tracheotomie, Fremdkörper-Extr.	360
Curettage, N.U., Cervix-Eingriffe, Ra-Einlage	220
Spontangeburten, geburtshilfliche Operationen	63
Narkoseeinleitung: Risikofälle, Knochenchir.-Lagerung, Appendektomie (+ SCh, 23 Fälle)	90
	1000

Die Abb. 10 zeigt die Altersverteilung bei unseren ersten 1000 dissoziativen Anaesthesien. Der jüngste Patient war 7 Tage, der älteste 91 Jahre alt.

Wie die Abb. 11 für jeweils 10 junge kreislaufgesunde Patienten demonstriert, unterscheidet sich die Einleitung mit Ketamine (links) von der mit Barbiturat (rechts) zur nachfolgenden $N_2O:O_2$; Fluothane-Narkose durch das Fehlen einer initialen Kreislaufdepression. Hierin sehen wir einen der Gründe für die guten Erfahrungen mit Ketamine zur Einleitung für Risikonarkosen (siehe auch Blutdruckverhalten bei Risikofällen: Tab. 1, Zeile 4. u. 8.).

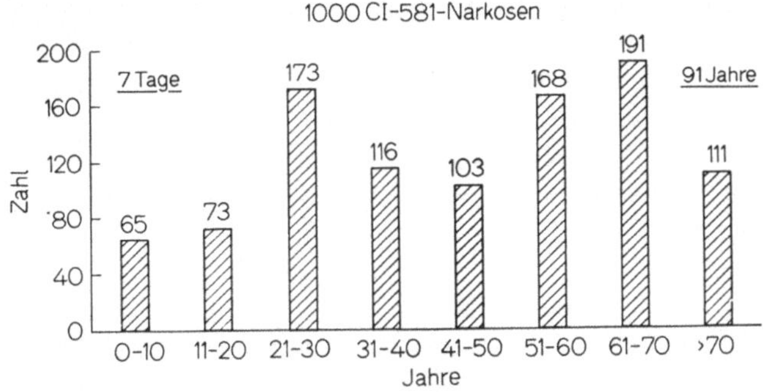

Abb. 10.   Patienten-Altersverteilung   der   ersten   1000 Ketamine-Anaesthesien

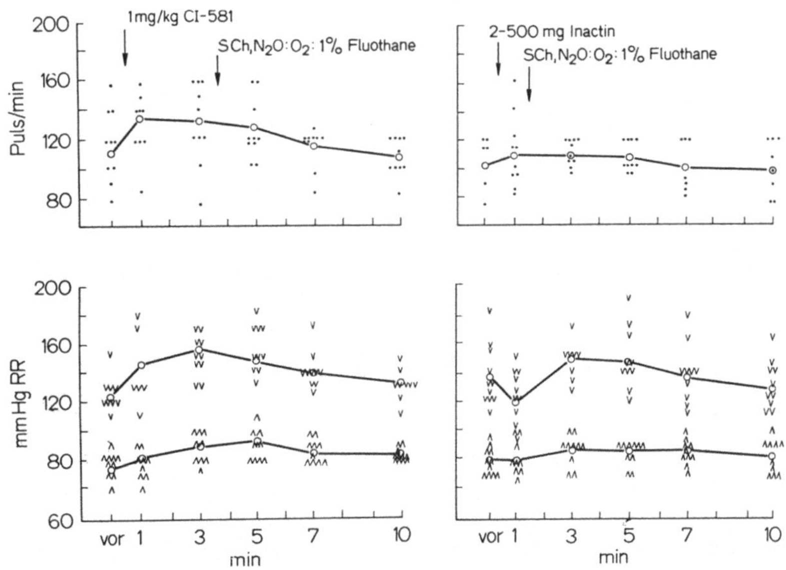

Abb. 11. Blutdruck- und Pulsfrequenzverhalten bei jeweils 10 kreislaufgesunden Patienten nach Einleitung mit 1 mg/kg Ketamine i.v. (links) und 200–500 mg Inactin i.v. (rechts) zur N$_2$O:O$_2$;1 Vol.-% Fluothane Relaxationsanaesthesie. o————o arithmetische Mittelwerte in jeder Zeitgruppe. Beachte die initiale Kreislaufdepression nach Barbiturateinleitung

9. Indikationen zur Anwendung von Ketamine

Fassen wir unsere Erfahrungen und die in der Literatur mitgeteilten Befunde zusammen, so ergeben sich für die Anwendung von Ketamine folgende Indikationen:

1. Chirurgische Eingriffe bis zu 30 min Dauer vor allem bei Kindern, alten Menschen und Patienten in schlechtem Allgemeinzustand (ophthalmologische Eingriffe, Otochirurgie, Chirurgie des Gesichts- und Halsbereichs, Zahnextraktionen, Abszeßincisionen im Mundbereich, Wundbehandlung bei Verbrennungsfällen, septische Chirurgie z. B. beim Diabetes, dringliche Frakturbehandlung und Wundversorgung, dringliche Erstversorgung im Schock, Tracheotomie, Drainagen und Verbandwechsel u. a.).

2. Endoskopische und diagnostische Eingriffe besonders unter erschwerten Umgebungsbedingungen für den Anaesthesisten und bei für die Anaesthesie schwierigen Körperhaltungen (Bronchoskopie, Bronchographie, Oesophago-Gastroskopie, Cystoskopie, Pneumocephalographie, Carotisangiographie, Myelographie, Laparoskopie, Herzkatheterismus).

3. Narkoseeinleitung für die länger dauernde große Riskiochirurgie bei Patienten in schlechtem Allgemeinzustand, im Schock und bei schweren Begleitkrankheiten.

4. Geburtshilfliche Chirurgie (Manualhilfen und manuelle Extraktionen, Forceps- und Vakuum-Extraktion, Sectio-caesarea-Einleitung im Schock).

Wir danken Frl. Ingrid Riecken für wertvolle technische Assistenz.

Summary

The paper deals with a 3 years experience in now more than 1600 cases with "Ketamine dissoziative anesthesia", based on experimental work about influence of the drug on circulation, myocardial force, respiration, blood gas balance, CO_2-response curves, ocular pressure, uterine contractility, blood sugar levels, spinal motricity, diaplacentar effects. We found the arterial blood pressure and heart minute volume moderately elevated, increase of heart frequency and no myocardial depression. There is evidence for the drug stimulating rhombencephalic vasomotor centers. Spontaneous respiration is only seldom depressed, blood gas analysis shows no marked alteration, pharyngeal and laryngeal reflexes are intact. CO_2-response curves are not depressed, in contrast for instance to barbiturates. The uterine contraction in labour is not affected, the foetal heart frequency not altered, we found the babies postpartal in good condition. There is no marked alteration of blood sugar levels neither in normal nor in diabetic patients.

Prominent indications for Ketamine anesthesia are: pädiatric and geriatric anesthesia, grafting in burned patients, interventions up to 45 min duration in poor risk patients, endoscopic and diagnostic examinations, obstetrical surgery, emergency anesthesia in shock patients, introduction for long lasting poor risk surgery.

Literatur

APGAR, V.: A proposal for a new method of evaluation of the newborn infant. Anesth. Analg. Curr. Res. **32**, 260 (1953).

BJARNESEN, W., and G. CORSSEN: CI-581: A new non-barbiturate short acting anesthetic for surgery in burns. Michigan Medicine, February 1967 (p. 177).

BLUMBERGER, K. J.: Die Untersuchung der Dynamik des Herzens beim Menschen. Ergebn. inn. Med. Kinderheilk. **62**, 424 (1942).

BREE, M. M., I. FELLER, and G. CORSSEN: Safety and tolerance of repeated anesthesia with ketamine (CI-581) in monkeys). Anesth. Analg. Curr. Res. **46**, 596 (1957).

BRINLING, I., T. D. SHOPIRO, and E. B. SIGG: Pharmacologic properties of a new nonbarbiturate anesthetic. Arch. int. Pharmacodyn. **134**, 126 (1962), **136**, 113 (1962).

McCARTHY, D.: Observations on the direct action of CI-581 on the myocardium as detected in the dog heart-lung preparation. Parke Davis Research Division 1966 (unpublished).

—, G. CHEN, D. H. KAUMP, and C. ENSOR: General anesthetic and other pharmacological properties of CI-581. J. New Drugs **5**, 21 (1965).

CHEN, G.: The effect of CI-581 on isolated heart. Parke Davis Research Division 1966 (unpublished).

— CI-581 and emesis. Parke Davis Research Division 1966 (unpublished).

—, C. ENSOR, and B. BOHNER: The neuropharmacology of 2-(O-chlorophenyl)-2-methylaminocyclohexanone hydrochloride. J. Pharmacol. exp. Ther. **152** 332 (1966)

— —, D. RUSSEL, and B. BOHNER: The pharmacology of 1-(1-phenylcyclohexyl)-piperidine-HCl. J. Pharmacol. exp. Ther. **127**, 241 (1959).

—, A. J. GLAZKO, and D. H. KAUMP: CI-581 revised laboratory summary. Parke Davis Research Division June 1967 (unpublished).

—, and J. K. WESTON: The analgesic and anesthetic effects of 1-(1-phenylcyclohexyl)piperidine-HCl on the monkey. Anesth. Analg. Curr. Res. **39**, 132 (1960).

CHODOFF, P., and J. G. STELLA: Use of CI-581, a phencyclidine derivate for obstetric anesthesia. Anesth. Analg. Curr. Res. **45**, 527 (1966).

COHEN, B. D., E. D. LUBY, G. ROSENBAUM, and J. S. GOTTLIEB: Combined sernyl and sensory deprivation. Comprehens. Psychiat. **1**, 345 (1960).

CORSSEN, G.: a) Pharmakologische und erste klinische Erfahrungen mit dem Kurznarkotikum CI-581. Tgg. Europ. Anästhesieges. Zürich 1965. –
b) Clinical use of CI-581. 2. European Congr. Anesthesiol. Kopenhagen 1966.–
c) Recent developments in the anesthetic management of burned patients. J. Trauma **7**, 152 (1967).

—, and E. F. DOMINO: Dissociative anesthesia: further pharmacologic studies and first clinical experience with the phencyclidine derivative CI-581. Anesth. Analg. Curr. Res. **45**, 29 (1966).

—, M. MIYASAKA u. E. F. DOMINO: Changing concepts in pain control during surgery: dissociative anesthesia with CI 581. Anesthesia Analg. **47**, 746 (1968).

Dill, W. A., T. Chang, L. Peterson, and A. J. Glazko: Metabolic disposition of CI-581 in laboratory animals. Parke Davis Research Division 1963 (unpublished).

Doenicke, A., J. Kugler, and M. Laub: Evaluation of recovery and street fitness by EEG and psychodiagnostic test safter anesthesia. Canad. Anaesth. Soc. J. 14, 567 (1967).

Domino, E. F., P. Chodoff, and G. Corssen: Pharmacological effects of CI-581, a new dissociative anesthetic, in man. Clin. Pharmacol. Ther. 6, 279 (1965).

Dowdy, E. G. and K. Kaya: Studies of the mechanism of cardiovascular responses to CI 581. Anesthesiology 29, 931 (1968).

Gött, U.: Zur Anästhesie mit Cyclohexaminen. Anaesthesist 9, 261 (1960).

Greifenstein, F. E., M. DeVault, J. Yoshitake, and J. E. Gajewski: A study of a 1-aryl-cyclohexyl-amine for anesthesia. Anesth. Analg. Curr Res. 37, 283 (1958).

Henatsch, H. D., D. Langrehr, F. J. Schulte u. H. J. Kaese: Eigenreflex Depressionen bei chemischer Muskelspindelerregung. Pflügers Arch. ges. Physiol. 274, 511 (1962).

Hoffer, A., and H. Osmond: The Hallucinogens. New York and London: Academic Press 1967.

Holldack, K.: Die Bedeutung der Umformungs- und Druckanstiegszeit. Dtsch. Arch. klin. Med. 198, 71 (1951).

Johnstone, M.: Die Verwendung von Sernyl in der klinischen Anästhesie. Anaesthesist 9, 114 (1960).

Ilett, K. F., B. Jarrot, S. R. O'Donnell, and J. C. Wanstall: Mechanism of cardiovascular actions of phencyclidine. Brit. J. Pharmacol. 28, 73 (1966).

Kaump, D. H., J. L. Schardein, R. A. Fisken, and T. F. Reutner: Local tolerance studies on CI-581 following intrarterial injection in rats and dogs. Parke Davis Research Division, Jan. 1967) unpublished).

Kloos, G.: Grundrisse der Psychiatrie und Neurologie. München: Müller u. Steinicke 1951.

Kreuscher, H.: Der Einfluß von Dehydrobenzperidol auf die Kontraktilität des Herzmuskels. In: Die Neuroleptanalgesie. Berlin-Heidelberg-New York: Springer 1966, S. 66.

—, u. H. Gauch: Die Wirkung des Phencyclidinderivates Ketamin auf das cardiovasculäre System des Menschen. Anaesthesist 16, 229 (1967).

Langrehr, D.: Zur Frage der Receptorspezifität endoanästhetischer Wirkungen am Beispiel des Benzononatin (Tessalon). Arch. pex. Path. Pharmakol. 245, 427 (1963).

— Klinische und experimentelle Erfahrungen mit der dissoziativen Anästhesie durch Ketamine. actuelle chirurgie 4, 71 (1969.

—, F. Adelstein u. H. L'Allemand: Zur Frage der Fluothane-Nrakose für chirurgische Eingriffe am Auge. Ophthalmologica (Basel) 153, 200 (1967).

—, P. Alai, J. Andjelkovic u. I. Kluge: Zur Narkose mit Ketamine (CI-581): Bericht über erste Erfahrungen in 500 Fällen. Anaesthesist 16, 308 (1967).

—, u. H. L'Allemand: Narkoseprobleme in der Allgemeinpraxis. Hippokrates 33, 452 (1962).

— — Über das Verhalten von Kreislauf und Atmung bei intravenösen Kurznarkosen mit 2-M-4-A. Anaesthesist 12, 325 (1963).

— u. I. Kluge: Zur Anwendung von Ketamine in der Kinderanästhesie. Zschr. Kinderchirurgie (im Druck) 1969.

LANGREHR, D. u. R. MUELLER: Die Bedeutung von CI-581 für die veterinärmedizinische Anästhesiologie unter besonderer Berücksichtigung von Zootieren. 1967. Prag, Verh. Internat. Symp. Zootierärzte.

—, u. N. PAMUKCUOGLU: Conferencia en las Jornadas de la Sociedad Alemania de Anesthesia. Berlin-Göttingen-Heidelberg-New York: Springer 1964.

— and W. STOLP: Ketamine for obstetric anesthesia. Anesthesia Analg. (in Vorbereitung).

LEAR, E., R. SUNTAY, I. M. PALLIN, and A. E. CHIRON: Cyclohexamine (CI-400): a new intravenous agent. Anesthesiology **20**, 330 (1959).

LONGO VINCENCO, G.: Contribution a l'etude des effets centraux des medicaments hallucinogenes et psychotomimetiques. Actualites Neurophysiologiques VII, Masson (Paris 1967), p. 203.

MEINERS, S.: Meßmethoden zur Analyse der Herz- und Kreislaufdynamik. 1. Freiburger Colloq. Kreislaufmessungen, Banaschewski 1958.

PODLESCH, I., u. M. ZINDLER: Erste Erfahrungen mit dem Phencyclidinderivat Ketamine (CI-581), einem neuen intravenösen und intramuskulären Narkosemittel. Anaesthesist **16**, 299 (1967).

ROBERTS, F. W.: A new intramuscular anesthetic for small children. Anaesthesia **22**, 23 (1967).

ROSENBAUM, G., B. D. COHEN, E. D. LUBY, J. S. GOTTLIEB, and D. YELEN: Comparison of sernyl with other drugs. A. M. A. Arch. gen. Psychiat. **1**, 651 (1959).

SCHOLLER, K. L., H. THIES, u. K. WIEMERS: Die Allgemeinanästhesie mit Cyclohexaminderivaten, klinische Beobachtungen und elektroencephalographische Untersuchungen. Anaesthesist **9**, 163 (1960).

STANLEY, V., J. HUNT, K. W. WILLIS and C. R. STEPHEN: Cardiovascular and respiratory function with CI 581. Anesthesia Analg. **47**, 760 (1968).

STEPHEN, C. R., and H. KING: CI-581: a new intravenous or intramuscular anesthetic. Anesthesiology **28**, 258 (1967).

STOLP, W., D. LANGREHR, u. K. SOKOL: Zur Anwendung von Ketamine in der geburtshilflichen Anästhesie. Z. Geburtsh. Gynäk. **169**, 198 (1968).

TELIVUO, L.: Clinical experience with CI 581. Abstr. 4. World Congr., Excerpta medica, p. 141 (1968).

TRABER, D. L., R. D. WILSON and L. L. PRIANO: Differentiation of cardiovascular effects of CI 581. Anesthesia Analg. **47**, 769 (1968); **48**, 248 (1969).

VIRTUE, R. W., J. M. ALANIS, M. MORI, R. T. LAFARGUE, J. H. K. VOGEL, and D. R. METCALF: An anesthetic agent: CI-581. a) Amer. Soc. Anesth. 41. Congress Bal Harbour (1967); b) Anesthesiology **28**, 823 (1967).

WASSNER, U. J.: Die untere Leistungsgrenze der Lunge. Berlin-Göttingen-Heidelberg: Springer 1961, p. 15ff.

WHEELOCK, R. H.: The effect of CI-581 on experimental ventricular tachycardia in dogs. Parke Davis Research Division 1966 (unpublished).

WILSON, R. D., R. J. NICHOLS, and N. R. McCOY: Dissociative Anesthesia in burned children. a) Amer. Soc. Anesth. 41. Congress Bal Harbour (1967); b) Anesth. Analg. Curr. Res. **46**, 719 (1967).

WINTERS, W. D., K. MORI, CH. E. SPOENER, and R. O. BAUER: The neurophysiology of anesthesia. Anesthesiology **28**, 65 (1967).

WIRTH, W., u. F. HOFFMEISTER: In: Die intravenöse Kurznarkose mit Epontol. Berlin-Heidelberg-New York: Springer 1965.

ZIPF, K. F.: Elektrophysiologische Untersuchungen zum Problem der Ausschaltung innerer sensibler Receptoren durch Localanästhetica. Arch. exp. Path. Pharmakol. **217**, 472 (1953); **218**, 113 (1953).

4*

Kreislaufanalytische Untersuchung bei Anwendung von Ketamine am Menschen*

Von **H. Kreuscher** und **H. Gauch**

Aus dem Institut für Anaesthesiologie der Universität Mainz
(Direktor: Prof. Dr. R. Frey)

Die kardiovasculären Effekte der herkömmlichen intravenösen Narkosemittel, also der Barbiturate und Thiobarbiturate, sind gekennzeichnet durch negativ-inotrope und chronotrope Wirkungen auf das Herz und durch Minderung des peripheren Widerstandes. Herabsetzung des Schlag- und Minutenvolumens einerseits, Blutvolumenverlagerung in das Niederdrucksystem und die periphere Strombahn andererseits bedingen Hypotonie. Diese bekannten und in der Regel unerwünschten Begleiterscheinungen der Barbiturate und Thiobarbiturate sind unter bestimmten Risikobedingungen gefürchtet, woraus sich eine Reihe von Kontraindikationen ihrer Anwendung ergeben. Nicht nur die Barbiturate und Thiobarbiturate sondern auch einige Inhalationsnarkotica, insbesondere das Halothan, haben ähnliche kardiovasculäre Effekte auch im klinisch üblichen Dosierungsbereich.

Wenn wir uns mit einem neuen Narkosemittel kritisch befassen wollen, dann gilt unser Augenmerk in erster Linie auf seine Wirkungseigenschaften auf das kardiovasculäre System, in zweiter Linie auf das respiratorische System. Darum haben wir Ketamine kreislaufanalytischen Studien am Menschen unterzogen.

Unsere Untersuchungen führten wir an gesunden jungen Männern im Alter von 20–27 Jahren durch. Wir verwendeten zur kontinuierlichen Analyse der Kreislaufparameter das bekannte Verfahren von BROEMSER und RANKE und zur Kontrolle die Farbstoffverdünnungsmethode mit Cardiogreen. Außerdem wurde der venöse Blutdruck gemessen. Ich darf die Methoden als bekannt voraussetzen und möchte sogleich die Ergebnisse unserer Versuche vorstellen.

Der Versuchsablauf ist auf der Abb. 1 dargestellt. Die Probanden mußten zunächst 30 min in Rückenlage ruhen. Während dieser Zeit wurden die verschiedenen Elektroden, Meßgeräte und Venenkatheter angelegt. Prämedikation mit 0,5 mg Atropin und 5 min später Aufzeichnung der

---

* Mit Unterstützung der Deutschen Forschungsgemeinschaft.

Kontrollwerte. 10 min nach der Prämedikation wurden die Ausgangswerte von Puls und Blutdruck kontrolliert. Wenn diese stabil geblieben
waren, erhielten die Probanden 1,5 mg/kg CI-581. 5 min nach der intravenösen Applikation wurden erneut Kreislaufanalysen einschließlich der
Farbstoffverdünnungsmethode aufgezeichnet. Im Anschluß daran erhielten
die Probanden Stickoxydul-Sauerstoff mit 1 Vol.-% Halothan. Nach 10 min
war bei allen Probanden ein steady-state erreicht und es wurden erneut
Kreislaufanalysen durchgeführt.

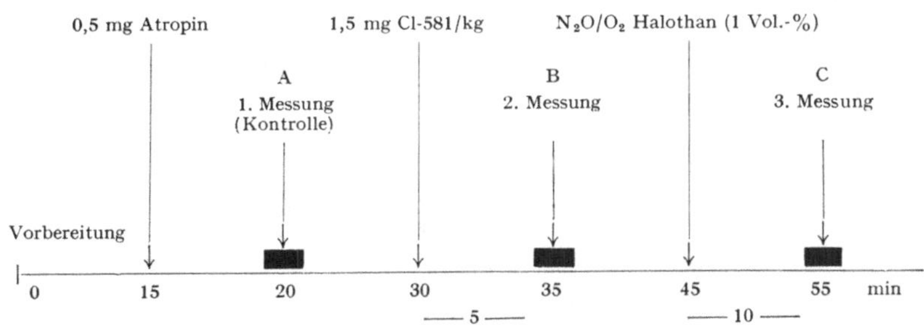

Ab. 1. Versuchsablauf

Ergebnisse

a) *Blutdruck:* Bei allen Probanden stieg der systolische und diastolische
Blutdruck innerhalb von 5 min nach der Ketamin-Injektion um durch-
schnittlich 31 mmHg (systol.) bzw. 24 mmHg (diastol.) an. 10 min nach
Applikation eines Halothan(1%)-N_2O-Sauerstoffgemisches kehrten die
Druckwerte wieder in ihre Ausgangslage zurück (Abb. 2 u. 3). Der venöse
Blutdruck stieg – mit einer Ausnahme – bei allen Probanden um durch-
schnittlich 6 cm H_2O innerhalb der ersten 5 min, fiel unter der anschließen-
den Halothan-Narkose jedoch nur um 2,3 cm H_2O (Abb. 4).

b) *Herzfrequenz:* Bei allen Probanden – jedoch wieder mit einer Ausnahme – stieg die Herzfrequenz nach der Injektion von Ketamine um
durchschnittlich 27 Schläge/min an und erreichte unter der anschließenden
Halothannarkose etwas tiefere Werte als unter Ausgangsbedingungen
(Abb. 5).

c) *Herzminutenvolumen:* Mit beiden Methoden gemessen erfuhr das
Herzminutenvolumen unter der Wirkung von Ketamine eine erhebliche
Steigerung um 2,76 l/min (74%) (BROEMSER-RANKE) resp. 3,81 l/min (77%)
(Farbstoffverdünnungsmethode) (Abb. 6 u. 7).

d) *Elastischer Widerstand:* Unter Ketamine stieg der Volumenelastizitäts-
modul von 776,5 dyn/cm⁵ auf 964,3 dyn/cm⁵ und erreichte unter der anschließenden Halothannarkose 662,6 dyn/cm⁵.

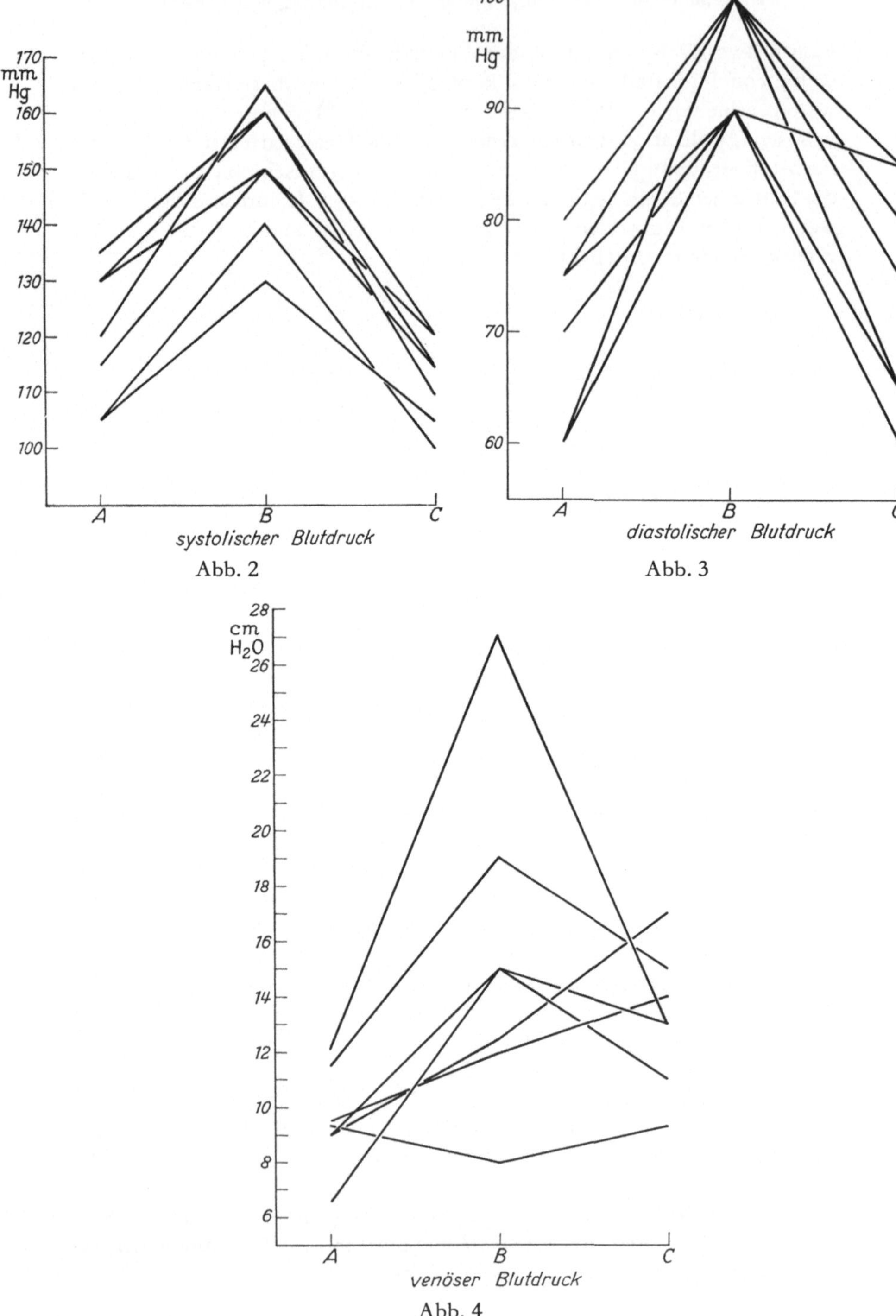

Abb. 2

Abb. 3

Abb. 4

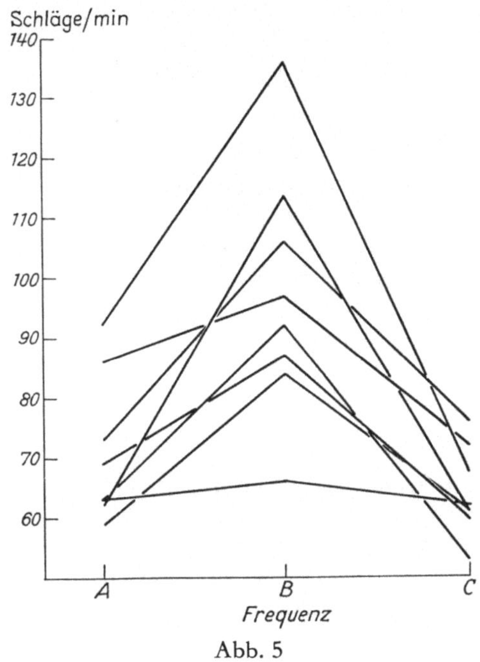

Abb. 5

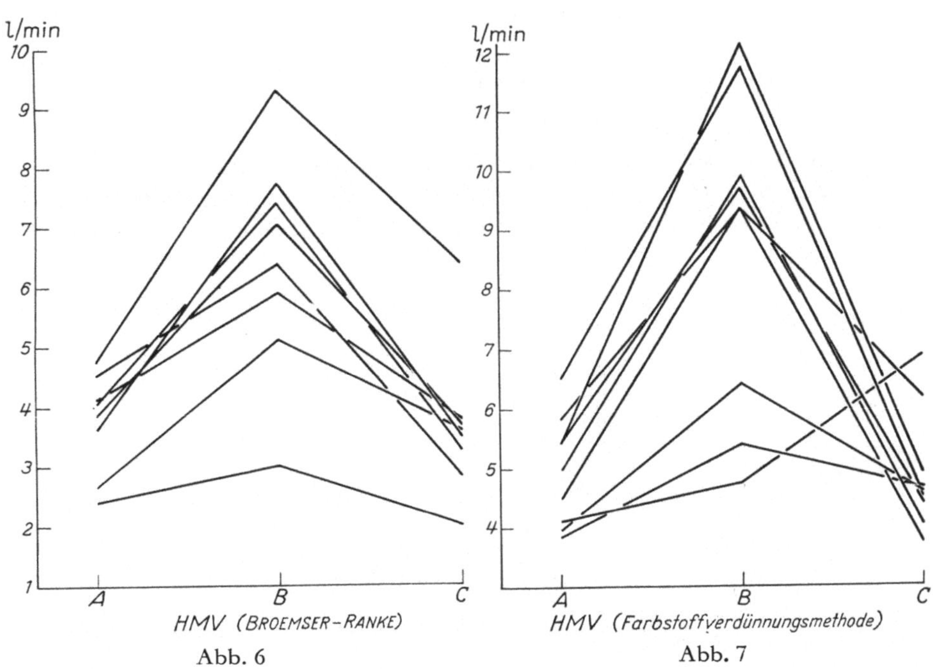

Abb. 6   Abb. 7

e) *Peripherer Widerstand:* Ketamine bewirkte einen Abfall von 2158 dyn/sec/cm^5 auf 1596/sec/cm^5. Unter der anschließenden Halothannarkose wurden die Ausgangswerte wieder erreicht.

Die Ergebnisse zeigen, daß unter den Bedingungen der Versuchsanordnung nach 1,5 mg/kg Ketamine intravenös regelmäßig eine deutliche positive inotrope und chronotrope Wirkung auf das Herz sowie eine Steigerung des elastischen und ein Abfall des peripheren Widerstandes beobachtet werden konnte. – Diese kardiovasculären Eigenschaften des Ketamine stehen im Gegensatz zu den eingangs erwähnten Wirkungen der Barbiturate und Thiobarbiturate.

Summary

Using two different methods (Broemser-Ranke and Stewart-Hamilton) investigations were performed on the cardiovascular effects of 1,5 mg/kg Ketamine, given intravenously each of 9 male volonteers (mean age: 23 years; weight: 74 kg). The functional cardiovascular parameters were recorded simultaneously. All measured and/or calculated values increased within 5 min after application of the drug:

Systolic blood pressure:	26%
Heart frequency:	38%
Venous blood pressure:	62%
Cardiac output:	74%
Module of volume elast.:	24%

The total vascular resistance decreased 26% from initial value. After application of Halothane (1%) in nitrous oxyde and oxygen during a period of 10 min, the increased values returned to the individual normal.

Literatur

Blumberger, K. J.: Ergebn. inn. Med. Kinderheilk. **62**, 424 (1942).
Broemser, Ph., u. O. Ranke: Z. Biol. **90**, 467 (1930).
Chan, T.: Fed. Proc. **24**, 268 (1965).
Chen, G., C. Ensor, D. Russell, and B. Bohner: J. Pharmacol. exp. Ther. **127**, 241 (1959).
—, J. Pharmacol. exp. Ther. **149**, 71 (1965).
Corssen, G., and E. F. Domino: Anesth. Analg. (N. Y.) **45**, 29 (1966).
Domino, E. F.: Int. Rev. Neurobiol. **6**, 303 (1964).
—, P. Chodoff, and G. Corssen: Clin. Pharmacol. Ther. **6**, 279 (1965).
Görr, U.: Anaesthesist **9**, 261-264 (1960).
Greifenstein, F. E., M. de Vault, J. Yoshitake, and J. E. Gajewski: Anesth. Analg. (N. Y.) **37**, 283–294 (1958).

HEGGLIN, R., u. W. RUTISHAUSER: Die Kreislaufdiagnostik mit der Farbstoff-verdünnungsmethode. Stuttgart: Georg Thieme 1962.

JOHNSTONE, M.: Anaesthesist 9, 114 (1960).

KOLLER, S.: Statistische Auswertungsmethoden. In: RAUEN, Biochemisches Taschenbuch. Berlin-Göttingen-Heidelberg-New York: Springer 1964.

McCARTHY, D. A., and G. CHEN: Fed. Proc. 24, 268 (1965).

MEYER, J. S., F. GREIFENSTEIN, and M. DE VAULT: J. nerv. ment. Dis. 129, 54 (1959).

SCHOLLER, K.-L., H. THIES u. K. WIEMERS: Anaesthesist 9, 163 (1960).

WEBER, A., u. K. BLUMBERGER: Freiburger Kolloquium über Kreislaufmessungen. München-Gräfelfing: Dr. E. Banaschewski 1958.

WIEMERS, K.: Anaesthesist 9, 186 (1960).

ZISSLER, J.: Arch. Kreisl.-Forsch. 19, 58 (1953).

Diskussion

Corssen: Da wir uns nach diesen Vorträgen dem klinischen Teil zuwenden, möchte ich die Gelegenheit wahrnehmen, noch auf einen experimentellen Versuch hinzuweisen, den wir in Zusammenarbeit mit unserem Tierarzt an der Universität von Michigan durchgeführt haben. Zur Frage der Toleranz beim Affen: Wie Dr. DILLON aus Los Angeles glauben auch wir, eine gewisse klinische Toleranz festgestellt zu haben, wenn z. B. Ketamine mehr als 10, 15 oder 20mal an demselben Patienten verabreicht wurde. Wir haben 3 Affen narkotisiert, 24mal in 48 Tagen, d. h. jeden 2. Tag haben wir den Affen 25 mg/kg intramuskulär gespritzt und haben dann die Zeit gemessen, während der Affe narkotisiert war. Nach der 1. Injektion von 25 mg/kg haben wir etwa 62 min Schlafzeit registriert. Nach 10 Injektionen – also nach 20 Tagen dieser Versuchsserie – sahen wir, daß die Schlafzeit schon auf fast 50 min abnahm, und am Ende dieser Versuchsserie, nach 24 Injektionen von je 25 mg/kg sahen wir, daß der Affe nur noch etwa 40 min in Narkose war. Diese Untersuchungen bestätigen unseren klinischen Eindruck, daß durch wiederholte Gabe von Ketamine eine gewisse Toleranz hervorgerufen wird. Klinisch ist diese Beobachtung vielleicht von geringerer Bedeutung, weil wir nur selten einem einzelnen Patienten mehr als 10 Anaesthesien verabreichen. Es kommt nur bei der chirurgischen Behandlung von Verbrannten vor, worüber wir heute Nachmittag und auch morgen noch hören werden. Diese Entwicklung der Toleranz ist außerdem klinisch von geringer Bedeutung, weil wir ja automatisch die Dosis erhöhen, um dieselbe Schlafzeit oder dieselbe Tiefe der Narkose zu erreichen. Da wir, wie wir von Herrn LANGREHR gehört haben, wissen, daß die therapeutische Breite von Ketamine erheblich ist, spielt es keine Rolle, ob wir z. B. 1 mg oder 2 mg nachspritzen. Der Effekt auf das kardiovasculäre und das Atemsystem ist bei diesen therapeutischen Dosen minimal.

Söhring: Herr LANGREHR, Sie haben vorher einmal von Akkomodationsstörungen, dann von Konvergierungsstörungen gesprochen und dann war auch die Rede von Fusionsstörungen. Nachdem damit das Thema der Straßenverkehrstüchtigkeit angesprochen ist, würde ich gerne wissen: Gibt es genaue Studien a) über die Flimmer-Verschmelzungsfrequenz und wie verhält sich diese, b) gibt es genaue Studien über Akkomodationsstörungen und c) wie verhält sich das Adaptationsvermögen nach Ketamine?

Langrehr: Wir haben die Patienten lesen und Formen erkennen lassen.

Schiller (Gießen): Ich habe eine Frage an Herrn KREUSCHER: Auch wir hatten uns bemüht, mit der WETZLER-BÖRGER- oder BROEMSER-RANKE-

Methode etwas messen zu können. Wir mußten aber diese Methode verlassen, weil die Patienten einen so großen Muskeltonus entwickelten, daß man normale Kurven nicht mehr aufnehmen konnte. Mich wundert, daß Herr Kreuscher bei seinen Versuchen so schöne Messungen erzielen konnte, und uns so schöne Ergebnisse vorstellen kann. Wir selbst mußten diese Methode verlassen und auf die Verdünnungsmethode umschalten, was wir nicht gerne taten. Im übrigen decken sich unsere Ergebnisse mit dem bisher Vorgetragenen, was Herzfrequenz, Blutdruck und Anspannungszeit betrifft.

Kreuscher: Ich kann Ihnen leider nicht sehr viel sagen, außer daß es bei uns ging, und Sie sehen an der guten Übereinstimmung mit den Ergebnissen der Farbstoff-Verdünnungskurve, die Sie ja auch gemacht haben, daß offensichtlich keine erheblichen Meßfehler durch Unruhe, Muskelspannung etc. zustandekamen. Ich muß allerdings sagen, daß wir für diese Untersuchungen ein gut eingespieltes Team zur Verfügung hatten und mit großer Sorgfalt die Druckabnehmer fixierten, wenn notwendig korrigierten und zwischendurch eichten. Es war sicher nicht ganz einfach, aber es ging.

Klaus: Ich möchte zu der ausgeprägten Wirkung auf das Herz- und Kreislaufsystem noch etwas fragen. Der Mechanismus scheint bisher noch nicht ganz geklärt zu sein, z. B. auch wie weit psychomimetischer Einfluß eine Rolle spielt. Aber zweifellos bewirkt doch wohl die ganz beträchtliche Zunahme der Herzfrequenz und des Druckanstieges eine Zunahme der Herzarbeit und damit auch eine Zunahme des intrakardialen Sauerstoffbedarfes. Wie weit ergeben sich daraus Kontraindikationen? Das dürfte doch bei bestimmten Personen- und Patientengruppen von großer Bedeutung sein, daß man keine Steigerung des intrakardialen Sauerstoffbedarfes hat.

Chen: In animals we have not done this kind of work. Of course, this problem will have to be investigated.

Klaus: I am quite sure that there is an increase in cardiac oxygen consumption but in fact, nobody has measured it.

Langrehr: Den kardialen Sauerstoffverbrauch zu messen wäre natürlich ideal. Der Gesamtsauerstoff-Verbrauch, den wir bei der Atemantriebskurve erfassen, steigt eher leicht an, fällt aber nicht ab wie bei anderen Narkoseformen.

Klaus: Meine Frage zielt darauf, wie gefährlich es ist, diese Substanz bei Patienten anzuwenden, die eine vorhandene oder drohende Coronarinsuffizienz haben, was man ja nicht in jedem Fall im voraus weiß.

Langrehr: Nun gut, wir haben keine Messungen, wir haben aber eine Erfahrung: Wenn ein Mensch nicht mehr zu anaesthesieren ist, weil er eine Herzinsuffizienz hat, acut oder chronisch, und er ante finem ist, können

Sie auf der Welt nach einer Anaesthesiemöglichkeit suchen. Sie haben eigentlich nur diese: Verwenden Sie Ketamine.

Frau **Podlesch:** Sie haben gesagt, daß der Blutdruckanstieg bei Patienten mit und ohne Prämedikation der gleiche sei. Nach unserer Erfahrung ist bei einer normalen Prämedikation der Blutdruckanstieg wesentlich geringer als bei einer Prämedikation, die nur aus Atropin besteht. Im Hinblick auf „coronarische Indikationen" haben wir keine Erfahrung. Wir wissen aber, daß bei „Kammerkindern" der Blutdruck nicht ansteigt, wenn wir Ketamine geben. Wahrscheinlich sind diese Kinder schon an der Grenze ihrer kardialen Leistungsfähigkeit. Wir können in diesen Fällen kein anderes Narkosemittel anwenden wegen des Blutdruckabfalles, denn diese Kinder kommen schon mit einem Druck von 80–90 systolisch auf den Tisch, und wenn man Ketamine injiziert, ändert sich eigentlich nichts an dem Druck. Wir haben diese Eigenschaft des Ketamins stets als einen Fortschritt betrachtet.

Langrehr: Zur Frage des Blutdruckverhaltens mit und ohne Prämedikation möchte ich sagen, daß es selbstverständlich Unterschiede gibt, denn es kann nicht gleichgültig sein, ob man von einer Atropin gesteigerten Herzfrequenz von 110 oder einer Herzfrequenz von 80 ausgeht. Trotzdem kommt es bei beiden zum Blutdruckanstieg, wenn auch das Ausmaß unterschiedlich sein mag. Wesentlich scheint mir aber zu sein, daß es überhaupt zu einer Steigerung des Blutdruckes kommt.

Kuschinsky: Herr LANGREHR, was Sie da vorhin sagten, möchte ich doch noch kritisieren: Was Sie als Erfahrung hinstellten, war doch nur ein Glaube! Aber Glaube ist nicht Wissenschaft!

Langrehr: Ich habe nicht gesagt, daß ich glaube, daß man diese Patienten mit Ketamine anaesthesieren könne, sondern ich habe gesagt, man kann sie anaesthesieren. Ich tat es jedenfalls.

Kuschinsky: Weil Sie daran glaubten!

Langrehr: Weil ich es glaubte!
Wenn Sie einen Patienten haben, der in einer außerordentlich schwierigen kardialen Situation ist, dann können Sie den Effekt von Ketamine folgendermaßen beschreiben: Es kommt zu keinem Blutdruckabfall, und der Patient hat keine Rhythmusstörungen, die er bei jedem Barbiturat-bedingten Druckabfall in derselben Situation entwickeln würde. Ich kann das nur als positiv auffassen Leider gibt es darüber keine Messungen.

Kuschinsky: Das war keine wissenschaftliche Antwort auf die Frage von Herrn KLAUS. Das meinte ich mit meiner Kritik. Es war die Antwort eines Praktikers.

Kreuscher: Ich darf vielleicht zur Frage von Herrn KLAUS noch sagen: Wir haben den Sauerstoffverbrauch am Gehirn gemessen. Dort bleibt er unverändert, bzw. steigt geringfügig an. Das gibt natürlich keine Auskunft darüber, was am Herzen passiert. Man müßte sich aber überlegen, ob beim

Risikopatienten diese Steigerung, die wir beim Gesunden sehen, überhaupt eintritt; oder ob nur der Abfall, z. B. der negativ-chronotrope Effekt anderer Narkosemitte ausbleibt.

Corssen: Dr. Elisabeth Dowdy von der Universität in Jackson/Mississippi hat im letzten Herbst in Las Vegas eine Arbeit präsentiert, in der sie merkwürdigerweise feststellte, daß beim Kaninchen das Ketamin einen negativ-inotropen Effekt aufweist. Sie ist jetzt dabei, das noch im einzelnen zu untersuchen, sie ist aber sicher, daß sie sich bei ihren Beobachtungen nicht geirrt hat. Sie hat dann gefordert, daß man im Hinblick auf die negativ-inotrope Wirkung des Ketamins bei dieser Species vorsichtig sein sollte bei der Anwendung von Ketamine bei Patienten mit drohender Coronarinsuffizienz oder angeborenen Herzfehlern. Sowohl Dr. Virtue als auch wir in Ann Arbor haben nachgewiesen, daß beim Menschen ohne Zweifel eine positiv-inotrope Wirkung vorhanden ist, und das entspricht genau dem, was Herr Kreuscher gesagt hat. Trotzdem hat Dr. Dowdy gefordert, daß man die angeborenen Herzfehler und die Coronarinsuffizienz als Kontraindikationen bei der Beurteilung der klinischen Eignung des Ketamins zu berücksichtigen habe.

Tetzlaff: Herr Kreuscher, Sie sprachen von der positiven inotropen und chronotropen Wirkung. Ist diese Beobachtung unter Umständen ein Adaptationsvorgang des Herzens auf den vermehrten venösen Rückfluß infolge der erhöhten Muskelspannung?

Chen: In isolated conditions we cannot show any positive chronotropic or inotropic effect. Only in unisolated conditions, can we see it.

Kreuscher: Der Anstieg des zentral-venösen Druckes könnte für Ihre Theorie sprechen. Ich glaube aber doch nicht, daß diese Frage so einfach zu beantworten ist. Man sollte die Pharmakologen noch einmal fragen, ob sie Untersuchungen gemacht haben über den Katecholaminspiegel vor und nach der Wirkung von CI-581. May I ask the pharmacologists: Did you perform investigations about the catecholamine excretion during the action of CI-581?

Chen: No, we have not!

Kreuscher: I think, this would be a very important investigation that we should perform, because this positive chronotropic and inotropic action on the heart-muscle and the oxygen-consumption of the heart muscle depend also upon the catecholamine-level in the blood.

Chen: This is a problem of the technique. We cannot detect the catecholamine in the heart.

Kreuscher: Thank you very much. Ich glaube, so lange dieses Problem nicht geklärt ist, können wir die Frage von Herrn Klaus, die ich für sehr wesentlich halte, nicht genügend exakt beantworten.

L'Allemand: Zur Frage der Katecholamine: Wir haben diese natürlich nicht direkt gemessen aber versucht, über die Fettsäuren und den Blutzucker

Aufschluß zu bekommen. Wenn wir die Untersuchungen von Herrn LANG-
REHR über das Verhalten des Blutzuckers zugrundelegen, so kann ich sagen,
daß wir die gleichen Ergebnisse haben. Das spricht etwas gegen einen
erhöhten Katecholaminspiegel. Genau so ist es mit den Fettsäuren. Wir
haben die Untersuchungen, deren Zahl nicht groß genug ist um hier End-
gültiges auszusagen, etwa so interpretiert: Wir glauben, daß der Katecholaminspiegel nicht erhöht ist; das ist allerdings nicht als Beweis zu werten.

Schirdewahn: Die klinischen Ergebnisse, die bisher vorgetragen wurden, schließen immer mit dem Satz, daß ein positiv-inotroper Effekt
vorhanden sei. Sind denn wirklich mit diesen Untersuchungen Aussagen
über eine positive Inotropie möglich? Denn wenn das Herzzeitvolumen
ansteigt, können wir doch noch nicht sagen, daß ein positiv-inotroper Effekt
vorliegt. Wenn die Herzfrequenz ansteigt und der Blutdruck nicht, ist das
auch noch kein Beweis dafür, daß dies ein positiv inotroper Effekt ist. Ich
meine, man sollte im Augenblick noch nicht sagen, daß Ketamine einen
positiv-inotropen Effekt habe, und man muß sich hüten, daraus zu schließen,
daß man Patienten mit Herzmuskelinsufffzienz oder Coronarinsuffizienz
damit narkotisieren kann. Die Theoretiker sollten uns sagen, wie man aus
diesen klinischen Ergebnissen tatsächlich eine positive Inotropie oder
Chronotropie erkennen kann.

Kuschinsky: Sie haben wirklich ganz recht; wenn man eine Treppe
hinaufsteigt, so hätte das Treppensteigen auch einen positiv-inotropen
Effekt, obgleich er nicht in jedem Fall therapeutisch günstig sein kann. Die
Frage ist also durchaus berechtigt. Man kann nur sagen, das Schlagvolumen
ist erhöht. Man kann aber nicht sagen, daß die Substanz eine positiv-
inotropen Effekt habe.

Klaus: Ich kann nur sagen, daß diese Effekte, die am Herz-Kreis-
laufsystem registriert wurden, wie Frequenzzunahme und Schlagvolumen-
vermehrung sich eigentlich auch ohne weiteres durch ein gesteigertes
venöses Angebot erklären ließen.

Kreuscher: Über den venösen Rückstrom sind meines Wissens keine
Volumenmessungen sondern lediglich Druckmessungen gemacht worden.
Bezüglich der positiv-inotropen Wirkung und ihrer Interpretation muß man
sich fragen, wie man diesen Parameter am Menschen messen kann. Das ist
natürlich außerordentlich schwierig. Sie können die Kontraktilität des
Herzmuskels und seine Veränderungen nicht direkt messen, sondern nur
aus der Steilheit des Druckanstieges während der isometrischen Kontrak-
tion kalkulieren. Dieses wurde mit einem von uns früher empfohlenen
indirekten Verfahren durch Herrn LANGREHR gemacht. Sie erinnern sich,
daß er kalkulativ die Steilheit der Druckanstiegskurve gemessen hat und
dabei ein gleichbleibendes Verhalten feststellte. Die Frage des Volumen-
angebotes und der daraus ableitbaren Leistung ist meines Erachtens noch
nicht ausreichend geklärt.

Zindler: Wenn man annimmt, daß der vermehrte venöse Rückstrom durch den erhöhten Muskeltonus bedingt ist, dann kann dieser Effekt nur ganz kurze Zeit dauern, denn es wird wahrscheinlich nicht mehr Blut mobilisiert. Wie lange dauert denn der Anstieg des Herzzeitvolumens?

Kreuscher: Nur wenige Minuten!

Langrehr: 10 bis 20 Minuten!

Zindler: Wo soll denn das venöse Angebot herkommen? Die Erhöhung des Muskeltonus ist nach 2 min beendet!

Schirdewahn: Dr. CHEN hat gezeigt, daß das Schlagvolumen nach 5 min gesteigert ist und nach 10 min schon die Ausgangslage wieder erreicht. Also länger als 5 min hält im Tierexperiment die Steigerung des Herzzeitvolumens offenbar nicht an.

Kreuscher: Das kann ich allerdings bestätigen. Auch bei unseren Versuchen war die Steigerung nur kurz.

Klaus: Mich wundert eigentlich, daß keine detaillierten pharmakologischen Untersuchungen an isolierten Herz-Lungen-Präparaten vorgenommen wurden, aus denen eindeutig zu klären wäre, ob indirekte oder direkte Wirkungen der Substanz auf den Herzmuskel vorhanden sind.

Droh: Ich hätte an Herrn KREUSCHER noch eine Frage: Es wurde diskutiert, ob die kardialen Effekte möglicherweise durch einen erhöhten venösen Rückfluß infolge des erhöhten Muskeltonus ausgelöst werden. Die Frage wäre doch einfach zu klären, wenn man die Patienten unmittelbar nach der Narkoseeinleitung mit einem Muskelrelaxans relaxiert.

Kreuscher: Wir haben bei einigen Fällen CI-581 zur endotrachealen Intubation unter Succinylcholin verwendet. Auch bei diesen Fällen, bei denen die Muskulatur total relaxiert war, konnten wir eine Drucksteigerung beobachten. Wir haben hier allerdings keine kontinuierlichen Messungen durchgeführt, sondern den Blutdruck in klinisch üblicher Weise intermittierend nach Riva-Rocci gemessen.

Droh: Wann haben Sie den Blutdruck gemessen, nachdem die Muskelfibrillationen abgeklungen waren?

Kreuscher: Jawohl, nach dem Abklingen!

Dangel: Haben Sie den intravenösen Wellendruck am curarisierten Patienten gemessen?

Kreuscher: Nein, der Wellendruck wurde nicht gemessen.

Gemperle: Am curarisierten Hund fanden wir nie einen erhöhten Venendruck.

Dissociative Anaesthesie mit Ketamine (CI-581)

Aus dem Department für Anaesthesie der Universität von Alabama
(Chairman: Prof. Dr. G. CORSSEN)
und dem Department für Pharmakologie der Universität von Michigan
(Chairman: Prof. Dr. M. SEEVERS)

Von **G. Corssen**, **M. Miyasaka** und **E. F. Domino**

Im Zusammenhang mit früheren Mitteilungen über pharmakologische und erste klinische Erfahrungen mit dem Phencyclidinderivat Ketamine (CI-581) [1, 2] haben wir vorgeschlagen, die von dieser Droge verursachte Narkose „dissoziative" Anaesthesie zu nennen. Auf Grund kürzlich durchgeführter elektroencephalographischer Untersuchungen im Hirn der Katze sind wir jetzt in der Lage, den experimentellen Beweis dafür zu führen, daß die Bezeichnung „dissoziative" Anaesthesie bei der Ketamine Narkose tatsächlich berechtigt erscheint.

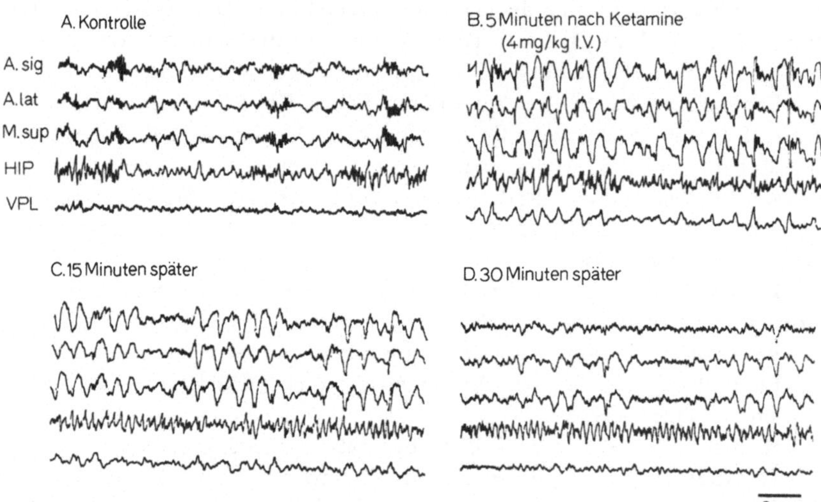

Abb. 1. Elektroencephalographische Effekte von Ketamine bei der Katze. Zeichenerklärung: A.SIG = Gyrus sigmoid anterior – Sensorische Motorregion des neocorticalen Systems, A.LAT = Gyrus lateral anterior – Assoziationsregion des neocorticalen Systems, M.SUP = Gyrus suprasylvii medialis – Assoziationsregion des neocorticalen Systems, HIP = Hippocampus – Limbisches System, VPL = Nucleus ventralis posterolateralis – Somatosensorischer Relay Nucleus des Thalamus

Bei 5 Katzen wurden permanente Elektroden in verschiedenen corticalen und subcorticalen Regionen eingepflanzt und die durch Ketamine verursachten Veränderungen der Hirnstromaktivität mit Hilfe konventioneller neurophysiologischer Methoden registriert.

Abb. 1, A zeigt die EEG Aktivität in den verschiedenen Hirnregionen der Katze im wachen Zustand (Erklärung der Abkürzungen siehe unter Abb. 1). Die drei oberen EEG-Ableitungen repräsentieren corticale Regionen, während die beiden unteren Ableitungen zu subcorticalen Zentren gehören.

Nach intravenöser Verabreichung von Ketamine (4 mg/kg) treten in den corticalen Bereichen *Delta*-Wellen auf (Abb. 1, B), die auch nach 15 min noch anhalten (Abb. 1, C), jedoch zu diesem Zeitpunkt rhythmisch von Wellen mit geringerer Voltspannung und schneller Aktivität unterbrochen sind. Auch das diffus projizierende thalamische System (VPL) zeigt mäßige *Delta*-Wellen-Aktivität 5 min nach der Ketamine-Injektion, die nach 15 min allmählich abklingt. Nach 30 min kehrt das EEG im cortico-thalamischen Bereich zur Ausgangslage zurück (Abb. 1, D).

Im Gegensatz zur *Delta*-Wellen-Aktivität in den cortico-thalamischen Regionen treten im Hippocampus (HIP) 5 min nach der Ketamine-Injektion *Theta*-Wellen auf (Abb. 1, B), die auf eine Aktivierung dieser Hirnregion hindeuten. Diese *Theta*-Wellen-Aktivität ist besonders ausgeprägt 30 min nach der Ketamine-Gabe, wenn die *Delta*-Aktivität im cortico-thalamischen Bereich zum Abklingen gekommen ist (Abb. 1, D).

Abb. 2 illustriert die durch Ketamine ausgelösten EEG-Veränderungen innerhalb corticaler Hirnanteile (Erklärung der Abkürzungen siehe unter

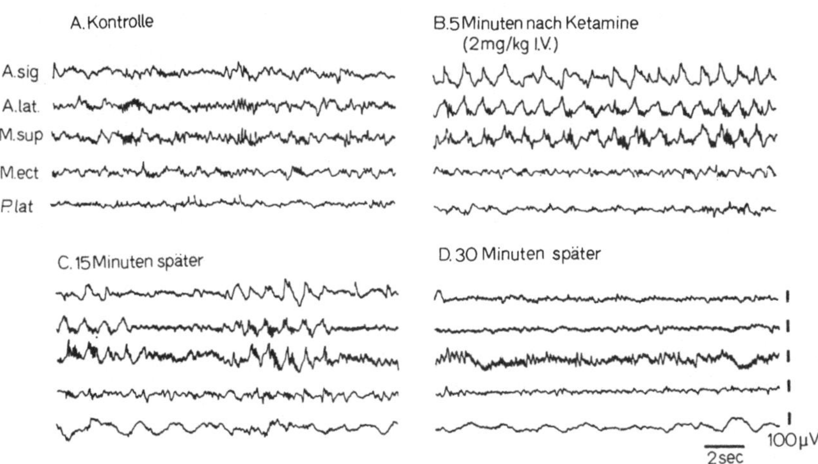

Abb. 2. Neocorticale regionale Unterschiede von Ketamineinduzierten EEG-effekten bei der Katze. Zeichenerklärung: M.ECT = Mittlerer Ectosylvischer Gyrus – Gehörrinde, P.LAT = Gyrus posterior lateralis – Sehrinde

Abb. 2). 5 min nach intravenöser Verabreichung von Ketamine (2 mg/kg) ist deutliche *Delta*-Wellen-Aktivität im Bereich der somatosensorischen Motorregion (A.SIG) und in den beiden Assoziationszentren (A.LAT, M.SUP) sichtbar (Abb. 2, B), während zu gleicher Zeit in der Gehörregion (M.ECT) sowie in der Sehrinde (P.LAT) keine wesentlichen Veränderungen der Hirnstromtätigkeit zu registrieren sind. Nach 15 min ist noch immer eine rhythmisch wiederkehrende *Delta*-Wellen-Aktivität zu beobachten, während auch zu diesem Zeitpunkt wenig Veränderungen im Hörzentrum und in der Sehrinde sichtbar sind (Abb. 2, C). Nach 30 min ist die EEG-Aktivität in allen Ableitungen zur Ausgangslage zurückgekehrt (Abb. 2, D).

Die Ergebnisse dieser EEG-Untersuchungen lassen den Schluß zu, daß Ketamine auf gewisse Hirnanteile, wie z. B. das cortico-thalamische System, einen depressorischen Effekt ausüben kann, während zu gleicher Zeit andere Hirnzentren, wie Teile des limbischen Systems (Hippocampus), durch Ketamine aktiviert werden können. Diese dissoziative Wirkung von Ketamine ist auch im Bereich der Hirnrinde selbst nachweisbar wie aus Abb. 2 ersichtlich ist.

Eine selektive Wirkung auf frontale Anteile der Hirnrinde konnte jetzt auch von uns in klinischen EEG-Studien mit Ketamine nachgewiesen werden [3].

Die mit Ketamine beobachtete dissoziative und selektive Wirkungsweise auf gewisse Hirnanteile ist von konventionellen Anaesthetica wie Chloroform, Äther, Halothan und Methoxyflurane nicht bekannt. Dies mag erklären, warum klinisch die durch Ketamine erzeugte Anaesthesie in vieler Hinsicht deutliche Unterschiede zu der von anderen Anaesthetica herbeigeführten Narkose aufzeigt.

Dissoziative Anaesthesie mit Ketamine ist gekennzeichnet durch komplette Analgesie, verbunden mit nur oberflächlichem Schlaf. Der Patient ist abgeschaltet („disconnected"). Alle Schutzreflexe wie Husten, Niesen, Schlucken, Lidschlag etc. sind erhalten und oft sogar gesteigert. Der Tonus der Masseter-Muskeln und der intraoralen Muskulatur, besonders der Zunge, ist unverändert oder gesteigert, so daß eine mechanische Verlegung der Atemwege praktisch ausgeschlossen ist. Das Kreislaufsystem ist stimuliert mit Anstieg des systolischen und diastolischen Blutdrucks und Erhöhung der Pulsfrequenz. Die Atmung ist nicht beeinflußt oder – nach schneller intravenöser Injektion – geringfügig und kurzdauernd gedämpft. Das Erwachen erfolgt ruhig und ohne Auftreten von Erregungszuständen, solange vermieden wird, den Patienten frühzeitig zu stimulieren. Übelkeit und Erbrechen werden selten während der Aufwachphase beobachtet.

Wir haben kürzlich an anderer Stelle über unsere Erfahrungen mit Ketamine bei über 1500 chirurgischen und diagnostischen Eingriffen berichtet [4]. Es soll daher hier nur zusammenfassend über die wichtigsten Indikationsgebiete der Ketamine-Anaesthesie, ihre Kontraindikationen, sowie Vorteile und Nachteile oder potentielle Gefahren berichtet werden.

Folgende *Indikationen* für die Anwendung von Ketamine scheinen uns nach $3^{1}/_{2}$jähriger klinischer Anwendung dieses Anaestheticums gegeben:

1. Kurzdauernde Risikoeingriffe in der septischen Chirurgie, chirurgische Behandlung schwerer Verbrennungen, Wundversorgung und Wechseln von Verbänden.

2. Pneumoencephalographie und verwandte diagnostische Manipulationen in der Neurochirurgie.

3. Herzkatheterisierung bei Patienten mit angeborenen oder erworbenen Herzdefekten.

4. Ophthalmologische diagnostische und kurzdauernde chirurgische Eingriffe.

5. Zahnextraktionen.

6. Diagnostische und kurzdauernde chirurgische Eingriffe in der Otologie, soweit diese nicht den Kehlkopf und Pharynx einschließen.

7. Kurzdauernde plastische Chirurgie an Kopf und Hals.

8. Geschlossene Frakturreposition mit Anlage eines Gipsverbandes.

9. Sigmoidoskopie und kleinere Eingriffe an Anus und Rectum.

10. Diagnostische und kleine chirurgische Eingriffe in der Urologie (mit Verwendung von Lachgas-Sauerstoff).

11. Dilatation und Currettage der Cervix (mit Verwendung von Lachgas-Sauerstoff).

12. Vaginale Entbindung und Kaiserschnitt (mit Verwendung von Lachgas-Sauerstoff).

13. Einleitung zur Kombinationsnarkose bei Patienten mit verminderter respiratorischer und kardialer Reserve.

Die Anwendung von Ketamine ist *kontraindiziert* bei:

1. Arteriellem Hochdruck (Blutdruck über 160/100 mmHg).

2. Schlaganfall in der Anamnese.

3. Eingriffe im Kehlkopf-, Schlund- und Bronchialbereich, ausgenommen, wenn ein endotrachealer Tubus gelegt ist und Muskelrelaxantien angewandt werden.

4. Abdominale und andere Eingriffe, die mit „visceralem" Schmerz verbunden sind, ausgenommen, wenn Ketamine mit Lachgas-Sauerstoff ergänzt wird.

5. Schwere Herzdekompensation.

Als eindeutige *Vorteile* der Ketamine-Anaesthesie seien genannt:

1. Tiefe Analgesie ohne signifikante Beeinträchtigung der Atmung.

2. Stimulierender Effekt auf das Kreislaufsystem.

3. Aufrechterhaltung der Schutzreflexe.

4. Freie Luftpassage ohne Anwendung von endotrachealem oder pharyngealem Tubus.

5. Kein toxischer Effekt auf lebenswichtige Organe wie Leber, Niere, Herz etc.

6. Ausgezeichnete Gewebeverträglichkeit, sowohl nach intravenöser wie auch nach intramuskulärer Verabreichung.

7. Große therapeutische Breite.

8. Übelkeit und Erbrechen während der Aufwachphase ist außerordentlich selten.

9. Antiarrhythmische Wirkung.

10. Amnesie.

Ketamine-Anaesthesie schließt die folgenden *Nachteile* ein:

1. Gelegentliche starke vasopressorische Wirkung, die besonders bei Patienten mit Hochdruckneigung zu beobachten ist.

2. Starke Salivation bei Fehlen von anticholinergischer Prämedikation.

3. Kumulative Wirkung nach wiederholter Verabreichung mit verlängerter Aufwachphase.

4. Psychotrope Wirkung, die sich besonders bei erwachsenen Patienten während des Erwachens manifestieren kann, wenn die dissoziative Wirkung von Ketamine noch nicht völlig abgeklungen ist und der Patient verbal oder taktil stimuliert wird.

5. Viscerale Schmerzen werden von Ketamine im Gegensatz zu somatischen Schmerzen ungenügend vermindert. Deshalb muß bei urologischen, gynäkologischen und allgemein-chirurgischen Eingriffen in der Bauchhöhle Lachgas-Sauerstoff als Zusatzanaestheticum gegeben werden.

6. Extrapyramidale Muskeltätigkeit, obgleich eine verhältnismäßig seltene Komplikation, kann bei ophthalmologischen und otologischen Eingriffen störend wirken.

Zusammenfassend darf festgestellt werden, daß Ketamine ein ungewöhnlich sicheres, wirkungsvolles und leicht zu verabreichendes neues Anaestheticum darstellt, das in seiner „dissoziativen" Wirkung auf das Zentralnervensystem eindeutige Unterschiede zu den bisher gebräuchlichen, konventionellen Anaesthetica aufweist. Mehr klinische Erfahrung mit diesem Anaestheticum ist notwendig, bevor sein Platz innerhalb der modernen Anaesthesiemittel und -methoden festgestellt werden kann.

Summary

Electroencephalographic recordings obtained from various cortical and subcortical regions of the cat before and after the administration of Ketamine suggest a selective, "dissociative" action of the drug. Ketamine exerts depressant effects on the cortico-thalamic system, while simultaneously stimulating parts of the limbic system (Hippocpamus). The documented dissociative action of Ketamine may explain, why, clinically, Ketamine-induced anesthesia differs markedly from anesthesia induced by conventional anesthetics.

On the basis of more than 1500 clinical administrations of Ketamine, it is concluded that Ketamine is an unusually safe, effective and easy to administer new anesthetic which may prove of definitive value in certain well defined surgical areas.

Literatur

1. CORSSEN, G., and E. F. DOMINO: Dissociative Anesthesia: Further Pharmacologic Studies and First Clinical Experience with the Phencyclidine Derivative CI-581. Anesth. Analg. **45**, 29 (1966).
2. DOMINO, E. F., P. CHODOFF, and G. CORSSEN: Pharmacologic Effects of CI-581, A New Dissociative Anesthetic in Man. J. clin. Pharmacol. Therap. **6**, 279 (1965).
3. CORSSEN, G., E. F. DOMINO, and R. L. BREE: EEG Effects of Ketamine (CI-581) in Children. Anesth. Analg. **48**, 141 (1969).
4. —, M. MIYASAKA, and E. F. DOMINO: Changing Concepts in Pain Control during Surgery: Dissociative Anesthesia – A Progress Report. Anesth. Analg. **47**, 746 (1968).

The Effect of Ketamine (CI-581) on the Cardiovascular and Central Nervous System

By **G. Szappanyos, A. Beaumanoir, G. Gemperle, M. Gemperle** and
P. Moret

Hôpital Cantonal, Dép. d'Anesthésiologie, Genève

The very promising clinical experiences with the new type of anesthetic agent, CI-581, stimulated our interest in further pharmacological studies concerning its action on the *cardiovascular system*.

The rapidity of the complete loss of sensation and consciousness and apparent lack of convulsive property prompted us to attempt to determine its site of action in the *central nervous system*.

A. Cardiovascular System

Subjects and Methods

The cardiovascular experiments were carried out in two series on dogs. In the first series, in order to have accurate details on the entire cardio-vascular system, dogs with open thorax were used. This method permitted us to measure different parameters, which are interesting to clinicians, such as the contractile force, cardiac output, rate, rhythm, irritability, coronary circulation, different pressures and peripheral resistance. The dogs were induced with Sodium Pentobarbital, intubated and their respiration controlled with an Engström respirator with Nitrous Oxide-Oxygen (60–40 percent).

In general, in this series we have measured:

1. The electrocardiographic recording of the cardiac frequency.

2. Different pressures: left ventricular, thoracic aortic, right ventricular, pulmonary arterial, left auricular and central venous pressure.

3. The cardiac output, continuously monitored with a special electro-magnetic square wawe flow meter (Carolina Med. Electr.) placed around the aorta. (This also permitted us to measure the left ventricular ejection speed.)

4. The isometric systolic tension of a segment of the left ventricle with the Walton-Brodie strain gauge system.

5. The rate of change of the left ventricular pressure ($dp./dt.$). This echang seems to be directly proportional to the contractile force of the heart.

6. The change in the length of the myocardial fibre at each contraction and, at the same time, with an amplification system, the slow variation of the cardiac volume.

7. Coronary sinus flow by a catheter, introduced into the coronary sinus.

8. Arterial, venous O_2 saturation, arterial pH and pCO_2.

9. Peripheral resistance (measured in dyn $\cdot$ sec $\cdot$ cm^{-5}).

In the second series, in dogs with intact thorax, we measured the following parameters:

1. Electrocardiographic recording of the cardiac frequency.

2. Aortic pressure by cannulation of the femoral artery and insertion of a catheter into the thoracic aorta.

3. Central venous pressure with a catheter introduced into the vena cava inferior via the formal vein.

4. Respiratory repercussions on the central venous pressure.

The CI-581 was given i.v. in doses varying from 1 to 10 mg/kg. The intervals between the repeated doses were 15 to 20 min and were only given if all the controlled parameters returned to the pre-injection levels. Before the administration of the drug, sufficient time was allowed to elapse to eliminate any additional effect of the given induction dose of Sodium Pentothal.

Results

a. Open Thorax Series. The remarkably fast analgetic effect of the drug, characterized by the immediate (20 to 25 sec) stabilization of the measured parameters, is well demonstrated. The varying cardiac rhythm, left ventricular and aortic pressure, and the instability of the changes in the length of the myocardial fibre at each contraction (déplacement) show the awakening of the animal. The maximum calculated peripheral resistance was 4300 dyn $\cdot$ sec $\cdot$ cm^{-5}. The i.v. injection of 3 mg/kg of the drug decreased markedly the peripheral resistance to 2500 dyn $\cdot$ sec$\cdot$ cm^{-5}, contrary to the findings of VIRTUE who has not seen this change (Fig. 1).

In contrast with the closed chest series, there was a decrease in the cardiac frequency of from 20 to 25 percent as a constant finding, with a decrease of the left ventricular pressure in conjunction with a 15 percent diminution of the aortic pressure. There was no change in the left auricular pressure, which would be a sign of cardiac insufficiency. The increase in the cardiac output is well demonstrated as an almost constant finding (7 out of the 10 experiments). The diminution of the rate of change of the left ventricular pressure (dp./dt.) indicated a decreased contractile force with an increase in the cardiac volume. This slight negative inotropic effect, also shown by CHEN G., McCARTHY D. and ENSOR C. R., was accompanied by cardiac dilatation and an increased venous return.

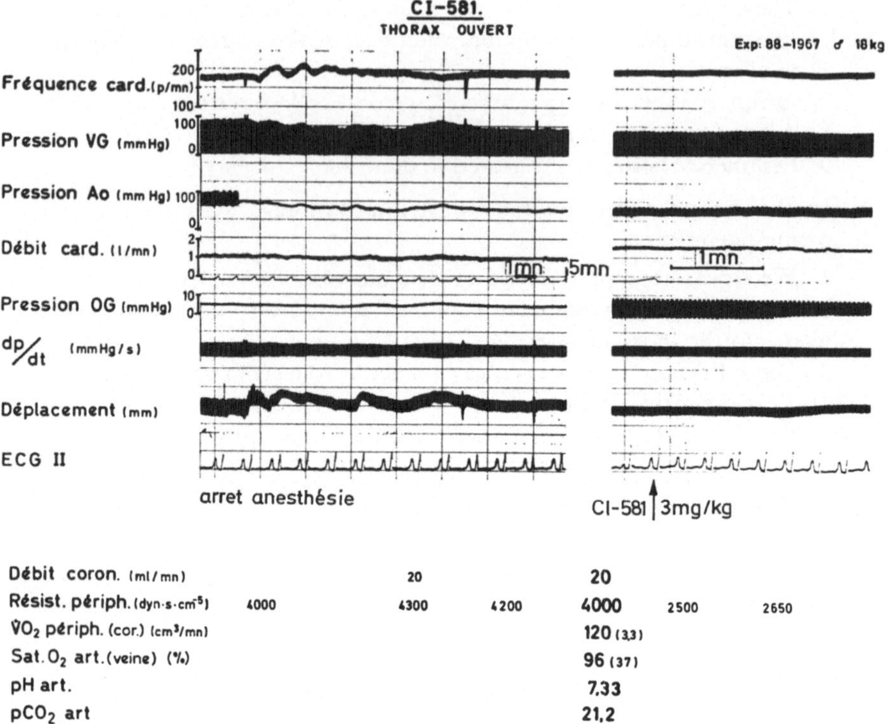

Débit coron. (ml/mn)		20		20		
Résist. périph. (dyn·s·cm⁵)	4000	4300	4200	4000	2500	2650
$\dot{V}O_2$ périph. (cor.) (cm³/mn)		120 (33)				
Sat. O_2 art. (veine) (%)		96 (37)				
pH art.		7,33				
pCO_2 art		21,2				

Fig. 1. Left – Shows the instability of the measured parameters after the arrest of conventional general anesthesia. Right – Shows immediate effect of the drug with the marked decrease of the peripheral resistance

These signs of reduced cardiac work were not the direct effect of the drug on the heart but were due to the marked decrease in the peripheral resistance, with excellent perfusion also proven by the increased Oxygen consumption (Fig. 2). (VO_2 peripheral of 120 to 152 cm³/min with increased venous saturation of from 37 to 47 percent.)

There was no significant change in the arterial O_2 saturation, arterial pH and arterial pCO_2. Repeated, successive and increasing i.v. doses (5–7–10 mg/kg respectively) injected at 20-min intervals showed cumulative effects on every measured parameter. It was interesting to see that the injection of Droperidol 2 mg/kg following the administration of the CI-581 further decreased the peripheral resistance (Fig. 3).

Signs of cardiac irritability with Epinephrine infusion could not be detected with the continuously monitored ECG.

If, following the injection of 5 mg/kg i.v. of CI-581, a Nor-Epinephrine infusion was started (3.5 mg/kg/min), the characteristic response of the

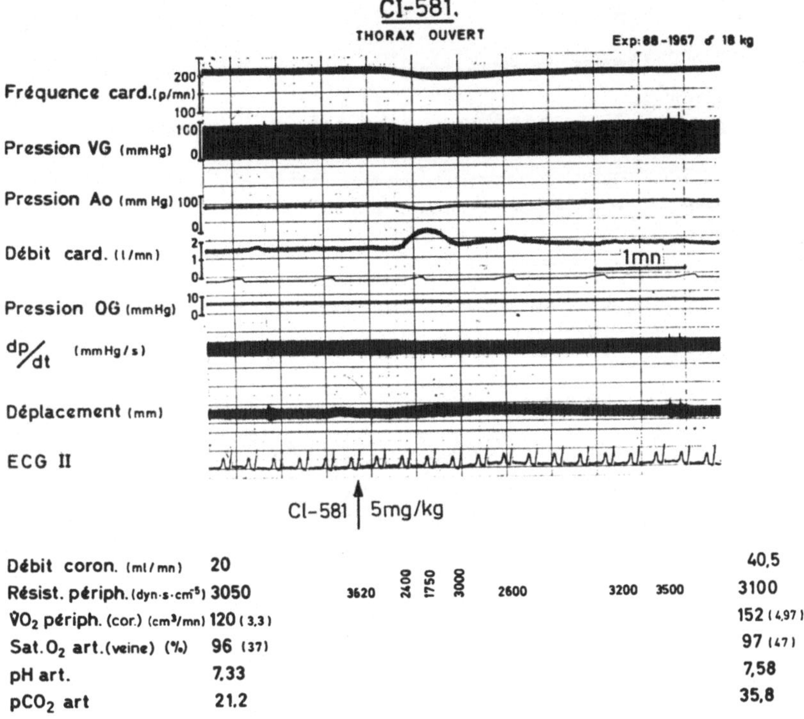

Débit coron. (ml/mn)	20									40,5
Résist. périph. (dyn·s·cm⁻⁵)	3050	3620	2400	1750	3000	2600	3200	3500		3100
V̇O₂ périph. (cor.) (cm³/mn)	120 (3,3)									152 (4,97)
Sat.O₂ art. (veine) (%)	96 (37)									97 (47)
pH art.	7,33									7,58
pCO₂ art	21,2									35,8

Fig. 2. Illustration of the reduced cardiac work as a result of the marked decrease in the peripheral resistance with excellent perfusion

heart, such as increased cardiac frequency as well as the left ventricular and aortic pressure, cardiac output, augmented peripheral resistance and contractile force were all seen. During the infusion, a repeated dose of 5 mg/kg i.v. of CI-581 was given and, interestingly enough, all the primary effects of the CI-581 were immediately but transiently seen, such as diminution of cardiac frequency with the left ventricular and aortic pressure also decreased, increased cardiac output, unchanged left auricular pressure, cardiac dilatation, and first diminished but then moderately increased contractile force with significant decrease of the peripheral resistance (Fig. 4).

b. Closed Thorax Series. With rapid injections (18 to 24 sec) there was an invariably increased heart rate, unchanged central venous pressure, and a marked, transient decrease (20 to 25 percent) of the aortic pressure, without modification of the ECG pattern. The doses injected were 1, 2, 3 and 5 mg/kg i.v. The transient, significant decrease of the aortic pressure lasted 50–55 sec. The preinjection normal parameter readings, except for the sinus tachycardia which was in most cases a longer lasting

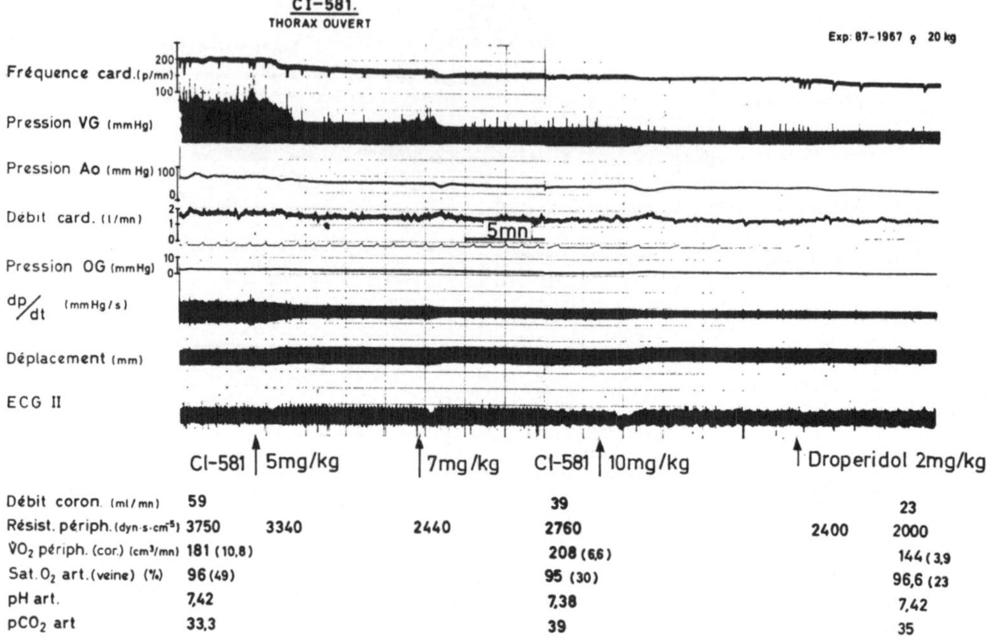

	CI-581 5mg/kg		7mg/kg	CI-581 10mg/kg		Droperidol 2mg/kg
Débit coron. (ml/mn)	59			39		23
Résist. périph. (dyn·s·cm⁻⁵)	3750	3340	2440	2760	2400	2000
V̇O₂ périph. (cor.) (cm³/mn)	181 (10,8)			208 (6,6)		144 (3,9
Sat. O₂ art. (veine) (%)	96 (49)			95 (30)		96,6 (23
pH art.	7,42			7,38		7,42
pCO₂ art	33,3			39		35

Fig. 3. The CI-581 injected in repeated, successive and increasing doses showing the cumulative effects

effect (4 out of 5), were reached in variable time (70 to 120 sec) not depending on the doses injected (Figs. 5, 6, 7).

With slow injections (100 sec), similar and even larger doses (5 to 10 mg/kg i.v.) produced only a slight augmentation of the cardiac rate (10–12 percent), an unchanged central venous pressure and an appreciably smaller decrease of the aortic pressure (5 to 10 percent) (Figs. 8, 9).

The duration of the moderate, transient decrease of the aortic pressure, in contrast to the series with rapid injection with identical dose of 5 mg/kg i.v., was much shorter (15 sec versus 50 sec). The repercussions of the respiration on the central venous pressure were clearly visible. With rapid injection there was a transient, brief period of slower respiratory rate with decreased amplitude lasting 50 to 55 sec. With slow injection, respiration remained adequate in rate and amplitude.

Conclusion

In basic research, if one wishes to study the effects of a drug on cardiac output, blood pressure, peripheral vascular resistance, heart rate, etc., one has to measure these parameters, as they are related events, simultaneously,

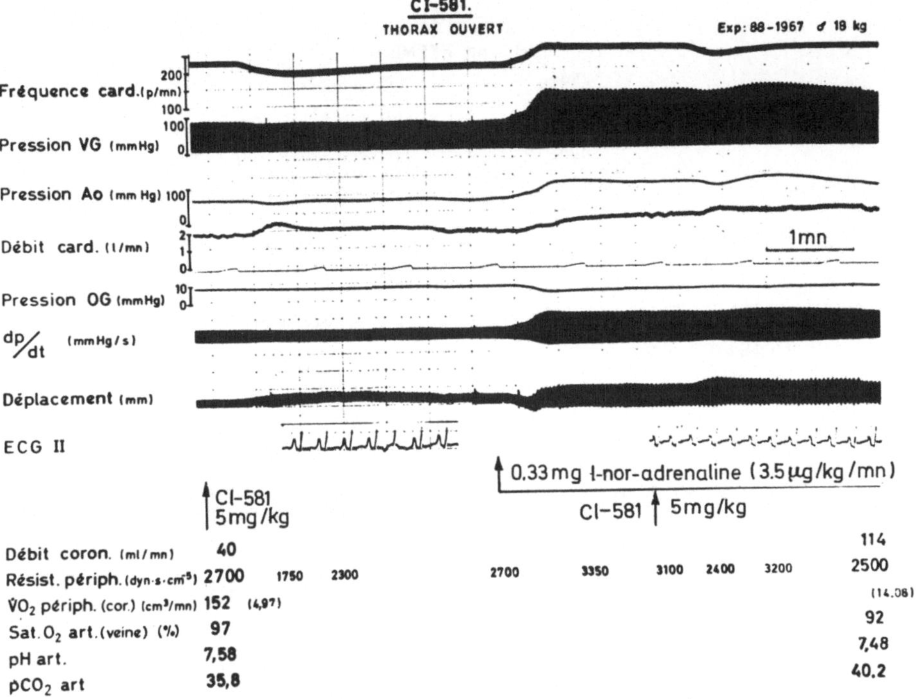

Fig. 4. The effect of the CI-581 during Nor-Epinephrine infusion

in the same animal. The variability of individual animals' response to drugs is great, and there are far too many factors unrelated to the drug (open and closed chest, controlled respiration, etc.), which affect response and are beyond the investigator's control.

These principles and problems could explain the difference in results obtained in our experiments compared to those of other investigators. However, our clinical studies confirm entirely the findings of the numerous centers involved in the research with the CI-581.

One of the important characteristics of CI-581 is its rapid and brief action with remarkable analgesic and anesthetic properties. Its toxicity in animal studies is very low but repeated, increasing doses showed cumulative effects on the cardiovascular system. In the open thorax series there was the consistent finding of decreased cardiac rate in contrast with the closed thorax series. This unexpected finding could be explained by the altered haemodyanamism in the open versus the closed thorax.

In the closed thorax series the biphasic response, consisting of a transitory depressor effect, followed by a more prolonged pressor effect, was influenced not by the amount of the drug but by the speed of injection, as

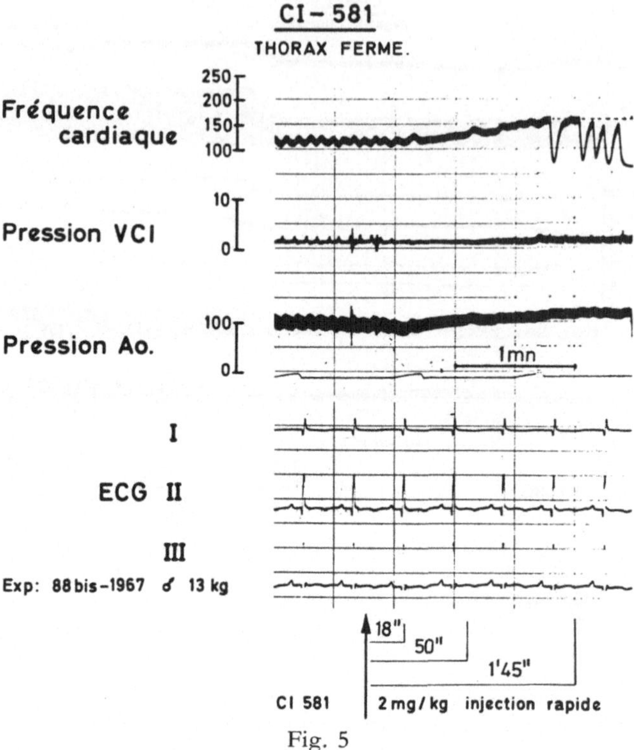

Fig. 5

Figs. 5, 6, and 7. Rapid injection of the CI-581 showing the effects on the cardiac
rate, aortic pressure, central venous pressure

observed also in humans by Corssen G. The CI-581 did not have an
Epinephrine-like arrythmia producing activity and, even under large doses
of Epinephrine infusion, we have not seen arrythmias on the ECG tracing.
The decreased contractile force, aortic pressure and left ventricular pressure
were not signs of a direct effect on the heart, but could be explained by the
spectacular diminution of the peripheral resistance with consecutive but
physiologic diminution of the cardiac work. A possible central effect on the
cardiovascular system of CI-581 might be demonstrated by its action under
Nor-Epinephrine infusion and, as we will see in the second part of this
experiment, by proving its possible site of action at the level of the caudal
brain stem, including the bulbar and pontine structures.

CI-581.
THORAX FERME
Fréquence cardiaque
250
200
150
100
Pression VCI
10
0
Pression Ao.
100
0
1mn
I
ECG II
III
Exp: 88bis-1967 ♂ 13 kg
18s
2 mn.
CI-581
3mg/kg
injection rapide

Fig. 6

CI-581.
THORAX FERME
Fréquence cardiaque
250
200
150
100
Pression VCI
10
0
Pression Ao
100
0
1mn
I
ECG II
III
Exp. 88bis-1967 ♂ 13 kg
18"
55"
5mg/kg CI-581
injection rapide
55"

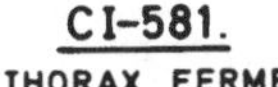

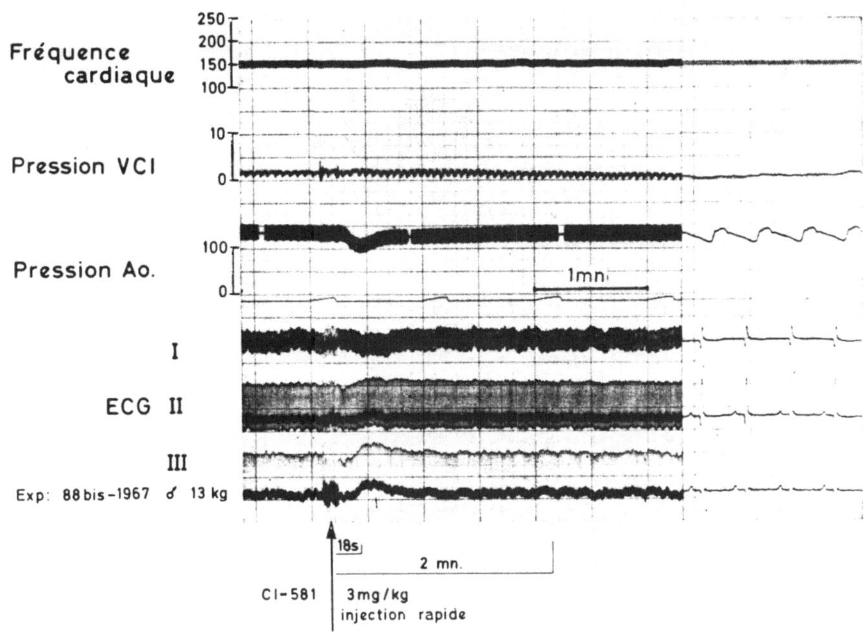

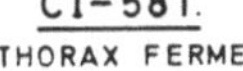

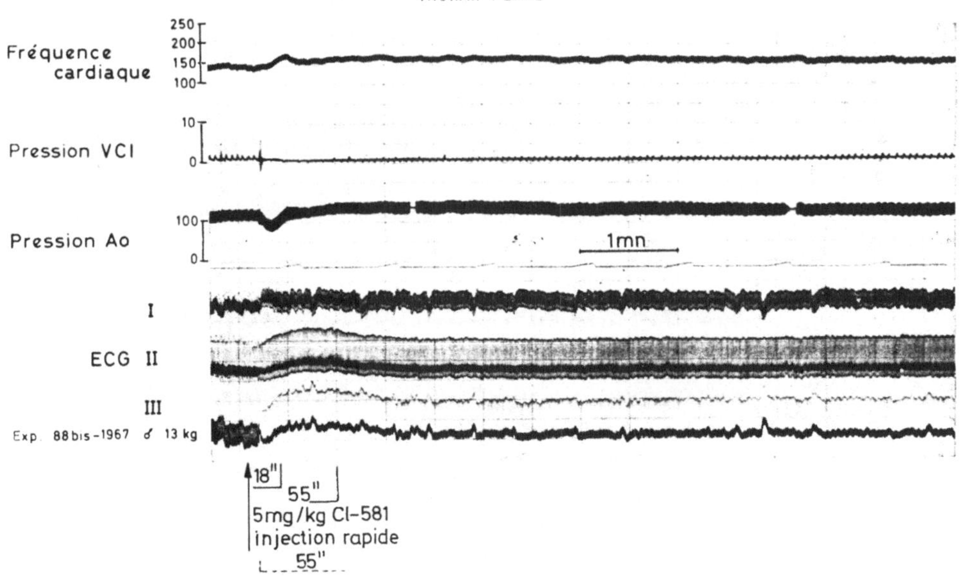

Fig. 7

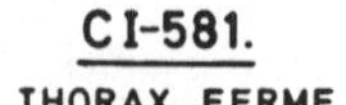

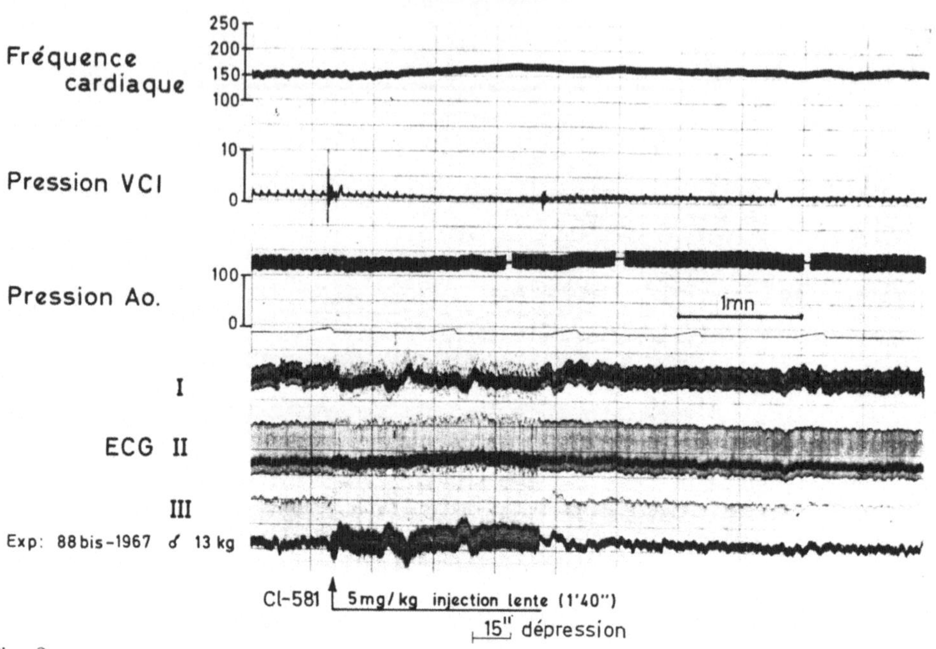

Fig. 8

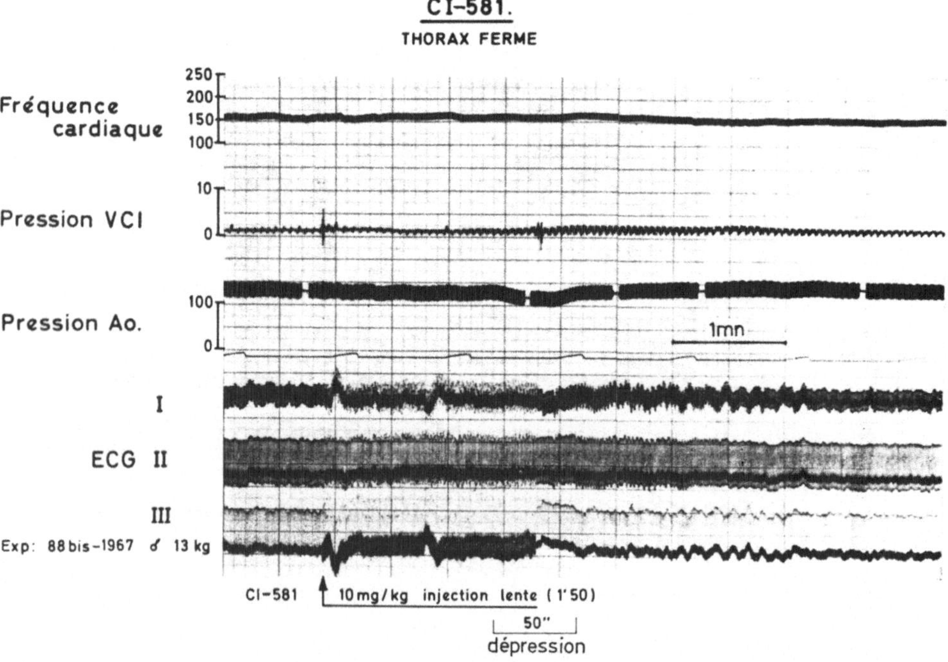

Fig. 9

Figs. 8 and 9. Slow injection of the CI-581 demonstrating that not the amount of the drug but the duration of the injection determines the cardiovascular and respiratory effects

B. Central Nervous System

Subjects and Methods

The experiments described in this work have been carried out on monkeys (Baboons from Senegal) and cats.

I. Monkeys. Monkeys chosen for this experiment were "Baboons from Senegal", known for their sensitivity to S.L.I. The animals belonged to a non-epileptic group (tests carried out in the I.N.P., C.N.R.S. – Marseille – Dr. NAQUET).

Electrodes were either implanted from two to four weeks before the experiments in the subcortical structures, or permanently connected to the dura mater. The product was injected intramuscularly to the awake animal. The doses varied from 5 mg/kg to 10 mg/kg. When several injections were given to the same animal, the intervals between each injection were of approximately two hours. The subcortical electrodes were of the Bickford's type, with 4 to 6 sources of recording. The structures explored were verified by histological examination after the death of the animal.

II. Cats. Three experimental series were carried out:

a) In chronically prepared animals, with electrodes connected to the dura mater, the injections were made with the animals awake and free to move in their cage.

b) In acutely prepared animals, all surgical procedures (endotracheal intubation, implantation of electrodes in the dura mater on one side, and limited craniotomy on the other side) were carried out under general ether anaesthesia. Respiration was controlled with a variable-speed mechanical respirator. Flaxedil was administered i.v. to insure immobility until the ether was eliminated and the first CI-581 injection was given. The recording of the activities of the subcortical structures was transmitted by bipolar electrodes, directed stereotaxically (Horsley-Clarke coordinates). The C.M., V.L., L.P., V.P.L., C.G.L., C.G.M.*, amygdala, hypocampus and substantia reticularis mesencephalica were explored during the effect of the product. The i.v. doses varied from 3 to 5 mg/kg.

c) Also in the acute preparation, the product was injected i.v. (3 to 5 mg/kg) after sectioning the brain-stem, at the levels: "encephale isolé", "retropontin", "prepontin", and "cerveau isolé".

---

* C.M.   – Centrum Medianum
  V.L.   – Nucleus Ventralis Lateralis
  L.P.   – Nucleus Lateralis Posterior
  V.G.L. – Nucleus Ventralis Posterio Lateralis
  C.G.L. – Corpus Geniculatum Laterale
  C.G.M. – Corpus Geniculatum Mediale

Results

I. Baboon Monkeys in Chronic Preparations (8 animals, 17 experiments) *EEG Changes.*

a) The electrocorticographic tracing was quickly modified after the injection of the product (8 mg/kg, i. m. and a characteristic increase of the fast activity was noticed. The topographic study of the cortical activities in the animal No. 157 with a dose of 8 mg/kg i.m. produced after 4 min an amplitude increase of the rolandic fast and the u (mu) activities. In 5 animals and 17 experiments, with doses varying from 5 to 10 mg/kg i. m., spikes appeared in the pre and post rolandic regions 2 min after the injections (Fig. 10).

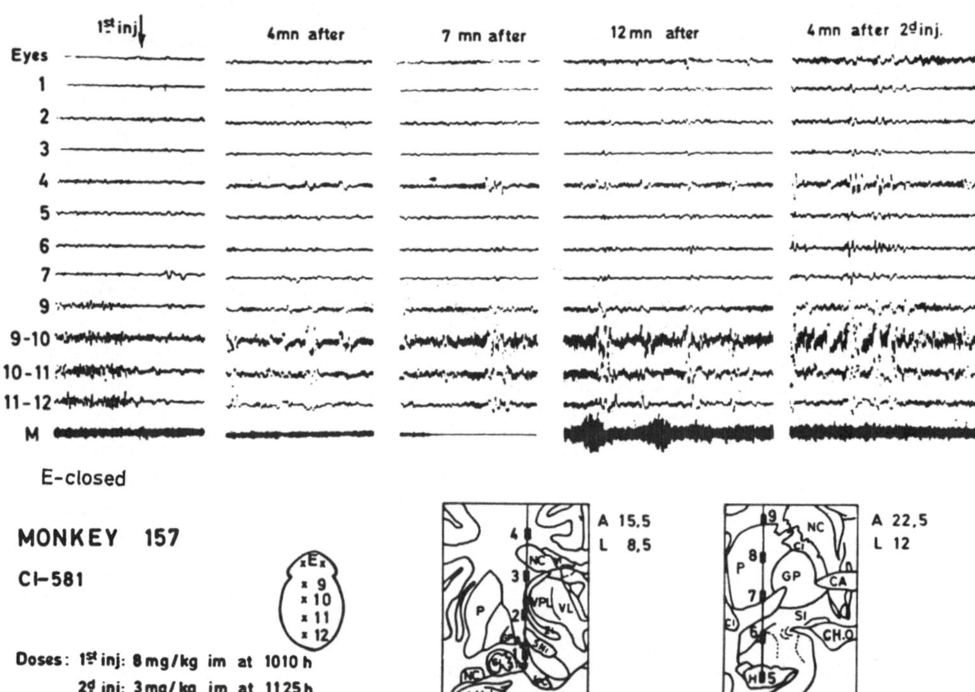

Fig. 10. Bipolar cortical (Bickford's type) electrodes and subcortical recordings. Note: 4 9–10 10–11. Characteristic increase of fast activities. After 7 minutes total hypotony. After 12 minutes hypertonicity (catatonic state) manifested by important spikes and waves with subcortical spikes. With the second injection the EEG changes appear more rapidly and the subcortical structures are more involved

In 7 experiments with doses of 5 to 10 mg/kg i.m., after 4 to 8 min a discharge of generalized spikes appeared on the whole explored neo cortex. In 2 animals, spikes and waves were observed between 5 and 8 min following the i.m. injections. These epileptic-like phenomenons have persisted 20 min in 1 animal and more than 1 h in the other. The epileptic-like discharges were controlled with Valium (Figs. 11, 12).

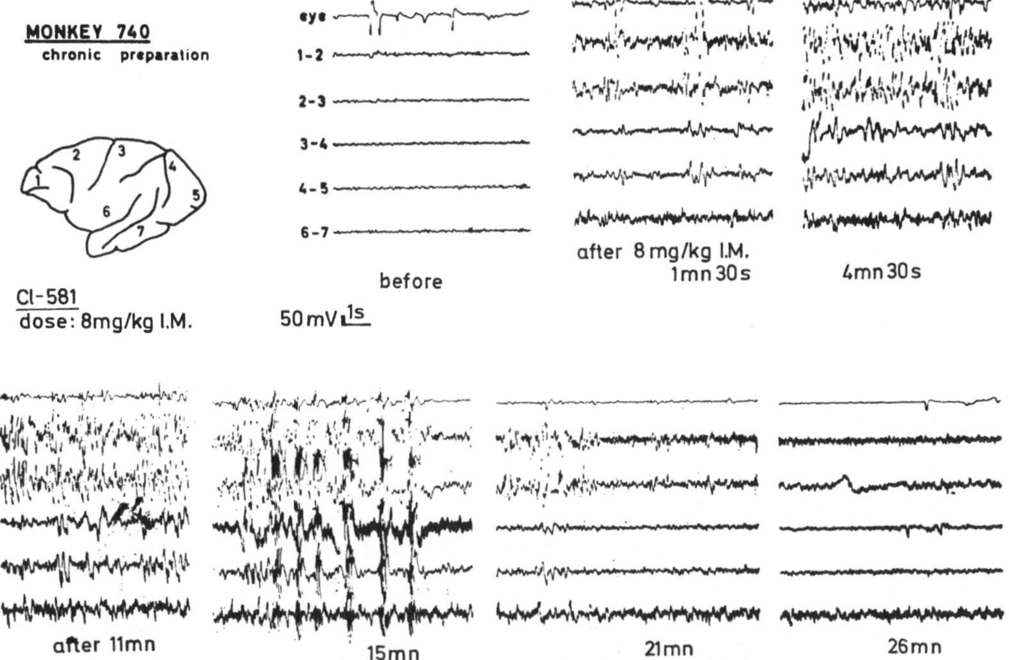

Fig. 11. Bipolar cortical recordings. Increase of the fast activities and after 4–8 minutes a discharge of spikes and waves appears on the whole explored neocortex. (Characteristic epileptic-like discharges.) Spikes and waves are recorded in the formatio reticularis, mesencephalic structures (following primary discharges of the rolandic cortex)

b) At the level of the explored subcortical structures (nucleus caudatus, hypocampus, nuclei amygdalae, putamen, subthalamus including the zona incerta reticularis, and nucleus of the thalamus) there were no important changes noticed during the different phases of the anaesthesia. Meanwhile, after 8 min, spikes and polyspikes were recorded on the cortex and the specific theta rhythm of the hypocampus disappeared. If epileptic-like discharges were obtained, spikes and wawes were recorded in the formatio reticularis and the mesencephalic structures. These discharges occurred after a brief latency period following the primary discharges of the rolandic cortex.

Changes in the Tonus. A few minutes after the injections, the tonic muscular activity – recorded with contact electrodes – was decreased and almost total hypotony ensued. Some animals had rhythmic movements of

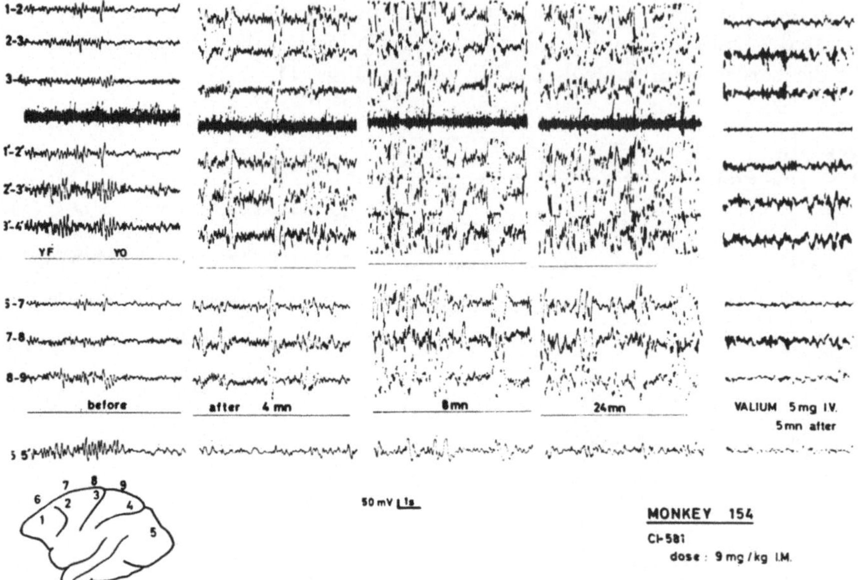

Fig. 12. Convulsive discharges after 4 minutes without muscular hypotony. The epileptic-like phenomenons persisted in 1 animal 20 minutes and more than 1 hour in the other. Effect of Valium on the convulsive activity

their tongue. In all cases (except one – Monkey 741, Fig. 13) following the hypotonic phase, a catatonic state was visible, manifested with important generalized spikes and waves (s. Fig. 1). In 2 animals, between 10 and 20 min following the injections in which the catatonic phase was not very noticeable, increased movements of the eyes were recorded (Fig. 13).

In the 2 animals with epileptic-like discharges, no jerk was recorded or observed while the anaesthetic effect of the drug lasted. Visible convulsions were not observed in either case.

Summary of the EEG Changes

a) In the first 2 min following the injection there was an increase or apparition of the rolandic beta rhythms.

b) Between the first and third minutes rolandic spikes and μ (mu) activities appeared.

c) After the fifth minute in many cases, but in a different time, generalized spikes were noted.

d) In 2 cases, characteristic epileptic-like discharges were seen without clinical manifestation during the anaesthetic action of the drug.

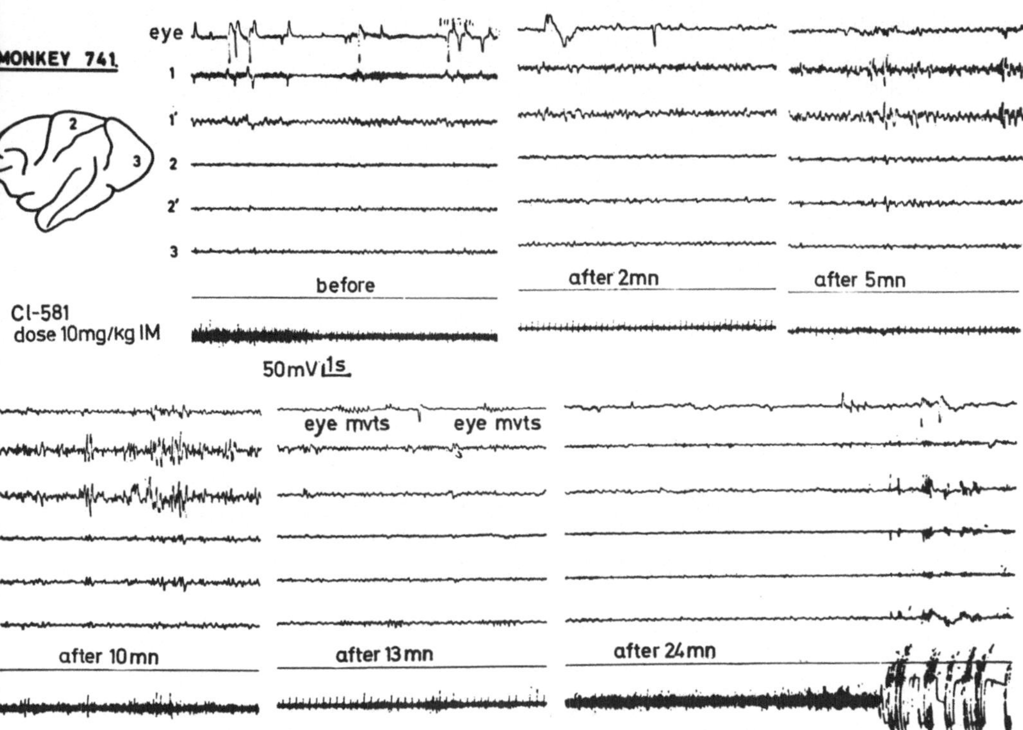

Fig. 13. Monopolar cortical recordings. 1 –2 – 3 – right hemisphere, 1' – 2' – 3' – left hemisphere. Increase of the fast rolandic activities. Rapid, interrupted ocular movements seen also in the paradoxical phase of the normal sleep

e) When the rolandic spikes appeared, the hypotonic phase was observed; preceeding or simultaneous with the apparition of the generalized spike discharges, the catatonic phase was noted (Fig. 14).

II. Cats

a) Animals in chronic preparation with electrodes implanted into the bone or in direct contact with the dura mater were used in this experimental series.

1. The EEG tracing showed only fast activity if the amount of drug used was less than 8 mg/kg i.m. With higher doses of 8–10 mg/kg, spikes and waves appeared.

2. Two minutes after the injection there was a visible muscular relaxation with the collapse of the animal if not held in position. This phenomenon

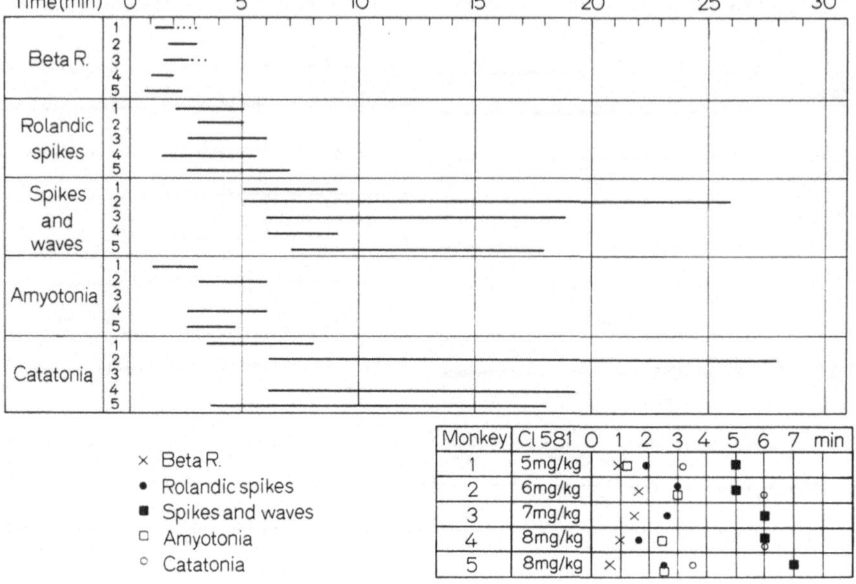

Monkey	Cl 581	0	1	2	3	4	5	6	7	min
1	5mg/kg		×□ ●		○		■			
2	6mg/kg		×	● □			■	○		
3	7mg/kg		×	●				■		
4	8mg/kg		× ●	□				■ ○		
5	8mg/kg	×		● □	○				■	

Fig. 14. Summary of 10, 11, 12, 13

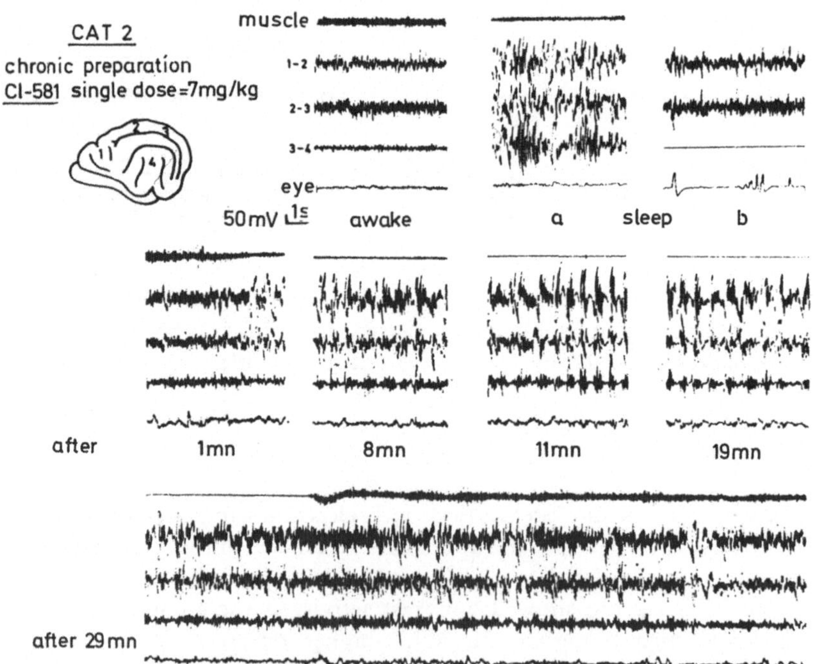

Fig. 15. Cortical bipolar recordings (cat). Above: Normal, awake animal and same animal during sleep (paradoxical phase of normal sleep). Below: After 1 min increase of fast rolandic activities. After 8 min apparition of spikes and waves (convulsive discharges). Remark: The fast activity persists after the anesthetic effect of CI-581 has worn off

was similar to what we had seen in the experiments in monkeys and was characterized by rolandic spike activities on the EEG tracing. The muscular tonus returned to normal when the anesthetic effect of the drug had worn off. The rolandic spikes disappeared simultaneously. However, the fast activity in some cases persisted a few minutes (4 to 20) after the cessation of the effect of the drug (Fig. 15).

b) In animals in acute preparation with electrodes implanted, the thalamus and mesencephalic reticular formation were studied.

1. The EEG tracings, concerning the fundamental cortical EEG activities, were the same in both acute and chronic preparations.

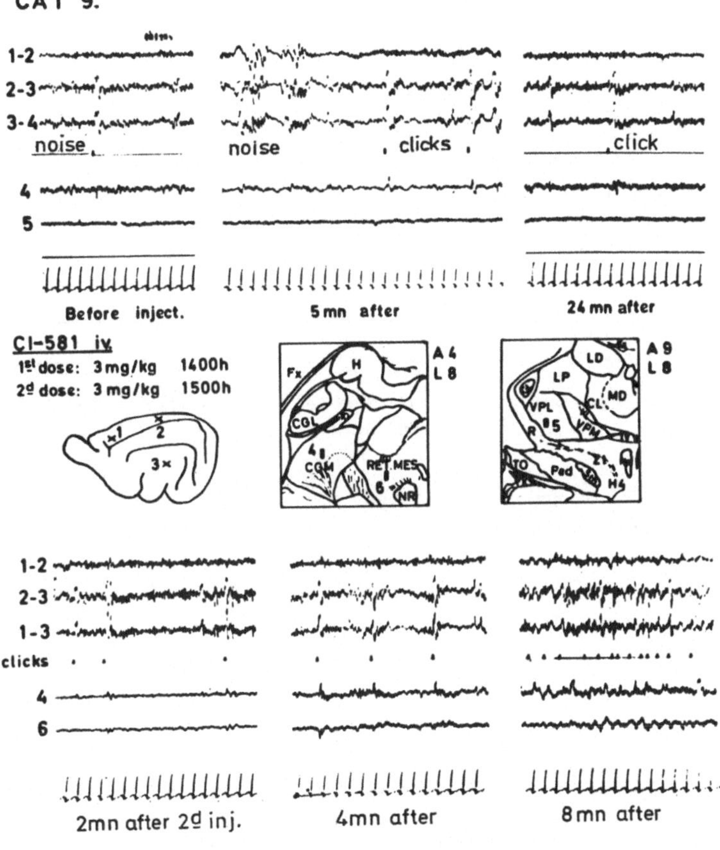

Fig. 16. Bipolar cortical and deep subcortical recordings. Increase of the voltage of the evoked potentials is evident in the accoustic cortex. Visual stimulation produced the same effect on the visual cortex. The increase of the voltage as a primary response is also present in the specific nuclei of the thalamus and with important doses in the mesencephalic reticular formation

2. In these experiments an increase in the voltage of the evoked potentials was evident in the accoustic cortex; if generalized spikes appeared, then these potentials were related in time with the noise heard in the room. The visual stimulation produced the same effect on the visual cortex.

The increase in the voltage, as a primary response, was present not only on the EEG tracing corresponding to the specific cortex but also in the specific nuclei of the thalamus and with important doses in the reticular formation. In our experiments, firing phenomenons could be elicited neither in the subcortical structures nor in the mesencephalic reticular formation. The CI-581 in doses between 5 and 9 mg/kg i.m. had no effect on the basic activity of the mesencephalic reticular formation, VPL, VL and CM, but did have an effect on the theta hypocampic rhythm (Fig. 16).

It was interesting to observe that in the acute cat preparations, in which Flaxedyl was used (although the first dose of the CI-581 was given after the effect of the Flaxedyl had worn off), only repeated doses of the drug could provoke generalized spike and wave discharges (Fig. 17).

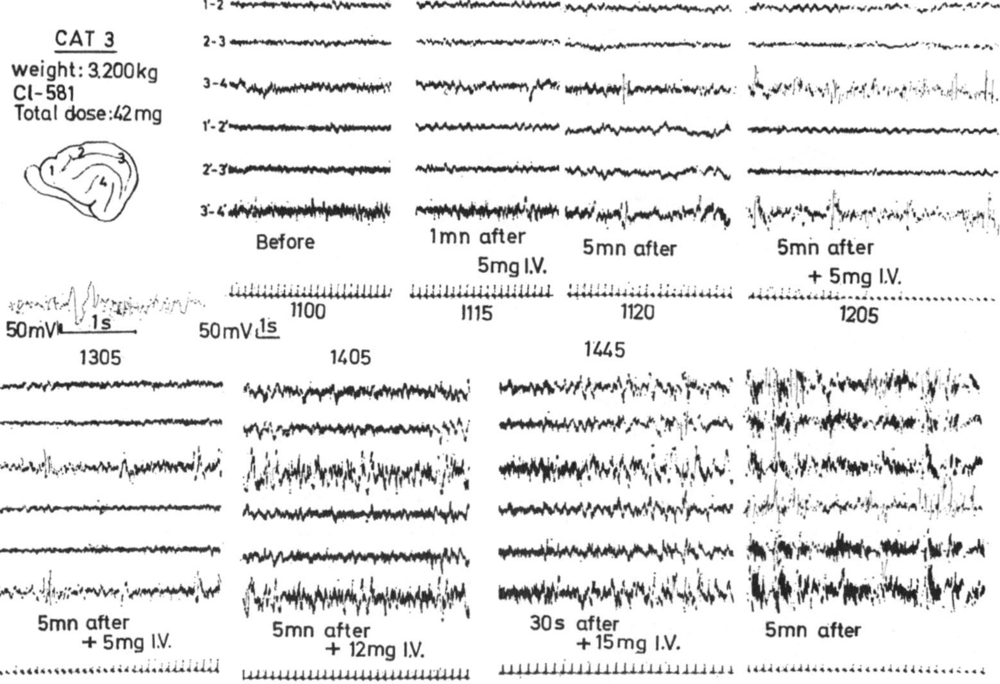

Fig. 17. Acute preparation (Flaxedyl used) bipolar cortical recordings. The interesting fact is that the convulsive activity appears only after large 42 mg. of total dose is injected

Effects on animals who had brain stem transections. The drug injected in doses from 3 to 5 mg/kg i.v. to cats with "encephale isolé" produced an increase in the cortical fast activities as well as an increase in the evoked potentials (Fig. 18 A and 18 B). In the same animals the cerebellar ablation did not modify the fast rhythms (Fig. 18 B); a section at the level of the mediopontine structures elicited slow bursts, but the fast activities also persisted (Fig. 18 C). If the transection was intercollicular, the EEG and ocular signs of slow sleep were obtained, but the fast activities of the neocortex were more difficult to observe (Fig. 18 D).

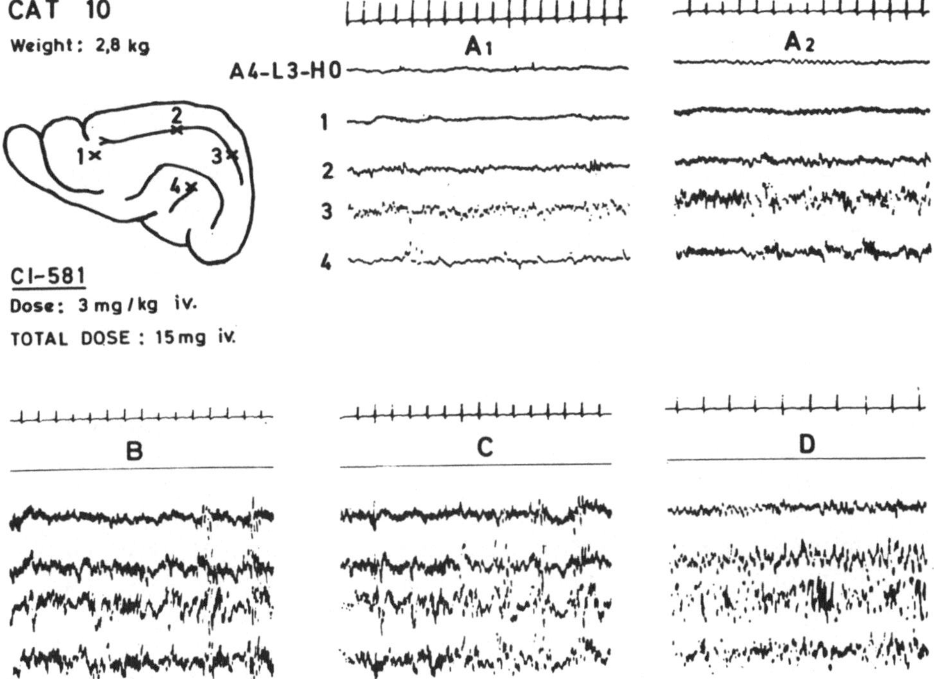

Fig. 18. (Brain stem transections). A-. Encephale isolé (increase of cortical fast activities and evoked potentials). A_2. Encephale isolé after 3 mg/kg i.v. injection C-581. B. After the ablation of the cerebellum (fast activities not modified). C. After mediopontin transection (slow bursts elicited but fast activity also persists). D. Cerveau isolé (intercollicular transection). The EEG and ocular signs of sleep (slow waves) seen, but the fast activities of the neocortex are more difficult to observe

Comments

These preliminary results incite more systematic experiments with the aim of studying the action of the CI-581, as recommended in M. BRAZIER's works (1963), on the three big neuronal systems: sensorial, non specific and limbic systems.

For the muscular effects, new experiments might determine the respective participation of the pheripheral and central system. Our studies permitted only confirmation of the central action of the drug. In effect, the modifications of the electro-cortical activities with the increase of fast rhythms were similar to the tracings seen when benzodiazepine was used. However, in certain animals (in cats with high doses or in baboon monkeys with anesthetic doses, known for their convulsive potentialities), contrary to the effect when, for example, Valium was injected, the CI-581 increased the muscular tonic activities and also elicited epileptic-like EEG discharges. In every case, in the first stage of the effect of the drug, slow rhythms associated with fast bursts did not appear, which one could see in the induction stage with Sodium Pentothal. With the exploration of the nucleus caudatum and anterior thalamus we could not see evidence of spindles and bursts, so characteristic during the hypnotic action of Sodium Pentothal.

The fact that the CI-581 might give spike and wawe activities only when the catatonic stage is reached is difficult to explain.

Perhaps we could suggest that the CI-581 decreases the convulsive threshold and provokes – in particular subjects – epileptic-like discharges seen only on the EEG tracing. These subjects would be more sensitive to this product than others and identical doses could produce a muscular hypertonic effect secondary to the liberation of the brain stem structures. This would appear when the cortex is in epileptic activity. However, our observations with the implanted electrodes were that the subcortical structures were not involved in the epileptic-like discharges. This finding is in perfect accord with NAQUET's and FISCHER WILLIAM's observations made during the spontaneous tonic – clonic seizures in the baboon monkeys (personal communications).

The primary central effect might only be a cortical effect; however, the intercollicular transections decreased the fast cortical activities which were always present after the retropontic transections. These findings are in favour of an action of the CI-581 at the level of the pontine structures.

Conclusion

The CI-581 is a drug with central action, appearing very rapidly after either i.v. or i.m. injections. This phenomenon is immediately characterized by a profound analgesia, but the electrocortical fast activities on the EEG tracings remain visible even after the effect of the drug has worn off. These findings can be explained with two different central sites of action of the drug:

1. The first impact is at the level of the caudal brain stem, including the bulbar and pontine structures (effect on the blood pressure, cardiac rhythm, ocular movements, dreams).

2. The other site of action could be the thalamo-cortical system (evidenced by the increase of the rolandic activity and the voltage of the evoked potentials).

The CI-581 has such wide, far reaching, multiple effects, most of which in humans, at least, are extremely desirable, that the interpretation and possible explanation of its action on the different but still related systems is almost impossible. The aim of this symposium is to present the accumulated factual research data and show not only the beneficial but also the undesirable side effects. We clinicians believe that raising doubts and creating controversy are the only ways to open up new territories in research and improve the qualities – by stimulating the minds of our highly esteemed pharmacologist colleagues – of this valuable new drug which, I hope, will stay in the armamentarium of the Anesthesiologist.

Summary

At this stage of our experiments it was possible to say that the administration of the CI-581:

1. Increased first the rolandic fast activities which, after a period of latency, became generalized.

2. Could evoke with important doses, but still within the accepted anesthetic dose range, in the cat and baboon monkey (with a possible epileptogenic potentiality, although screened for the experiments), spike and wave discharges.

3. Increased the voltage of the specific response to accoustic and visual stimulations.

4. Elicited rapidly obvious tonus modifications:

a) amyotonia, a few minutes after the injection, with concurrent increase in the rolandic activities;

b) in the monkeys 5 to 10 min following the injections and increase of the muscular tonus that often appeared when spikes and wawes were recorded on the EEG tracings.

Zusammenfassung

Vielseitige Untersuchungen verschiedener Parameter des kardiovasculären Systems und des zentralen Nervensystems wurden untersucht. Folgende Eigenschaften des Ketamine wurden hierbei festgestellt: Starker analgetischer Effekt mit stabilisierender Eigenschaft auf die gemessenen Parameter, deutliche Abnahme des Druckes im linken Ventrikel und in der Aorta, Ansteigen des Herzschlagvolumens, Zunahme des Herzvolumens, Abfall des peripheren Widerstandes, Abnahme der Coronardurchblutung, Zunahme des Sauerstoffverbrauchs in Verbindung mit der Vaso-Dilatation. Die Sauerstoffsättigung, der pH und der pCO_2 im arteriellen Blut veränderten sich nicht signifikant. Eine direkte Wirkung auf das Herz konnte nicht festgestellt werden. Die gleichzeitige Adrenalininfusion verursacht keine Herzrhythmusstörungen. Wiederholte Injektionen ansteigender Dosen im 10–15 min-Intervall führen zu einer Kumulation der Wirkung. Die Applikation von Dehydrobenzperidol nach Ketamine führt zu einer weiteren Verminderung des peripheren Widerstandes. Im EEG der Katze und bei Affen fanden sich Zeichen konvulsiver Aktivität bei Dosen von 6–10 mg/kg Ketamine.

Bibliography

Part 1

Cardiovascular system

1. BJARNESEN, W., and G. CORSSEN: CI-581: a new non-barbiturate short-acting anesthetic for surgery in burns. Mich. Med. **66**, 177 (1967).
2. BONIFACE, K. L., O. J. BRODIE, and R. P. WALTON: Resistance strain – gauge arches for direct measurement of heart contractile force in animals. Proc. Soc. exp. Biol. (N. Y.) **84**, 263–266 (1953).
3. BROWN, J. M.: Anesthesia and the contractile force of the heart. Anesth. Analg. Curr. Res. Nov.-Dec. 1960, vol. **39/6**, 487–498.
4. CHEN, G.: Evaluation of phencyclidine-type cataleptic activity. Arch. int. Pharmacodyn. **157**, 193 (1965).
5. —, et al.: The neuropharmacology of 2-(o-chlorophenyl)-2-methylamino-cyclohexanone hydrochloride. J. Pharmacol. exp. Ther. **152**, 332 (1966).
6. —, D. McCARTHY, and C. R. ENSOR: Studies on the cardiovascular effect of 2-(o-chlorophenyl)-2-methylamino-cyclohexanone. HCl (CI-581) in laboratory animals. Memo of January 12, 1966 to Dr. Bratton.
7. The effect of 2-o-chlorophenyl-2-methylamino-cyclohexanone. HCI (CI-581) on isolated heart. Memo of May 23, 1966 to Dr. Bratton.
8. CORSSEN, G., and E. F. DOMINO: Dissociative anesthesia: further pharmacologic studies and first clinical experience with the phencyclidine derivative CI-581. Anesth. Analg. **45**, 29 (1966).
9. — — Dissociative anesthesia: further pharmacologic studies and first clinical experience with the phencyclidine derivative CI-581. Anesth. Analg. **45**, 29 (1966).
10. DOMINO, E. F., et al.: Human pharmacology of CI-581, a new intravenous agent chemically related to phencyclidine. (Abstract 771) Fed. Proc. **24**, 268 (1965).
11. — — Pharmacologic effects of CI-581, a new dissociative anesthetic, in man. Clin. Pharmacol. Ther. **6**, 279 (1965).
12. KUAMP, D. H.: Preclinical toxicological studies on CL-369 (CI-581). Memo of December 10, 1963 to Dr. Bratton.

13. — N.D.A. toxicological studies on CL-369 (CI-581); Acute toxicity in dogs. Memo of January 5, 1965 to Dr. Bratton.
14. — Local tolerance studies on CI-581 following intraarterial injection in rats and dogs. Memo to Dr. Bratton, January 20, 1967.
15. KING, C. H., and C. R. STEPHEN: A new intravenous or intramuscular anesthetic. Anesthesiology **28**, 258 (1967).
16. KREUSCHER, H., and H. GAUCH: (The effect of phencyclidine derivative Ketamine (CI-581) on the human cardiovascular system.) (Ger) Anaesthesist **16**, 229 (1967).
17. McCARTHY, D. A., and G. M. CHEN: General anesthetic action of 2-(o-chlorophenyl)-2-methylaminocyclohexanone HCl (CI-581) in the rhesus monkey. (Abstract 769) Fed. Proc. **24**, 268 (1965).
18. —, et al.: General anesthetic and other pharmacological properties of 2-(o-chlorophenyl)-2-methylaminocyclohexanone HCl (CI-581). J. New Drugs **5**, 21 (1965).
19. —, G. CHEN, and C. R. ENSOR: Pharmacologic studies on CI-581. Memo of December 16, 1963 to Dr. Bratton.
20. McCARTHY, D.: Effect of CI-581 on epinephrine-induced cardiac arrhythmias in dogs anesthetized with methoxyflurane. Memo of May 31, 1966 to Dr. Bratton.
21. — Direct depressant effect of CI-581 on the myocardium as detected in the heart-lung preparation. Memo of May 31, 1966 to Dr. Bratton.
22. McLEAN, J. R.: CI-581 and heart norepinephrine. Memo of February 17, 1966 to Dr. Chen.
23. MORET, P. R., R. MEGEVAND, et M. GEMPERLE: Action de diverses amines vasoactives sur la fonction cardiaque normale et pathologique; choc cardiogénique principalement. 4é ass. ann. de la Soc. Suisse d'Angéïologie, Bâle. Bibl. Cardiol. (Basel) Vol **17**, 45–74 (1966).
24. RUSHMER, R. F.: Cardiovascular dynamics. Philadelphia: Saunders 1961.
25. VIRTUE, R. E. et al.: An anesthetic agent: 2-orthochlorophenyl-2-methylamino cyclohexanone HCl (CI-581). Anesthesiology **28**, 823 (1967).
26. WHEELOCK, R. H.: The effect of CI-581 (CL-369, AA-460) on experimental ventricular tachycardia in dogs. Memo of April 29, 1966 to Dr. Bratton.

Part 2

Central nervous system

1. BRAZIER, M. A. D.: Studies of evoked responses by flash in man and cat. Jasper, H. H., Proctor, L. D., Knighton, R. S., Noshay, W. C. and Costello, R. T.: Reticular formation of the brain. Boston: Brown and Co. 151–158, 1958.
2. BREMER, F.: „Cerveau isolé" et physiologie du sommeil. C. R. Soc. Biol. **118**, 1241–1242 (1935).
3. GAPTAUT, H., R. NAQUET, R. POIRE, and C. A. TASSINARI: Treatment of status epilepticus with diazepam (Valium). Epilepsia **6**, 167–182 (1965).
4. GREEN, J. D., and D. S. MAXWELL: Hippocampal electrical activity. 1. Morphological aspects. Electroenceph. clin. Neurophysiol. **13**, 837–846 (1961).
5. HERNANDEZ-PEON, R., J. A. ROJAS-RAMIREZ, J. J. D'FLAHERTY, and A. L. MAZZUCCHELLI-O'FLAHERTY: An experimental study of the anticonvulsive and relaxant actions of Valium. Int. J. Neuropharmacol. **3**, 405–412 (1964).

6. Jouvet, M.: Telencephalic and rhombencephalic sleep in the cat. The nature of the sleep. A Ciba Foundation symposium. London: Churchill, 188–208, 1961.
7. Killam, K. F., E. K. Killam, and R. Naquet: An animal model of light sensitive epilepsy. Electroenceph. clin. Neurophysio. **22**, 497–513 (1967).
8. Lanoir, J.: Etude neurophysiologique comparative de quatre drogues psychotropes. Thèse Marseille, 212, 1967.
9. —, R. Plas, et R. Naquet: Etude neurophysiologique comparée de trois drogues psychotropes. J. Physiol. (Paris) **55**, 281–282 (1963).
10. Naquet, R., K. F. Killam, J. Bimar, C. Gareyte, et M. Jutier: Analyse spectrale des activités électrographiques recueillies chez Papio papio (à paraître), 1967.
11. — —, E. K. Killam, J. Lanoir, et J. Engel: Cycle veille-sommeil de deux espèces animales placées dans des conditions expérimentales diverses. Rev. neurol. **115**, 443–483.
12. Passouant, P., et J. Cadilhac: Les rythmes thêta hippocampiques au cours du sommeil. Passouant, P.: Physiologie de l'hypocampe. Paris, C.N.R.S., 331–347, 1962.

Klinische Beobachtungen mit Ketamine unter besonderer Berücksichtigung von Kreislauf und Atmung

Von **F. Böhmert** und **W. F. Henschel**

Aus der Anaesthesie-Abtlg. der städt. Krankenanstalten Bremen (Direktor OMR. Dr. W. F. Henschel) und der Anaesthesie-Abtlg. des Zentralkrankenhauses Bremen „Links der Weser" (Direktor: OMR. Dr. F. Böhmert)

Bei der Erprobung neuer intravenöser Kurznarkotica interessiert neben der anaesthesiologischen Wirksamkeit in erster Linie deren Einfluß auf die wichtigsten Vitalfunktionen, insbesondere von Kreislauf und Atmung. Für eine oberflächliche Betrachtung der Kreislaufsituation gibt die einfache Messung des Blutdruckes und Kontrolle des Pulses bei einer größeren Zahl von Patienten einen gewissen Anhalt. So sahen auch wir analog zu anderen Untersuchern nach der Injektion von 1,5 mg CI-581 pro Kilogramm Körpergewicht bei einer Injektionsgeschwindigkeit von 15–20 sec eine Ascendenz des systolischen und auch des diastolischen Blutdruckes, sowie einen geringfügigen Anstieg des Pulses mit einem Maximalwert bei 2 bis 4 min. Erst im Laufe von 20 min gingen diese Werte wieder in die Nähe des Ausgangswertes zurück. Für eine lückenlose und exaktere Beurteilung der Kreislaufverhältnisse reichen diese Untersuchungen natürlich nicht aus.

Zur Erfassung zusätzlicher kreislaufdynamischer Größen führten wir bei 10 Patienten 2,5 und 20 min nach der Anaesthesie mit CI-581 physikalische Kreislaufanalysen mit der sphymographischen Methode unter Benutzung der Formeln von Broemser und Ranke während der Narkose mit CI-581 durch. Wir kamen dabei zu folgenden Ergebnissen (Abb. 1).

Der elastische Widerstand (E') stieg von 884 auf 1223 dyn/cm⁵ 2 min nach der Anaesthesie und betrug nach 20 min noch 1034 dyn/cm⁵. Der periphere Widerstand stieg von 600 auf 1575, nach 5 min auf 2012 dyn/ sec/cm⁵ um danach erst wieder langsam abzusinken. Das Schlagvolumen des Herzen (Vs) erfuhr eine geringe Steigerung nach 2 min, ging aber nach 5 min wieder auf den Ausgangswert zurück. Infolge der Pulsfrequenzerhöhung stieg das Herz-Minutenvolumen (Vm) nach 2 min um 75% und war nach 20 min noch 10% über dem Ausgangswert. Herzarbeit (HA) und Herzleistung (HL) waren dementsprechend erhöht. Der arterielle Mittel-druck stieg von 84,26 auf 106 mmHg und betrug nach 20 min noch 99,4 mmHg.

Unsere Untersuchungen stimmen danach mit denen von Kreuscher und Gauch weitgehend überein. Im Gegensatz zu ihnen haben wir jedoch einen Anstieg des peripheren Gesamtwiderstandes nach der Injektion von CI-581 gemessen. Jedenfalls dürfte aber die kardiovasculäre Wirkung von CI-581 der von Katecholaminen gleichen.

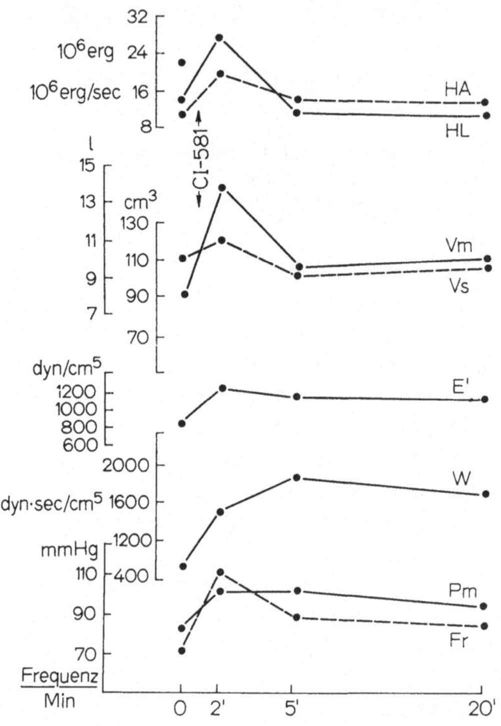

Abb. 1. Kreislaufanalysen nach Injektion von CI-581 (Mittelwerte von 10 Pat.)

Von gleichgroßer Bedeutung ist das Verhalten der Atmung. Bei oberflächlicher Betrachtung der Atemgrößen beobachteten wir ein Absinken der Atemfrequenz in den ersten Minuten nach der Injektion von CI-581. Eine genauere Aussage könnte allerdings erst dann gemacht werden, wenn die verschiedenen Ventilationsgrößen wie alveoläre Totraumventilation, Atemminutenvolumen usw. bestimmt werden. Von entscheidender Bedeutung dürfte jedoch die vergleichende Analyse der Blutgase sein. So haben wir auch bei 10 Patienten mit der Mikromethode nach Astrup 2, 5 und 20 min nach der Injektion von 1,5 mg CI-581 pro Kilogramm Körpergewicht pH, pCO_2 ,pO_2 und das Standardbicarbonat bestimmt. Die Ergebnisse erbrachten keine eklatanten Unterschiede (Abb. 2).

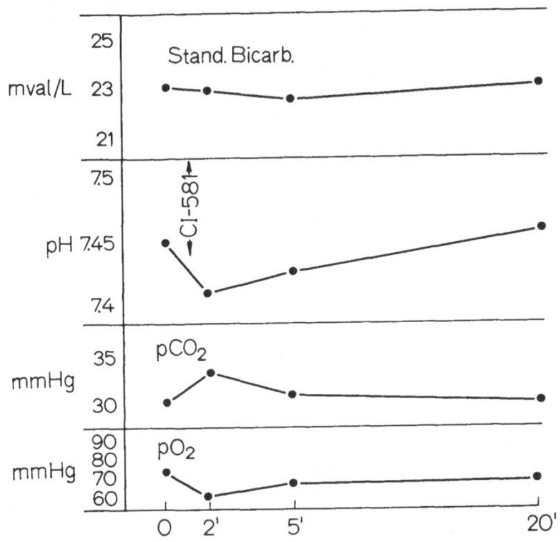

Abb. 2. Blutgasanalyse nach Injektion von CI-581 (Mittelwerte von 10 Pat.)

Bei der Betrachtung der Mittelwerte sehen wir, daß mit der Abnahme der Atemfrequenz auch die Blutgase eine geringfügige Änderung erfahren. Der Kohlensäuredruck stieg um 3 mmHg, während der Sauerstoffdruck um 13 mmHg abfiel. Das Standardbicarbonat blieb praktisch gleich. Entsprechend erfuhren die pH-Werte eine leichte Verschiebung zur sauren Seite hin. Schon nach 5 min näherten sich die Blutgase jedoch wieder den Ausgangswerten, um sich nach 20 min wieder zu normalisieren. An Hand dieser Untersuchungen können wir aussagen, daß 2 min nach der Injektion von CI-581 Atemveränderungen im Sinne einer respiratorischen Acidose auftreten, diese aber schon nach 5 min wieder zur Norm zurückkehren. Die respiratorische Acidose bewegt sich jedoch in Grenzen. Der Anstieg des Kohlensäuredruckes blieb bei allen unseren Patienten im Normbereich, so daß wir glauben sagen zu können, daß nach der Injektion von 1,5 mg CI-581 pro Kilogramm Körpergewicht keine nennenswerten pathologischen Atemstörungen zu erwarten sind.

Fassen wir unsere Untersuchungen über die Wirkung von CI-581 auf Kreislauf- und Atemfunktion des Menschen zusammen, so sind wir in Übereinstimmung mit KREUSCHER und LANGREHR. Die stimulierende Wirkung von CI-581 auf das kardiovasculäre System kann sich nur bei Hypertonikern und hyperthyreoten Patienten nachteilig auswirken, gereicht aber bei hypotoner Kreislaufsituation zum Vorteil. Die kaum ins Gewicht fallenden Atemstörungen – wenn man überhaupt von Störungen sprechen kann – stehen einer Anwendung von CI-581 nicht entgegen und dürften bei der entsprechenden Dosierung keine Gefahr bedeuten.

Auf Grund unserer klinischen Erfahrungen bei 150 Patienten haben wir die Indikation für eine Anaesthesie mit CI-581 weitgehend einschränken müssen. Positiv hervorzuheben ist die anaesthesiologische und analgetische Wirkung bei kurzdauernden Eingriffen. Bei einer großen Zahl unserer Patienten haben wir jedoch in der Aufwachphase zum Teil erhebliche Halluzinationen und verschiedenartige psychische Reaktionen beobachtet. Manche Patienten gaben diese Erlebnisse sogar erst nach einigen Tagen an, nachdem sie unmittelbar nach der Anaesthesie noch keine negativen Aussagen gemacht haben. Diese Beobachtungen haben wir praktisch bei allen Patienten im jugendlichen und mittleren Alter anstellen können. Ca. 80% dieser Patienten empfanden die Narkose als ausgesprochen unangenehm. Viele hatten sehr unangenehme Träume während der Anaesthesie und auch in der Aufwachphase. Ein ganz geringer Prozentsatz der Patienten betrachtete die Narkose wiederum als ein angenehmes Ereignis gegenüber anderen Anaesthesieformen, denen sie sich unterziehen mußten. Bei alten Menschen – ungefähr über 60 Jahre – traten die oben genannten Erscheinungen nur selten auf. Jedenfalls in so geringem Maße, daß eine weitere Anwendung als durchaus gerechtfertigt erscheint. Zumal die eingangs geschilderten positiven Eigenschaften seitens Kreislauf und Atmung gegenüber anderen Anaesthetica sichtliche Vorteile bringen. So haben wir bei sehr alten Patienten z. B. auch mittlere Eingriffe wie Appendektomien und Herniotomien bei inkarzerierten Hernien bis zu 45 min Operationsdauer mit CI-581 durchgeführt.

Auch bei diagnostischen Eingriffen, wie Bronchoskopien, Bronchographien, Oesophaguskopien o. a., haben wir CI-581 bei alten Patienten mit gutem Erfolg angewandt.

Nach unserer Meinung kann CI-581 bei richtiger Indikationsstellung durchaus im Bereich unserer anaesthesiologischen Möglichkeiten einen Platz finden.

Summary

We have considered the effect upon the circulatory and respiratory systems after a single injection of Ketamines by operations of short duration. We used 10 patients to make comparative circulatory analyses using the method of Broemser and Ranke. The result were identical with those obtained by Kreuscher. In accordance with other researchers we have also found a constant raise of systolic and diastolic blood pressures. The analyses of blood-gases, 2, 5 and 15 min after the injection of Ketamine showed no significant changes. The authors concluded that

Ketamines can be used by operations of short duration by children and by patients over sixty years of age and that they have showen certain advantages in comparison with other anaesthetics. One can stress here especially the stimulating effect on the cardiovascular system. By younger patients is the use of Ketamine not advisable because of the frequent observed halucinations during the waking period.

Diskussion

Zindler: Ich frage mich oft, ob die Untersuchungen mit der Methode von Boemser-Ranke überhaupt sinnvoll sind. Vielleicht kann uns Herr Kreuscher dazu etwas sagen, weil er parallel zu dieser Methode Farbstoffverdünnungskurven aufgezeichnet hat. Wenn so wichtige Untersuchungen, die für Indikation und Kontraindikation entscheidend sind wie peripherer Widerstand und elastischer Widerstand, völlig unterschiedlich ausfallen, dann scheint entweder das eine oder das andere nicht richtig zu sein.

Kreuscher: Die Kreislaufanalyse nach Broemser-Ranke hat den Nachteil, daß sie eine rein kalkulative Methode ist, mit der man auf indirekte Weise auf bestimmte nicht direkt gemessene Kreislaufparameter schließt. Die Methode hat den großen Vorteil, daß man kontinuierlich messen und somit jede Phase des zu prüfenden Zeitablaufes erfassen kann. Wir haben aus diesem Grunde versucht, die physikalische Kreislaufanalyse mit der Farbstoffverdünnungsmethode zu untermauern, und wie Sie gesehen haben, konnte man doch eine weitgehende Übereinstimmung finden, jedenfalls in der Tendenz der ermittelten Werte. Die Absolutwerte, und das sollte man vielleicht hervorheben, können unterschiedlich sein. Bezüglich des peripheren Widerstandes würde ich sagen, daß man – soweit er nach der kalkulativen Methode von Broemser-Ranke errechnet wurde – vorsichtig sein sollte. Etwas verläßlicher ist vielleicht der auf diese Weise errechnete elastische Widerstand.

Zindler: Ich glaube, daß diese Frage sehr wichtig ist in bezug auf die Erarbeitung eventueller Kontraindikationen bei kreislaufinsuffizienten Patienten.

I would like to ask Dr. Szappanyos to this question. You have some remarkable findings e. g. a considerable decrease of the total peripheral resistance. On the other hand you said, there is a decreased cardiac work, if I saw it correctly. But your oxygen consumption increased at the same time. And one other question is: Did you use a wall straingauge?

Szappanyos: Yes, we did use a straingauge.

Zindler: Could you say just a few words about this matter? Did you use it in congested heart failure, or do you think this is too dangerous?

Szappanyos: Most of the patients had some cardiac problems with that poore risk, and we have not seen any effect to it, if we use it in small doses.

Zindler: You saw a decreased cardiac work but an increased oxygen consumption, is that possible?

Szappanyos: Well, decreased cardiac work is an ordinary response to an increased peripheral resistance, but the consumption of oygen goes up, which is due to a dilation and increased cardiac output due to the increased venous return.

Zindler: Does the heart work more or less - you said both? –

Szappanyos: Yes. Our findings are different in closed chest and open chest patients.

Zindler: Well, you saw in open chest bradycardia and in closed chest increase of the pulse rate.

Langrehr: Wenn man den Kreislauf untersucht, muß man die Befunde bei Katzen, Hunden und Menschen unterschiedlich beurteilen. Katzen und Hunde haben ein Blutdruckverhalten, das sich immer von dem des Menschen unterscheidet. Diese Tiere haben bei den Experimenten entweder Schwankungen oder Abfälle des Druckes. Dieses Phänomen haben wir beim Menschen nie gesehen. Er reagiert nicht mit Schwankungen sondern mit einem steten Blutdruckanstieg und niemals mit einem initialen Druckabfall. Offensichtlich reagiert der Kreislauf von Hund und Katze anders. Vielleicht könnte das eine Erklärung dafür sein, daß wir unterschiedliche periphere Resistenzen finden. Soweit ich es jetzt übersehe, haben wir doch beim Menschen immer einen Anstieg des gesamtperipheren Widerstandes beobachtet. Lediglich Herr KREUSCHER hatte einen leichten Abfall beobachtet.

Kugler: Wir müssen doch auch beim Menschen die verschiedenen Phasen beobachten! Auf den Bildern von Herrn SZAPPANYOS sahen wir, daß er während der ersten 3 min nach der Injektion mißt, Herr KREUSCHER mißt 5 min nach der Injektion und Herr HENSCHEL 2,5 und 20 min nach der Injektion. Dazwischen kann doch viel passieren. Wenn Sie nun erklären, daß es in der Zwischenzeit Schwankungen gibt, die nicht erfaßt wurden, wurde doch der Broemser-Ranke nicht kontinuierlich registriert sondern in Intervallen.

Frau **Podlesch:** Ich möchte noch etwas zum Blutdruckverhalten des Menschen sagen. Herr LANGREHR, Sie haben auch nur einen Wert angegeben, der nach 1 min gemessen wurde. Wenn man aber innerhalb der ersten Minute mißt, hat man einen leichten Blutdruckabfall.

Langrehr: Ich muß einräumen, daß ähnliche Beobachtungen 40 sec nach Beendigung der Injektion gemacht wurden. Die Möglichkeit besteht also, daß innerhalb der ersten Minute Druckabfälle eintreten können. Unsere erste Messung war in der Regel 60 sec nach Beendigung der Injektion, weil wir die Kreislaufzeit von 20–30 sec berücksichtigen wollten. Und von diesem Zeitpunkt ab fanden wir bei unseren Messungen, die wir in relativ kurzen Minutenabständen durchführten, keinen Druckabfall, sondern einen kontinuierlichen Anstieg.

Soehring: Ich glaube, es gibt nicht nur Unterschiede zwischen den genannten Versuchstieren und dem Menschen sondern auch Unterschiede in der Methodik. Bei Versuchstieren wird im allgemeinen kontinuierlich gemessen. Ein großer Teil der klinisch durchgeführten Untersuchungen erfolgte aber diskontinuierlich oder, wie man heute in idealer Weise sagt „digital". Wenn ich diesen Einwand hier mache, dann deshalb, weil Sie die aus dem Tierexperiment bekannten Wellen (wie sie von MEYER und HERING im vorigen Jahrhundert schon beschrieben wurden) unter diesen Bedingungen nicht immer reproduzieren können.

Nun zur Frage der Broemser-Ranke-Methode: Diese Methode hat einen kardinalen Fehler, nämlich den, daß sie Konstanzen zeigt, die keine sind. Wenn man sich klar macht, daß das System der elastischen Fasern und der glatten Muskulatur eine Adaptation im Elastizitätsmodul kontinuierlich auch Belastungen verursachen kann, ist es völlig unmöglich, solche Faktoren einzusetzen, die nicht stimmen. Ich bin daher auch der Meinung, daß die hier gemessenen Werte zumindest sehr kritisch zu betrachten sind.

Corssen: Ich möchte Ihnen anhand der Befunde, die wir bei einem Gefangenen durch kontinuierliche Messungen gewonnen haben zeigen, daß sowohl der systolisch wie auch der diastolische arterielle Blutdruck kontinuierlich ansteigt. Nach Gabe von 1 mg/kg CI-581 steigt der Druck sofort an. Kein initialer Blutdruckabfall, wie ihn offenbar andere Autoren gesehen haben. Wir haben bei über 20 Gefangenen kontinuierlich arterielle Blutdruckanalysen durchgeführt und haben bei keinem einen Abfall des systolischen oder diastolischen Druckes gesehen. Wie auch Herr LANGREHR feststellte, sahen wir einen stetigen Druckanstieg bis ungefähr 10 min und anschließend einen allmählichen Abfall. Wenn man auf dem Höhepunkt des arteriellen Druckanstieges eine 2. Injektion verabfolgt, sehen wir allerdings nur in wenigen Fällen einen weiteren Druckanstieg. Im allgemeinen wird ein Plateau erreicht.

Zindler: Wenn Sie zu einem späteren Zeitpunkt injizieren, wird wahrscheinlich wieder ein Druckanstieg vorhanden sein?

Corssen: Ja!

Zindler: Wichtig ist auch der Hinweis von Herrn SZAPPANYOS auf die Injektionsgeschwindigkeit. Bei schneller Injektion erreichen wir mit einem hohen Blutspiegel auch erhebliche Veränderungen. Haben Sie nun schnell oder langsam injiziert?

Corssen: Wir haben 30 sec injiziert.

Elektroencephalographische Untersuchungen bei Ketamine und Methohexital

Von **J. Kugler, A. Doenicke, M. Laub und H. Kleinert***

Aus der Neurophysiologischen Abteilung (Leiter: Priv.-Doz. Dr. J. Kugler) der Nervenklinik (Kom. Direktor: Prof. Dr. M. Kaess) und der anaesthesiologischen Abteilung (Leiter: Priv.-Doz. Dr. A. Doenicke) der Chirurgischen Poliklinik der Universität München (Direktor: Prof. Dr. F. Holle)

In den letzten Jahren haben mehrere Autoren barbituratfreie Narkosemittel zu Kurznarkosen vorgeschlagen, darunter auch Cyclohexaminderivate (Corssen 1965, Scholler et al. 1960). Die guten Erfahrungen bei Narkosen an Kindern mit diesen Präparaten führten zu der Frage, ob das zuletzt synthetisierte CI-581 auch zu Kurznarkosen bei Erwachsenen geeignet sei. Wir haben uns der experimentellen Prüfung des Präparates an gesunden, freiwilligen Versuchspersonen gewidmet, um die üblichen Nebenwirkungen der Stressfaktoren vor, während und nach Operationen zu umgehen, um die unverfälschte Wirkung des verabreichten Pharmakons untersuchen zu können. Dazu bedienten wir uns klinischer, neurologischer und neurophysiologischer bzw. elektroencephalographischer Kontrollmethoden.

Methode

CI-581 und Methohexital wurden zu Narkosen an 12 gesunden Versuchspersonen im Alter von 22 bis 30 Jahren intravenös verabreicht. Bei 6 Personen wurde zuerst die Methohexital-Narkose und 14 Tage später die CI-581-Narkose durchgeführt, bei 6 Personen erfolgte zuerst die CI-581- und danach die Methohexital-Narkose. Die Dosis von 2 mg/kg des CI-581 wurde im allgemeinen in $1^1/_2$ min und die des Methohexital binnen 30 sec injiziert. Außer Atropin wurde keine Prämedikation gegeben.

10 min vor der Injektion wurde die EEG-Ableitung begonnen und nach CI-581 bis zur 120. min, nach Methohexital bis zur 60. min nach der Injektion fortgesetzt; weiter wurde 4, 6 und 8 Std nach der CI-581-Injektion und 2, 4, 6 und 8 Std nach der Methohexital-Injektion das EEG jeweils durch 30 min registriert.

---

* Mit Unterstützung der Deutschen Forschungsgemeinschaft.

Tabelle 1. *Die Narkose- und Schlafstadien, modifiziert nach* Loomis

Schlafstadien							
Stadienbezeichnung						EEG-Muster	
Gibbs	K. Dement, französ. Autoren	Loomis	Verhalten Wachheit	A_0	Roth	führendes Kennzeichen Normvariante	Reaktion Lidschlußeffekt
very slight sleep	I	A	Ermüdung	A_1		α diffus	Lidschlußeffekt
				A_2	1	α spärlich	
			Nullstadium	B_0	2a	flache ϑ	fehlt
		B	Einschlafen	B_1	2b	σ klein	
				B_2	2c	σ hoch	Vertex-Wellen
light sleep	II	C	leichter Schlaf	C_0		hohe ϑ, 30 % t	
				C_1	3	hohe ϑ, 50 % t	K-Komplex
				C_2		hohe ϑ, 80 % t	
moderately deep sleep	III	D	mittlerer Schlaf	D_0		δ, 30 % t	breite K-Kompl.
				D_1	4	δ, 50 % t	
				D_2		δ, 80 % t	δ-Aktivität
very deep sleep	IV	E	tiefer Schlaf	E	5	δ kontinuierlich	fehlt
early morning sleep	V		Periode der Augenbewegungen	PAB		A_1–B_2	fehlt (B^0) oder
	I/REM = rapid eye movements					Augenbewegungen	Vertex-Wellen

Die bipolare Ableitung des EEG erfolgte auf 8 Kanälen eines Hellige-Neuro-skript von paramedian angeordneten Elektrodenreihen. Die Papiergeschwindig-keit betrug 7,5 mm/sec. Zusätzlich wurden das EKG, das Okulogramm und ein Mechanogramm registriert. Anhand des EEG wurde in 40-sec-Perioden die Narkose- oder Schlaftiefe visuell geschätzt und in einer graphischen Übersicht dargestellt.

Die Bestimmung der Narkose- und Schlafstadien erfolgte gemäß einer Modifikation der Einteilung von Loomis (Tab. 1).

Ergebnisse

Sowohl während wie auch nach der Narkose zeigte der Ablauf des EEG Unterschiede zwischen CI-581 und Methohexital.

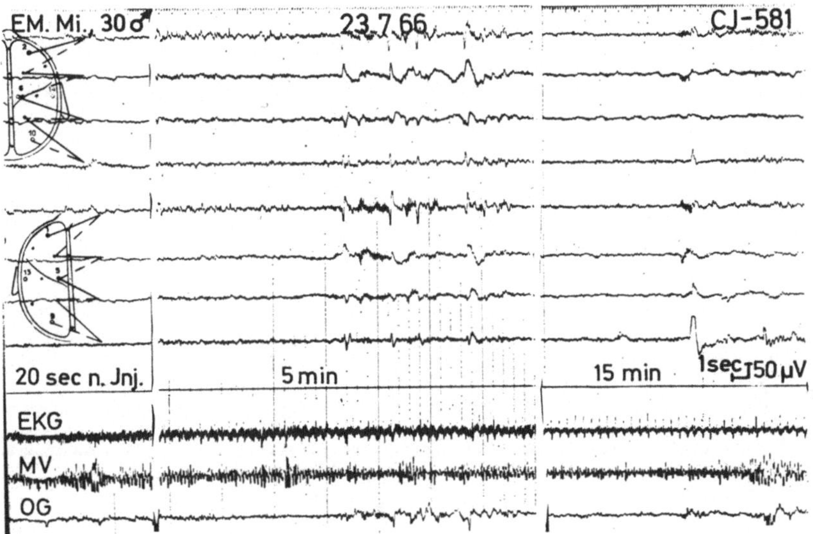

Abb. 1. EEG, EKG, Mikrovibrationen (MV) und Okulogramm (OG) in den ersten Minuten nach der Injektion von 2 mg/kg Körpergewicht CI-581 bei einer gesunden Versuchsperson (Em. Mi., 30 Jahre). Das EEG zeigt in der 5. min das Vorherrschen einer etwa 30 Mikrovolt hohen 5–7/sec Theta-Aktivität (Papier-geschwindigkeit 7,5 mm/sec). Dazu gesellen sich bei dieser Versuchsperson in der 5. min vorübergehend bilateral-synchrone, steile, langsame Wellen

CI-581 führte zum Auftreten einer mittelhohen Theta-Aktivität (Abb. 1). Bei allen unseren Versuchspersonen wurde mit Beginn in der 2. bis 5. min eine Serie von rhythmischen, bilateral-synchronen Komplexen aus langsamen und steilen Wellen sichtbar. Bei einem von den 12 Unter-suchten war diese Serie von Komplexen verhältnismäßig kurz, bei den anderen dauerten sie in der Regel 3½ min (Abb. 2). Rhythmik und Form

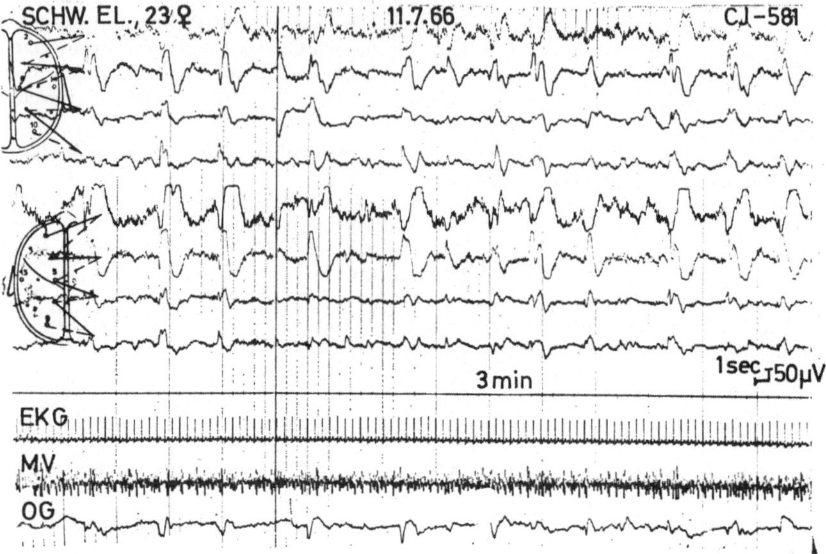

Abb. 2. Im EEG das Auftreten annähernd rhythmischer, steiler und langsamer Wellen in der 3. min nach Beginn der Injektion von CI-581 bei einer gesunden Versuchsperson (Schw. El., 23 Jahre)

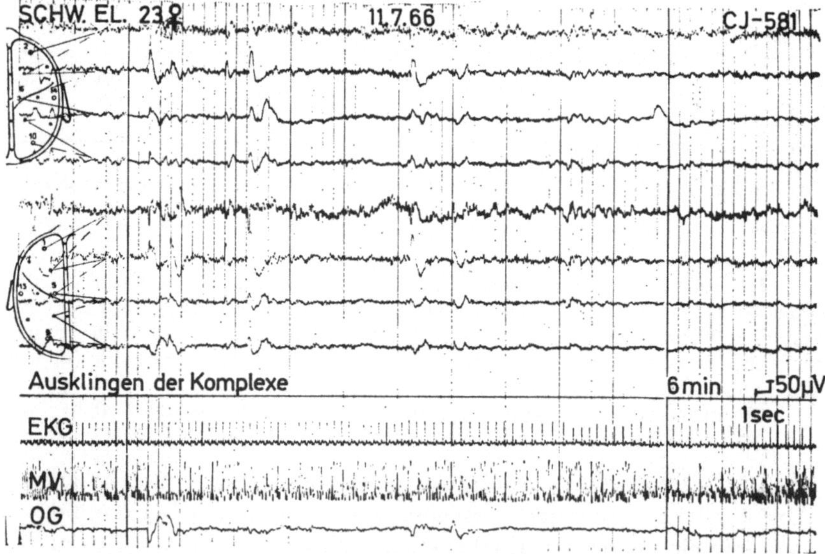

Abb. 3. Im EEG das Ausklingen der Serie von steilen und langsamen Wellen in der 6. min nach Beginn der Injektion von CI-581 bei einer gesunden Versuchsperson (Schw. El., 23 Jahre)

dieser Komplexe erinnern an die EEG-Veränderungen, wie man sie bei akuten, toxischen Encephalosen beobachten kann. Zwischen den Komplexen
und nach ihrem Ausklingen dominiert in der Hintergrundtätigkeit unverändert mittelhohe Theta-Tätigkeit (Abb. 3). Nach den ersten Spontanbewegungen oder Weckreaktionen, die im Mittel in der 15. min eintraten, wurde
die Theta-Tätigkeit niedrig. In der 25. min änderte sich meist das psychische
Verhalten der Versuchspersonen und ihre Kurven wurden allgemein flach,
jedoch weiterhin bis zur 60. min durch Serien von Theta-Wellen unterbrochen. Anschließend wurde bis zur 90. min nach der Injektion das Ausgangsverhalten mit Blockade der occipitalen Alpha-Tätigkeit bei psycho-
sensoriellen Reizen wieder hergestellt (Abb. 4). Im weiteren Verlauf bis zur
9. Std ergab sich keine Abweichung vom normalen Kurvenverlauf.

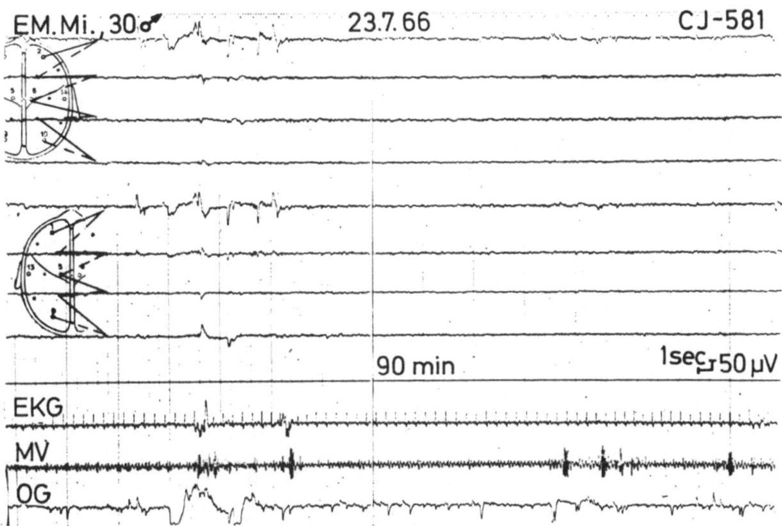

Abb. 4. Im EEG 90 min nach der Injektion von CI-581 Angleich der Aktivität
an das Ausgangsverhalten mit kleiner 9–11/sec-Aktivität bei einer gesunden
Versuchsperson (Em. Mi., 30 Jahre). Im Okulogramm Nystagmus

Verglichen damit zeigte sich nach Methohexital nach der 30. sec das
Eintreten von rascher und in der 45. sec das Eintreten von hoher, langsamer
Aktivität (Abb. 5). Die langsame Tätigkeit klang nach wenigen Minuten
wieder aus, doch konnte bis zur 20. min kleine, rasche Aktivität oder weit
streuende Alpha-Aktivität bestehen bleiben (Abb. 6). In den späteren
Kontrollen kam es bisweilen zum Auftreten von Nachschlafstadien (Abb. 7),
wie wir sie bereits in früheren Untersuchungen nach Thiobarbituraten und
N-methylierten Barbituraten beschrieben haben.

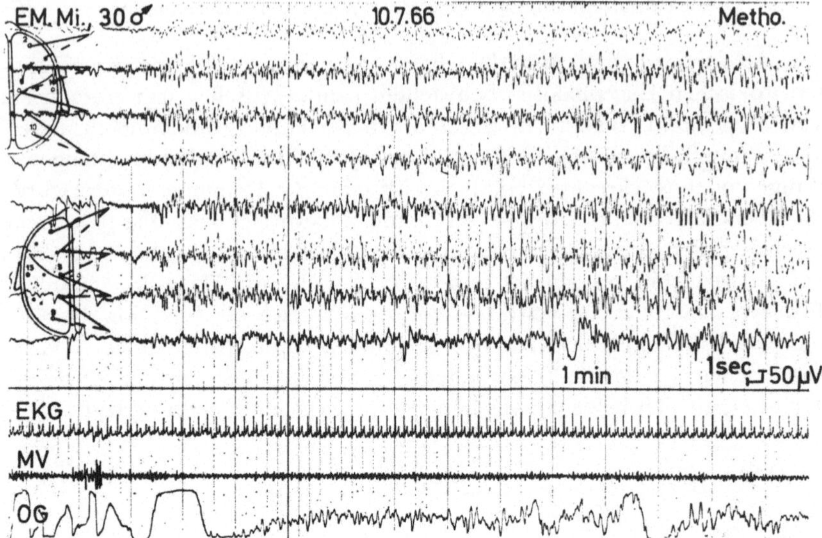

Abb. 5. Im EEG 30 sec nach Beginn der Injektion von 2 mg/kg Körpergewicht Methohexital bei einer gesunden Versuchsperson (Em. Mi., 30 Jahre). Rascher Übergang in hohe, langsame und überlagernde, raschere Aktivität

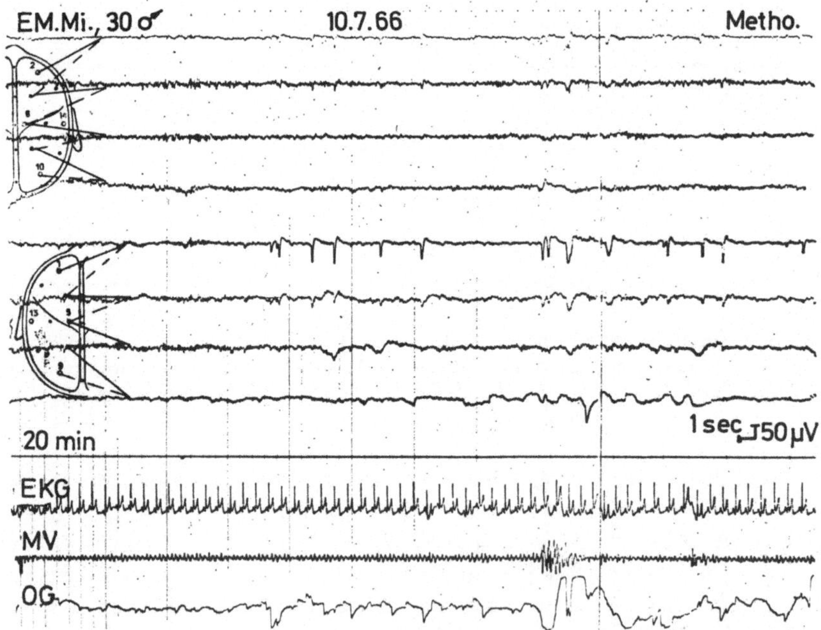

Abb. 6. Im EEG 20 min nach Methohexital-Injektion bei einer gesunden Versuchsperson (Em. Mi., 30 Jahre) diffuse, rasche Aktivität

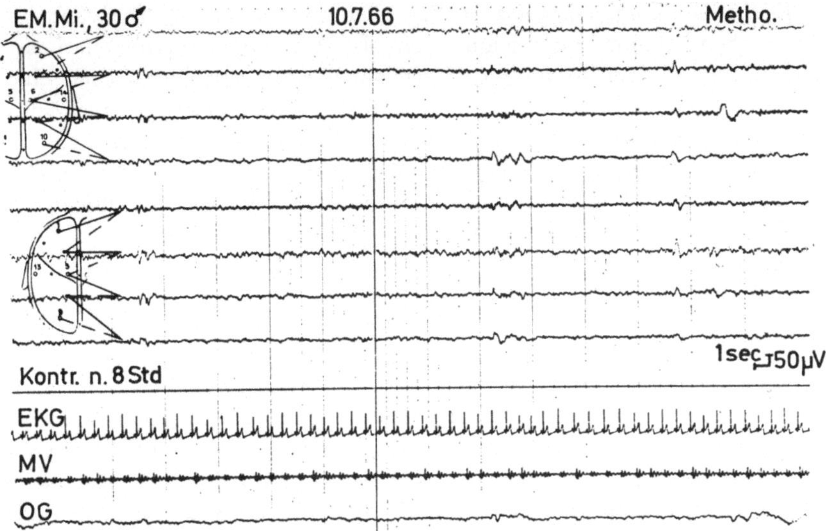

Abb. 7. Im EEG 8 Std nach Methohexital-Injektion neuerliches Auftreten von diffuser, langsamer Aktivität mit Vertexwellen und kleinen Sigmaspindeln, entsprechend leichten bis mittleren Schlafstadien

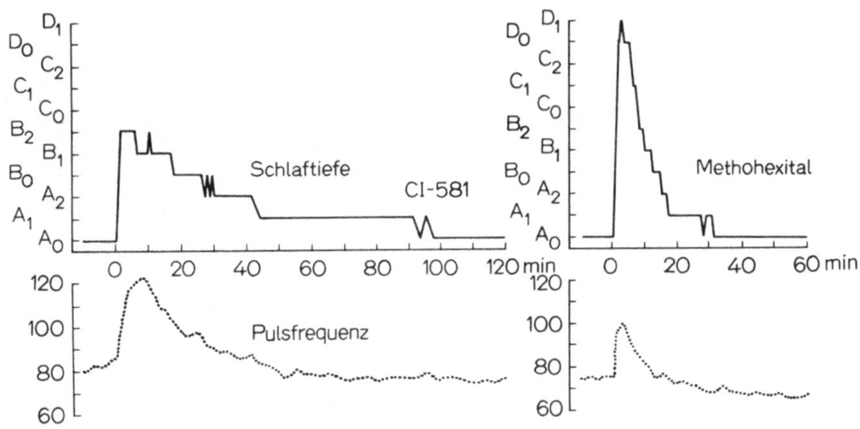

Abb. 8. Ablauf der Narkose- und Schlafstadien (obere Kurve) und der Pulsfrequenzänderungen (untere Kurve) nach CI-581 (linker Bildteil) und Methohexital (rechter Bildteil). Länger anhaltende Schläfrigkeit nach CI-581 als nach Methohexital, dabei jedoch geringere Schlaftiefe. Nach CI-581 stärkere initiale Tachycardie als nach Methohexital, im weiteren Verlauf Absinken der Pulsfrequenz unter das Ausgangsverhalten nach beiden Injektionen

Die Ablaufsfolge der aus allen Befunden gemittelten elektroencephalographischen Schlafneigung zeigte nach CI-581 das Fehlen tiefer Narkosestadien, wie sie nach Methohexital erreicht wurden und nach CI-581 eine länger anhaltende Wirkung als nach Methohexital (Abb. 8). Das mitregistrierte EKG erlaubte eine übersichtliche Darstellung des zeitlichen und qualitativen Verhaltens der Herzfrequenz. Etwa 6 Std nach der CI-581-Injektion kam es ebenso wie nach Methohexital zu neuerlichem, flüchtigen Auftreten von Schläfrigkeitsstadien.

Diskussion

Unsere Beobachtungen zeigen übereinstimmend mit Virtue u. Mitarb. als ungewöhnliches Kennzeichen der CI-581-Wirkung eine kontinuierliche, monomorphe, langanhaltende, mittelhohe Theta-Aktivität über der gesamten Konvexität. Diese Aktivitätsform ist nicht in die Schemata der bekannten Narkoseverläufe einzuordnen, zeigt erhebliche Unterschiede gegenüber den Barbiturateffekten und ist in ähnlicher Weise ansonsten nur bei Dehydrobenzpyridol bekannt.

Bei annähernd gleicher Dosis scheint die Injektionsgeschwindigkeit die Ursache für Unterschiede im Ablauf der EEG-Aktivität gegenüber den Befunden von Virtue zu sein: Virtue hat bei keiner seiner 7 gesunden Versuchspersonen eine Ablaufsfolge rhythmischer Komplexe beschrieben, wie wir sie bei allen 12 Versuchspersonen feststellen konnten. Dagegen hat Virtue bei 15 sec Injektionsdauer in einem Fall kurze Perioden sehr flacher, unregelmäßiger Aktivität zwischen hohen Gruppen von langsamen Wellen gefunden, die den tiefen Stadien von flüchtigen, exogenen Intoxikationen entsprechen, wogegen wir ein solches Ereignis nicht feststellten.

Die Gruppen rhythmischer Komplexe zeigen sehr starke Ähnlichkeit mit den von Scholler u. Mitarb. bereits bei den anderen Phencyclidin-Derivaten in geringerem Ausmaß beobachteten Veränderungen. Sie scheinen somit auf der Wirkung der allen Derivaten gemeinsamen Grundsubstanz zu beruhen, in ihrem Ausmaß neben den bereits angegebenen Unterschieden von Dosis und Injektionsgeschwindigkeit von der unterschiedlichen Struktur der Derivate abzuhängen.

Die traumhaften Erlebnisse, die bei allen 12 Versuchspersonen vorkamen, sind in die Beobachtungen über die psychoexperimentellen Untersuchungsergebnisse von Doenicke u. Mitarb. einbezogen.

Summary

Ketamine (2 mg/kg) was given intravenously in 12 healthy volunteers. The injection time was 1.5 min. For comparison methohexitone-anaesthesia was given to each volunteer at another day. In the EEG medium voltage theta waves occur until 60 min after application of Ketamine. This activity is untypical and not agreeable to a known schema.

Between 2 and 5 min after injection the EEG showed rhythmic bilateral-synchroneous complexes of slow and sharp waves. These changes are similar to those in acute toxic encephalosis.

Literatur

CORSSEN, G.: Pharmakologische und erste klinische Erfahrungen mit dem Kurz-narkotikum CI-581. Tagg. Europ. Anaesthesieges. Zürich 1965.

DOENICKE, A., J. KUGLER, and M. LAUB: Evaluation of Recovery and "Street Fitness,, by EEG and Psychogiagnostic Tests after Anaesthesia. Canad. Anaesth. Soc. J. **14**, 567–583 (1967).

KUGLER, J.: Elektroenzephalographie in Klinik und Praxis. Stuttgart: Georg Thieme-Verlag 1966, 2. Auflage.

SCHOLLER, K. L., H. THIES, u. K. WIEMERS: Die Allgemeinanästhesie mit Cyclohexylaminderivaten, klinische und elektroenzephalographische Unter-suchungen. Anaesthesist **9/5**, 163–168 (1960).

VIRTUE, R. W., J. M. ALANIS, M. MORI, R. T. LAFARGUE, J. H. K. VOGEL, and D. R. METCALF: An Anesthetic Agent: 2-Orthochlorophenyl, 2-Methyl-amino Cyclohexanone HCl (CI-581). Anesthesiology **28**, 823–833 (1967).

Diskussion

Wiemers: Ich möchte als Ergänzung zu den Befunden von Herrn KUGLER noch einige Untersuchungsergebnisse zeigen, die wir bei Anwendung der bereits bekannten Präparate CI-400 (Sernyl) und des Präparates CI-421 erhielten und bereits 1960 in der Zeitschrift „Der Anaesthesist" publizierten. Diese Präparate waren damals noch von niemand anderem klinisch erprobt worden. Ich weiß auch nicht, ob sich später noch jemand damit befaßt hat. Im Prinzip haben wir damals ganz ähnliche Veränderungen gefunden wie jetzt mit Ketamine. Wir haben damals bei je 25 Patienten Elektroencephalogramme bei Anwendung von CI-400 und CI-421 aufgezeichnet und fanden dabei zum Teil kontinuierliche Verlangsamungen der Frequenz und überwiegend von Zwischenwellen. Teilweise war aber, abweichend davon, eine ausgesprochene Gruppenbildung zu sehen. Steile Abläufe mit langsamen Nachschwankungen, die in rhythmischen, regelmäßig auftretenden Gruppen zu sehen waren. Vorwiegend bei jüngeren Patienten fanden wir eine auffallende Beta-Aktivierung, die teilweise zu ganzen Gruppen zu Beta-Krampfspitzen führten. Diese Erscheinung wurde bisher bei Ketamine nicht beschrieben. Wir konnten außerdem sehen, daß diese Veränderungen mit steilen Abläufen und enormen Amplitudenvergrößerungen durch die Injektion von 50 mg Thiopental unterdrückt werden können. Es handelt sich also um Veränderungen, die durch Barbiturat zu beeinflussen sind.

Szappanyos: I want to express my opinion about the observations concerning "spikes and waves" complexes: For me, they are not "spikes and waves", that are complexes of sharp and slow waves as you can find in certain forms of pathologic conditions. And therefore I am against the term "epilectic condition"! It is only a peculiar form of discharge in the brain which has nothing to do with an epileptic seizure. I am not a specialist in EEG but we have never seen in our material epileptic convulsions.

Zindler: Ich glaube, das sind Diskussionen für Spezialisten, die sie untereinander austragen sollten. Es wurde von 1000 Patienten berichtet, von denen 4 richtige epileptische Anfälle gehabt hätten. Was würden Sie da empfehlen, Barbiturate oder Valium?

Corssen: CI-581!

Wir hatten 2 Fälle von „epileptic seizure" im Zusammenhang mit unseren pneumo-encephalographischen Studien bei 96 Patienten. 2 Patienten kamen bereits mit Krampfanfällen in den Röntgenraum. Ein Säugling hatte bereits seit 3 Wochen, d. h. schon in utero, Epilepsie, bis es dann zur pneumoencephalographischen Untersuchung kam. Das andere war ein 4 oder 5 Jahre altes Kind. In beiden Fällen, d. h. in einem nach einer intramuskulären Injektion von 5 mg/Pfund im anderen Fall nach einer intravenösen Injektion von 1 mg/Pfund hörten die epileptischen Anfälle auf. Sie begannen 20 min nach der intramuskulären Injektion und 8 min nach der intravenösen Applikation von CI-581. Ich möchte aber doch noch die Ausführungen von Herrn Kugler bestätigen. Ich finde, daß der Ausdruck „epileptic spikes" tatsächlich unangebracht ist. Ich weiß auch nicht, ob Sie wirklich einen elektroencephalographischen Experten zur Interpretation Ihrer Kurven hinzugezogen haben. Wir haben das getan und haben von unserem Experten gelernt, daß es sich um spikes-ähnliche Veränderungen handelt.

Szappanyos: We asked Professor Naquet from Marseille, who is well known and he said: they are epileptic forms of spikes.

Vergleichende Untersuchungen über die Analgesie bei Kurznarkosen mit Ketamine, Thiopental und Propanidid

Von **H. Nolte, H. Teuteberg, J. Dudeck, W. Münchhoff** und **K. Rumpf**

Aus den Instituten für Anaesthesiologie der Universität Mainz (Direktor: Prof. Dr. R. FREY) und des Zweckverbandes Stadt- und Kreiskrankenhaus Minden (Chefarzt: Priv.-Doz. Dr. H. NOLTE), dem Institut für Medizinische Dokumentation und Statistik (Direktor: Prof. Dr. S. KOLLER) und der Universitäts-Nervenklinik (Kom. Direktor: Prof. Dr. K. H. SCHIFFER) der Universität Mainz

Unter den ersten Berichten über klinische Erfahrungen mit Ketamine fanden sich bei einigen Autoren [1, 2, 6, 9] Hinweise auf die ausgezeichneten analgetischen Eigenschaften dieses Mittels sowohl bei intravenöser als auch bei intramuskulärer Anwendung. Zur Prüfung dieser Angaben haben wir versucht, vergleichbare Aussagen über die Dauer der Analgesie nach klinisch gebräuchlichen Dosen von Ketamine, Thiopental und Propanidid zu machen, sowie eine Beziehung zwischen der Analgesie und Ansprechbarkeit des Probanden zu finden.

Die Dosis der intravenös applizierten Narkotica betrug für Ketamine 2 mg, für Thiopental 4 mg und für Propanidid 7 mg pro Kilogramm Körpergewicht bei einer Injektionsdauer von 1 min.

Methode

Die Versuchsanordnung war so gewählt, daß die 3 zu untersuchenden Substanzen jeder Versuchsperson injiziert wurden. Bei einer derartigen Versuchsanordnung ist zu erwarten, daß die Ergebnisse von der Reihenfolge der Applikation beeinflußt werden.

Der Versuchsplan wurde deshalb so aufgebaut, daß an je 9 männlichen und 9 weiblichen Versuchspersonen alle 6 möglichen Permutationen der Reihenfolge der Medikamente in gleicher Häufigkeit und innerhalb der Geschlechter jedes Medikament mit gleicher Häufigkeit an 1., 2. und 3. Stelle getestet wurden (Tab. 1).

Tabelle 1. *Versuchsanordnung der vergleichenden Untersuchung über die Analgesie bei Anaesthesien mit Ketamine, Thiopental und Propanidid*

Nummer des Versuchs	Männliche Versuchspersonen Reihenfolge d. Präparate			Nummer des Versuchs	Weibliche Versuchspersonen Reihenfolge d. Präparate		
1	C	B	A	2	C	A	B
3	B	A	C	4	A	B	C
5	A	C	B	6	A	C	B
7	B	C	A	8	B	A	C
9	C	A	B	10	B	C	A
11	A	B	C	12	C	B	A
13	C	A	B	14	C	B	A
15	B	C	A	16	A	C	B
17	A	B	C	18	B	A	C

A = Propanidid   7 mg/kg KG,
B = Thiopental   4 mg/kg KG,
C = Ketamine   2 mg/kg KG,

Die Auswertung erfolgte nach einem partiell-hierarchischen Modell einer mehrfachen Varianzanalyse mit den 3 Faktoren Geschlecht, Versuchsperson und Medikamente. Außerdem wurden für alle Parameter der Mittelwert und die einfache Standardabweichung berechnet.

Der Versuchsablauf war standardisiert. Die Ansprechbarkeit wurde durch Anruf des Probanden und die Analgesie durch Schmerzstimulation mit einem Federdruckalgesiemeter bei gleichbleibender Reizstärke am Oberschenkel getestet.

Anruf und Schmerzstimulation wurden nach dem Ende der Injektion des jeweiligen Medikamentes in Abständen von 1 min regelmäßig wiederholt. Zur Überwachung wurde das EKG, die Pulsfrequenz und der Blutdruck laufend registriert (Abb. 1).

Nach dem Wiedereintreten von Bewußtsein und Schmerzempfinden wurde eine Befragung der Probanden nach evtl. Traumerlebnissen angeschlossen, über die noch an anderer Stelle berichtet werden wird.

Ergebnisse

Die mittlere Dauer bis zum Auftreten von Abwehrbewegungen und bis zur vollen Schmerzreaktion war bei Ketamine am längsten. Sie betrug 13,3 bzw. 15 min. Bei Thiopental und Propanidid dauerte es 2,7 bzw. 3,7 min bis zur ersten Schmerzreaktion und 3,94 bzw. 4,72 min bis zur vollen Schmerzempfindung. Eine gesicherte Geschlechterdifferenz bestand nicht.

Die volle Ansprechbarkeit kehrte bei Ketamine nach 9,7, bei Thiopental nach 3,1 und bei Propanidid nach 3,2 min zurück (Tab. 2 u. Abb. 2).

Ketamine hat in der hier angewandten Dosierung eine eindeutig längere Wirkung auf den Verlust von Schmerzempfindung und Bewußtsein. Besonders auffallend ist der Zeitunterschied zwischen der Rückkehr von

Bewußtsein und Schmerzempfindung. Nach Wiederkehr der vollen Ansprechbarkeit dauerte die Analgesie im Mittel für Ketamine noch 5,3, für Thiopental und Propanidid jedoch nur noch 0,84 bzw. 1,52 min an. Diese Zeitunterschiede sind statistisch signifikant.

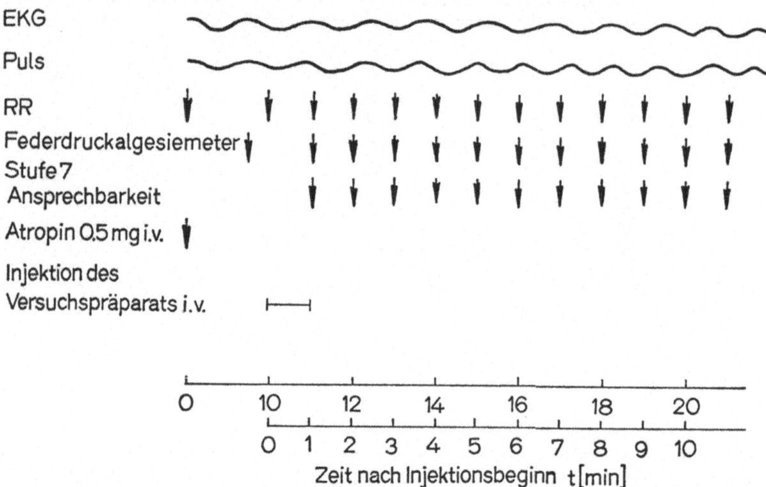

Abb. 1. Versuchsablauf der vergleichenden Untersuchung über die Analgesie bei Anaesthesien mit Ketamine, Thiopental und Propanidid

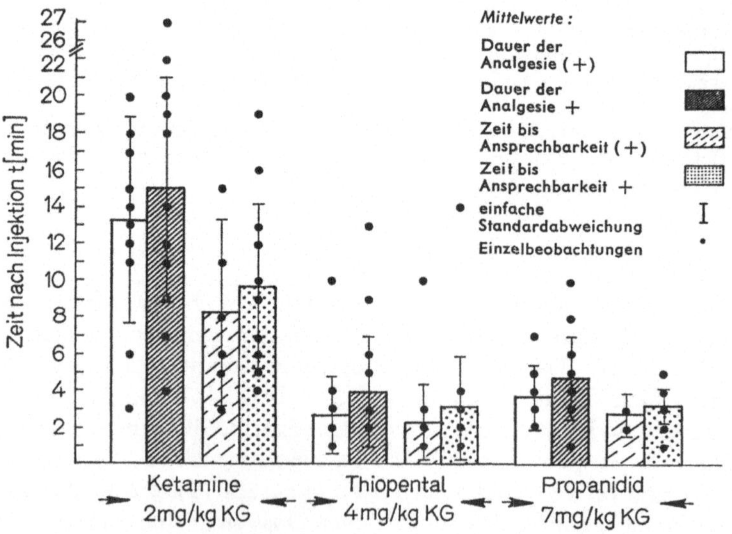

Abb. 2. Analgesiedauer und Länge des Bewußtseinsverlustes bei Anaesthesien mit Ketamine, Thiopental und Propanidid

Tabelle 2. *Dauer in Minuten bis zum Wiederauftreten von Schmerzempfindung und Bewußtsein bei Anaesthesien mit Ketamine, Thiopental und Propanidid*

Wiederauftreten von:	Ketamine Mittelwert	Maximalwert Minimalwert	SD	Thiopental Mittelwert	Maximalwert Minimalwert	SD	Propanidid Mittelwert	Maximalwert Minimalwert	SD
Schmerzempfindung (+)	13,30	$\frac{20}{3}$	±5,60	2,70	$\frac{10}{7}$	±2,11	3,70	$\frac{7}{2}$	±1,75
Schmerzempfindung +	15,00	$\frac{27}{7}$	±6,06	3,94	$\frac{13}{1}$	±3,04	4,72	$\frac{10}{1}$	±2,24
Bewußtsein (+)	8,33	$\frac{15}{3}$	±5,05	2,28	$\frac{10}{1}$	±2,08	2,72	$\frac{3}{1}$	±1,13
Bewußtsein +	9,70	$\frac{19}{4}$	±4,46	3,10	$\frac{14}{1}$	±2,84	3,20	$\frac{5}{1}$	±0,92

8*

Zusammenfassung

Es läßt sich aussagen, daß die früher berichteten Beobachtungen über analgetische Eigenschaften des Ketamine zu Recht bestehen. Die Dauer der Analgesie übertrifft die Dauer des Bewußtseinsverlustes bei intravenöser Anwendung des Präparates deutlich. Unter Berücksichtigung der hier verwendeten Dosierung der 3 untersuchten intravenösen Anaesthetica ist das Ketamine dem Thiopental und Propanidid besonders in bezug auf die analgetischen Eigenschaften deutlich überlegen.

Summary

The good analgesic properties of Ketamine as reported in the literature can be confirmed by this study. The duration of analgesia is much longer than the duration of unconsciousness with the intravenous administration of the drug. With respect to the dosage of the three intravenous anaesthetics used in this study Ketamine has much better analgesic properties than Thiopentone and Propanidid.

Literatur

1. Corssen, G., and E. F. Domino: Anesth. Analg. 45, 29 (1966).
2. — Münch. Med. Woch. 26, 1428 (1967).
3. —, and W. J. Bjarnesen: Amer. Ass. Nurse Anesthetists 34, 416 (1966).
4. Chodoff, P., and J. G. Stella: Anesth. Analg. 45, 527 (1966).
5. Dobkin, A. B., and J. P. Su: Clin. Pharmacol. Ther. 7, 648 (1966).
6. King, C. H., and C. R. Stephen: Anesthesiology 28, 258 (1967).
7. Kreuscher, H., u. H. Gauch: Anaesthesist 16, 229 (1967).
8. Stöker, L.: Dtsch. zahnärztl. Z. 21, 1241 (1966).
9. Virtue, R. W., J. M. Alanis, M. Moti, R. T. Lafargue, J. H. K. Vogel u. D. R. Metcalf: Anesthesiology 28, 823 (1967).

Use of Ketamine as Monoanesthetic in Clinical Anesthesia, Acid-Base Status and Oxygenation

By **G. Rolly**

University of Ghent, Akademisch-Ziekenhuis, Gent

I. Clinical experience

CI-581* was used in a 1% solution for intravenous injection and in a 5% solution for intramuscular injection. Due to the semi experimental nature of the drug, only patients in good or fair physical condition were scheduled for this anesthesia. In order to evaluate the drug as completely as possible, only interventions in which CI-581 could be used as mono-anesthetic were anticipated.

A total of 150 patients, 96 males and 54 females, were anesthetized with CI-581. Age, physical condition, site of intervention and duration of intervention are shown in Tables 1, 2, 3 and 4. The premedication consisted of atropine alone, or combined with pethidine (Dolantine) and promethazine (Phenergan), all given according to weight and condition of the patient (Table 5). The other patients were not premedicated at all.

Table 1. *Age and sex distribution*

Total number of patients	<5 Y.	5–15 Y.	15–65 Y.	>65 Y.	♂	♀
150	35	26	84	5	96	54

Table 2. *General physical condition and weight*

Total number of patients	General physical condition				Weight Mean 45,01 kg
	good	sufficient	moderate	bad	
150	102	27	14	7	(4,09–98 kg)

* CI-581 was generously supplied by Parke, Davis and Co. (Belgium).

Table 3. *Type of surgical intervention*

1. Endoscopic and radiological examinations   12
2. Eye surgery   21
3. Neurosurgical interventions (Holter-drainage)   9
4. O. R. L. surgery   4
5. Plastic surgery   49
6. Orthopedic and traumatologic surgery   7
7. Minor general surgery   48

Table 4. *Duration of surgical interventions (n = 150)*

minutes:	≤5	6–15	16–30	31–60	61–90	>90	Mean
n:	15	36	39	27	18	15	39,37 (1–160)

Table 5. *Premedication*

Type	Number of patients	Sedation satisfactory	unsatisfactory
Atropine	16	Not applicable for sedation	
Atropine Dolantin	71	63	8
Atropine Dolantin Phenergan	11	10	1
Dolantin	2	1	1

Of 150 patients, 18 received CI-581 in a 1 to 2 mg/kg dose by i.v. injection; 132 patients had the drug in a 3 to 7 mg/kg dose by i.m. injection. Several patients received a second or a third dose, in order to prolong or to deepen anesthesia and analgesia (Table 6). In 27 cases local anesthesia was routinely performed as prophylaxis against bleeding, to immobilize the eye, or for other purposes. In 9 cases CI-581 had to be supplemented by general anesthesia to have good operating conditions.

Table 6. *Number of CI-581 injections (n = 150)*

1 dose			2 doses			3 doses		
i.v.	i.m.	total	i.v.	i.m.	total	i.v.	i.m.	total
10	80	90	4	43	47	4	9	13

With i.v. administration of CI-581 the onset of operability after the start of injection was 90 sec; with i.m. injection it was 281 sec (Table 7). The rapid action of this drug given by i.m. route, was one of the reasons to prefer this last way of administration. An interesting phenomenon is noticed in Table 7. The mean interval between the first injection and operability was longer in the group of patients receiving 2 or 3 injections. A second and a third injection were only given when necessary. One could consider, if this difference in the interval to operability does not express a lesser degree of sensibility to CI-581 anesthesia in these patients.

Table 7. *Duration until onset of operability after the first injection*

Administration	Number of injections	Number of patients	Seconds until onset of operability
i.v. (n = 18)	1	10	70,5 (30–180)
	2	4	73,7 (60–95)
	3	4	157,5 (120–240)
		mean:	90,0 (30–240)
i.m. (n = 132)	1	80	261,7 (60–1020)
	2	43	313,7 (120–600)
	3	9	300,0 (120–600)
		mean:	281,3 (60–1020)

In evaluating the further results of our study, a distinction must be made between patients receiving CI-581 alone, or with local anesthesia, and those receiving additional general anesthesia. The first and second group are combined for evaluating our data. The duration of analgesia in 86 patients was 72 min; the time-interval between injection and reaccessibility or complete reorientation was 79 and 107 min respectively (Table 8).

The systolic bloodpressure during CI-581 anesthesia shows a maximum rise of 10 to 25% of the initial value in 43% of all patients, and of 25 to 50% in 30% of the patients. Only in 9% of all cases no raise or sometimes a decrease was noticed (Fig. 1). The rise of the bloodpressure is age dependent, as its frequency is lesser in the age group between 6 and 15 years, and even more decreased below the age of 6 years (Fig. 2). The rise of the maximum systolic bloodpressure is more marked after i.v. injection, than after i.m. administration. Diastolic bloodpressure and pulse frequency follow the same pattern (Fig. 1).

Table 8. *Range and mean of duration of analgesia, until reaccessibility and until complete reorientation*

Number of injections	Number of patients	Duration of analgesia (min)		Duration until reaccessibility (min)	
		Range	Mean	Range	Mean
1	48	2–270	60,81	6–165	61,27
2	34	5–200	81,71	16–190	94,91
3	4	75–160	123,00	105–200	154,25
Total	86	2–270	71,96	6–200	78,89

Number of injections	Duration until compl. reorientation (min)	
	Range	Mean
1	8–315	90,37
2	28–250	121,41
3	132–220	191,00
Total	8–315	107,31

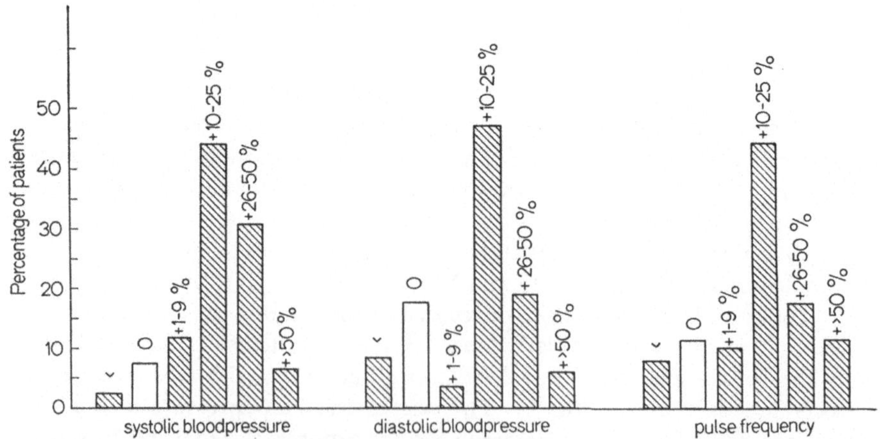

Fig. 1. General pattern of systolic and diastolic bloodpressure and pulse frequency

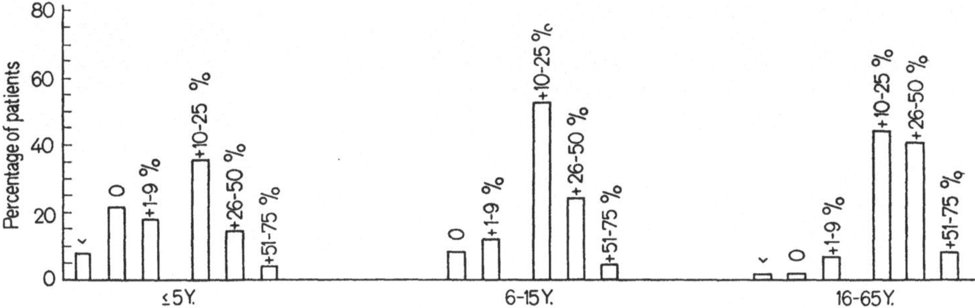

Fig. 2. Systolic bloodpressure according to age of patients

The respiratory frequency and the respiratory pattern are not markedly influenced (Table 9). More sensitive examinations were done in some patients, and these results are reported below.

Table 9. *Mean of respiratory frequency*

Number of patients	Preinjection	Maximum during anesthesia	Minimum during anesthesia
150	21,5 (12–60)	25,2 (12–80)	18,3 (3–42)

CI-581 seems to be a poor agent for muscular relaxation, as only in 25% of all cases relaxation existed. Analgesia was very good or suffient in 90% and too small in 10% of all cases. This last figure is high, but somewhat incorrect due to our search to minimize to the extreme the dosage of the drug.

Local tolerance of the drug was very good. Seven patients, all adults and receiving CI-581 as monoanesthetic, were excited and constituted a problem for postanesthetic management. 35 patients reported dreaming, which was pleasant in 14 cases and rather unpleasant or alarming in 18 cases. General side effects were mild or moderate (blurred vision, unvoluntary movements vomiting or nausea). Severe vomiting occured 6 times.

II. Measurements

1. Method. 10 patients were completely evaluated for acid-base balance and oxygenation. Intermediate lasting ophtalmologic interventions (retinal coagulation) were choosen. A plastic indwelling needle was introduced percutaneously in the radial artery before induction of anesthesia, and permitted intermittant sampling of arterial blood.

PH, Paco$_2$, standard bicarbonate and base excess were determined with the micro Astrup method, using the Siggaard Andersen nomogram. PaO$_2$ was determined with the PO$_2$ microelectrode of Radiometer. All determinations were done at a temperature of 37,5°C. As the temperature of the patients was always during the whole experiment 37 $\pm$ 0,75°C, no correction was made for temperature.

PA O$_2$ was calculated by the alveolar air formula:

$$PAO_2 = PIO_2 - \frac{PACO_2}{R} + PACO_2 \cdot \frac{1-R}{R} \cdot FI\,O_2$$

Paco$_2$ was substituted for PACO$_2$:

$$PAO_2 = PIO_2 - \frac{PaCO_2}{R} + PaCO_2 \cdot \frac{1-R}{R} \cdot FI\,O_2$$

A respiratory quotient (R) of 0,8 was assumed. The alveolar-arterial Po$_2$ difference (AaDo$_2$) was calculated (PAO$_2$ − PaO$_2$).

The blood oxygen saturation (SaO$_2$) was calculated, using the values of PaO$_2$, pH, Base Excess, according to the slide rule of SEVERINGHAUS (SEVERINGHAUS 1965).

2. Results. 10 patients were evaluated for acid-base status and oxygenation after i.m. administration of ketamine. It was possible to have 7 patients with complete and comparative values at different moments of time:

a) before anesthesia;
b) 1–15 min after injection;
c) 16–30 min after injection;
d) 31–60 min after injection;
e) 61–90 min after injection (Table 10).

The mean values are shown in Table 11. Paco$_2$ was rising from 40,5 mmHg to 45 mmHg. PH decreased from 7,37 to 7,33. The metabolic fraction of acid-base balance, evaluated by standard bicarbonate and base excess, was unchanged. The extremely light acidosis was entirely due to the slight respiratory depression.

As oxygenation is concerned, immediately after injection a fall of Pa$_{O2}$ is noticed, with a gradual retablishment. The bloodsaturation reflects the same variation. The Aa$_{DO2}$ is increasing as Pa$_{O2}$ falls and is decreasing when Pa$_{O2}$ increased.

The depression of respiration is generally very moderate (Figs. 3–5). Only on 2 occasions Paco$_2$ values higher than 50 mmHg were noticed among 56 determinations (Fig. 6). Occasionally an important desaturation is unexpectedly present just after injection without marked influence on Pa$_{CO2}$ (Fig. 7). Another time the desaturation was combined with a respiratory depression in the course of anesthesia (Fig. 8).

Table 10. *Values of* PaO_2, SaO_2, $PaCO_2$, pH, *standard bicarbonate and base excess of 7 patients*

Case nr.	a) before injection						b) 1–15 min after injection						16–30 min after injection					
	PaO_2	SaO_2 %	$PaCO_2$	pH	St.Bic.	B. E.	PaO_2	SaO_2 %	$PaCO_2$	PH	St.Bic.	B. E.	$PaCO_2$	SaO_2 %	$PaCO_2$	pH	St.Bic.	B. E.
86	58	89	33	7,37	19,5	−5,2	59	89	33	7,38	20	−5	63	90	41	7,33	20,5	−4
52	78	95,5	40	7,39	23,5	−0,5	36	66	44	7,36	23,5	−0,5	67	92	46	7,35	23,5	−0,5
47	72	94	36	7,38	21,5	−3	67	93	36	7,38	21,5	−3	66	93	35	7,38	21	−3,5
43	84	96	46	7,36	24	0	68	91,5	55	7,31	24	0	80	95,5	54	7,38	25	+1
38	84	96	46	7,36	24	0	84	96	43	7,38	24	0	82	96	43	7,37	23	−1
96	99	97	42	7,36	22,5	−2	99	97,5	42,5	7,32	21	−4	85	95,5	42,5	7,32	21	−4
130	80	96	41	7,39	24	0	56	87	47	7,33	25,5	0,5	63	90	43	7,33	21,5	−3

Case nr.	31–60 min after injection						61–90 min after injection					
	PaO_2	SaO_2 %	$PaCO_2$	pH	St.Bic.	B. E.	PaO_2	SaO_2 %	$PaCO_2$	pH	St.Bic.	B. E.
86	68	92	38	7,34	20	−5	73	94	38	7,35	20,5	−4
52	68	93	46	7,35	23,5	−0,5	69	93	44	7,36	23,5	−0,5
47	69	93	42	7,34	21,5	−3	69	93	42	7,34	21,5	−3
43	80	95	55	7,33	25	+1,5	80	95	55	7,33	25	+1,5
38	82	95,5	46	7,35	23	−1	83	95,5	50	7,33	23	−0,5
96	83	95,5	41,5	7,34	21,5	−3	90	96	42,5	7,32	21	−4
130	68	92	44	7,32	21,5	−3	77	95	44	7,32	21,5	−3

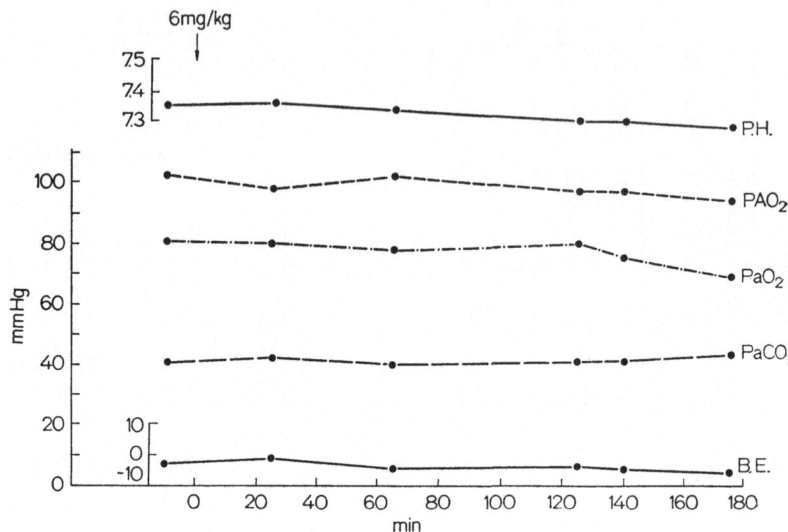

Fig. 3

Premedication: 75 mg Dolosal   Case Nr. 99   45 Y.
               0,5 mg Atropine   78 kg

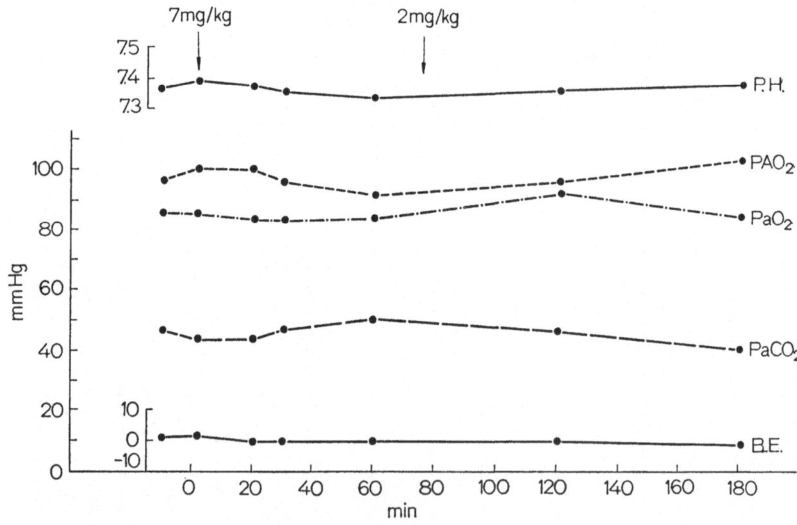

Fig. 4

Premedication: 75 mg Dolosal   Case Nr. 38   22 Y.
               0,5 mg Atropine   69 kg
               25 mg Phenergan

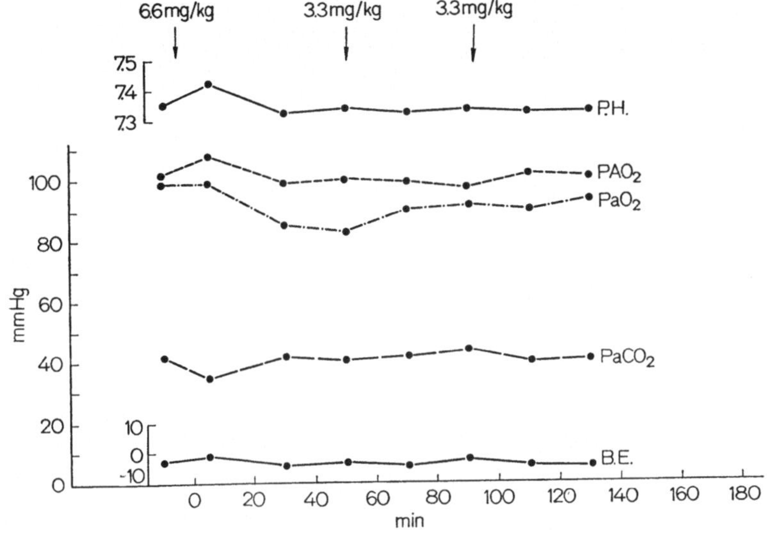

Fig. 5

Premedication: 75 mg Dolosal   Case Nr. 96   60 Y.
                0,5 Atropine   60 kg

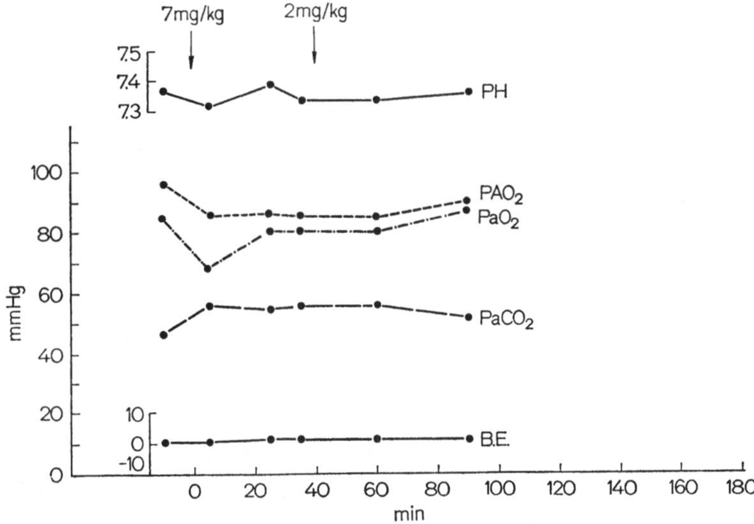

Fig. 6

Premedication: 100 mg Dolosal   Case Nr. 43   21 Y.
                25 mg Phenergan   69 kg
                0,5 mg Atropine

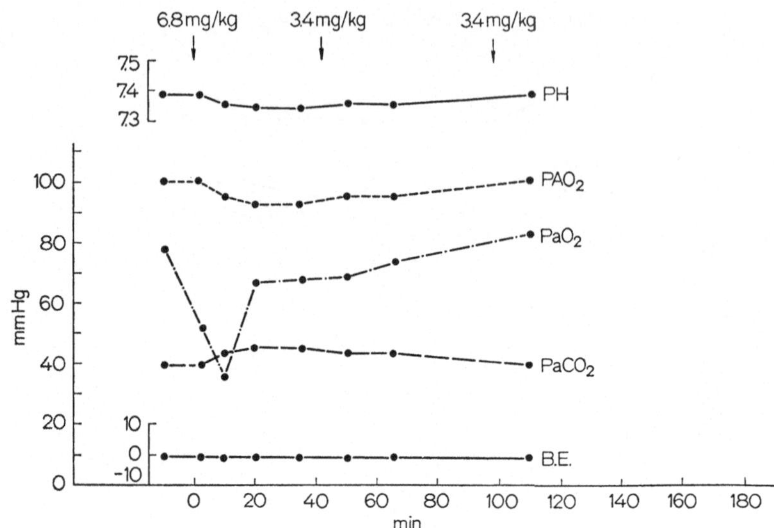

Fig. 7

Premedication: 100 mg Dolosal   Case Nr. 52   58 Y.
                0,5 mg Atropine   73 kg
                25 mg Phenergan

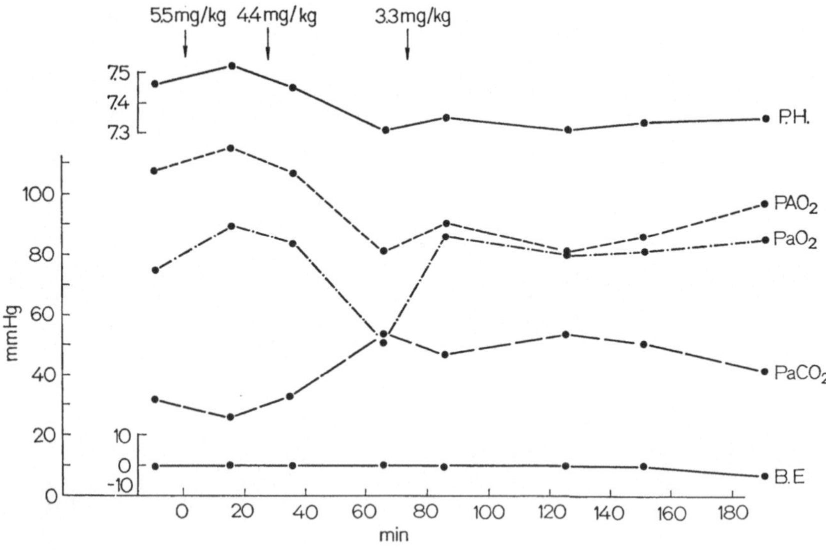

Fig. 8

Premedication: 100 mg Dolosal   Case Nr. 152   57 Y.
                0,5 mg Atropine   45 kg
                25 mg Phenergan

The fall of Pa_{O_2} was more pronounced after a heavy premedication. Age seems to be also an important factor, as the majority of decreased Pa_{O_2} values were present in the age group above 50 years.

Table 11. *Mean values of 7 patients (with both extremes)*

	Before injection	1–15 min after injection	16–30 min after injection
PaO_2	79,3 mmHg (58–99)	68,4 mmHg (36–99)	72,3 mmHg (63–85)
SaO_2	94,7 % (89–97)	91,4 % (66–97,5)	93,1 % (90–95,5)
$PaCO_2$	40,5 mmHg (33–46)	42,9 mmHg (33–55)	43,5 mmHg (35–54)
pH	7,37 (7,36–7,39)	7,35 (7,31–7,38)	7,35 (7,32–7,38)
Stand. Bic.	22,7 mEq/l (19,5–24)	22,8 mEq/l (20–24)	22,2 mEq/l (20,5–25)
Base Excess	−1,4 mEq/l (−5,5—0)	−1,8 mEq/l (−5—0)	−2,1 mEq/l (−4 — +1)

	31–60 min after injection	61–90 min after injection
PaO_2	74,2 mmHg (68–83)	77,3 mmHg (69–90)
SaO_2	93,7 % (92–95,5)	94,2 % (93–96)
$PaCO_2$	44,6 mmHg (38–55)	45,0 mmHg (38–55)
pH	7,34 (7,32–7,35)	7,33 (7,32–7,36)
Stand. Bic.	22,3 mEq/l (20–23,5)	22,3 mEq/ l (20,5–23,5)
Base Excess	−2 mEq/l (−5 — +1,5)	−1,9 mEq/l (−4 — +1,5)

III. Discussion

Ketamine was initial presented as a short acting anesthetic. According to our experience and our criteria, this drug cannot be classified as short acting, as its action prolongs over 60 min (Table 8). Its rapid onset of action makes it otherwise a usefull drug, especially for i.m. administration. The more moderate action on blood pressure and pulse frequency of the drug given by i.m. injection, is a further argument for preferring this route of administration.

The absence of relaxation limits the use of CI-581 as monoanesthetic to superficial surgery; this type of surgery, and especially plastic surgery, seems to be one of the best indications for this drug. The hallucinations however are side-effects not to be neglected; they can be suppressed by the use of barbiturates (CORSSEN G., DOMINO E. F. 1966); in this study, in order to evaluate the drug completely, this association has not been used. Hallucinations have not been seen in children; they may finally be the best age group for this drug.

Respiration is in general not depressed in our experience, after i.m. injection and during a prolonged anesthesia (90 min). In the literature however reports exist of hypoxemia after i.v. administration of the drug: O_2 saturation of 70% (DOMINO E. F., CHODOFF P., CORSSEN G. 1965); Pa_{O_2} of 62 mmHg (LANGREHR et al. 1967; PODLESCH et al. 1967). After i.m. administration a similar hypoxaemia can exceptionally also exist (Fig. 8); a progressive desaturation of 87% and 69%, with Pa_{O_2} of 51 and 36, was induced immediately after induction, but disappeared very soon. This example proves that even after intramuscular administration, unexpected respiratory depression and desaturation is possible.

IV. Zusammenfassung

Das neue Phencyclidinderivat CI-581 (Ketamine) wurde bei 150 Patienten untersucht. Die Applikation erfolgte entweder intravenös (1–2 mg/kg) oder intramuskulär (3–7 mg/kg). Analgesie und Bewußtlosigkeit traten 90 (i.v.) bzw. 281 (i.m.) sec nach Injektionsbeginn ein. Die Analgesie dauerte durchschnittlich 72 min. Systolischer und diastolischer Blutdruck sowie die Pulsfrequenz stiegen an. Die Muskelentspannung war gering, die Analgesie in 90% der Fälle gut. Ketamine wurde gut vertragen mit Ausnahme von Wachträumen oder Halluzinationen, die bei 18 Patienten auftraten. Bei 10 Patienten, die eine langdauernde Anaesthesie mit wiederholten Dosen von Ketamine für ophthalmologische Eingriffe erhielten, wurde der Säure-Basen-Haushalt, die Sauerstoffsättigung und der Sauerstoffpartialdruck im arteriellen Blut untersucht. Bei den meisten Patienten wurde nach der Injektion eine respiratorische Acidose mit Erniedrigung des Sauerstoffpartialdruckes beobachtet. Auf eine mögliche Korrelation dieser Veränderungen mit der verabreichten Prämedikation wurde hingewiesen.

References

1. CHEN, G., A. J. GLAZKO, and D. KAUMP: Report from the pharmacology department, Parke Davis Research Laboratories, February 4, 1965.
2. CORSSEN, G., and E. F. DOMINO: Dissociative Anesthesia: Further pharmacologic studies and first clinical experience with the Phencyclidine derivative CI-581 – Anesth. Analg. 45, 29 (1966).

3. Domino, E. F., P. Chodoff, and G. Corssen: Pharmacologic effects of CI-581, a new dissociative anesthetic, in man. Clin. Pharmacol. Ther. **6**, 279 (1965).
4. McCarthy, D. A., G. Chen, D. H. Kaump, and C. Ensor: General anesthetic and other pharmacological properties of 2-(o-chlorophenyl)-2-methyl-aminocyclohexanone HCl (CI-581). J. of New Drugs **5**, 1340 (1965).
5. Podlesch, I., u. M. Zindler: Erste Erfahrungen mit dem Phencyclidinederivat Ketamine (CI-581), einem neuen intravenösen und intramuskulären Narkosemittel. Anaesthesist **16**, 299–303 (1967).
6. Langrehr, D., P. Alai, J. Andjelkovic, u. I. Kluge: Zur Narkose mit Ketamine (CI-581): Bericht über erste Erfahrungen in 500 Fällen. Anaesthesist **16**, 308–318 (1967).

Untersuchungen über den Einfluß von Ketamine auf Humorale Systeme des Menschen

Von **S. Fuchs** und **H. Kreuscher**

Institut für Anaesthesiologie der Universität Mainz (Direktor: Prof. Dr. R. Frey)

Im Rahmen unserer Untersuchungen mit Ketamine versuchten wir festzustellen, ob eine klinisch übliche Dosis von Ketamine bei intravenöser Applikation einen Einfluß auf den Säure-Basen-Haushalt, den Sauerstoffpartialdruck und den Blutzucker hat. Außerdem wurde das Verhalten der Serum-Transaminasen kontrolliert.

Methodik

Die Versuche wurden an 10 Probanden beiderlei Geschlechts im Alter zwischen 23 und 30 Jahren durchgeführt. Es handelte sich um Personen mit gesunden kardiovasculären und respiratorischen Systemen.

Die Blutzuckerwerte wurden nach Hagedorn-Jensen bestimmt. Die Untersuchung der GOT und GPT im Serum erfolgte mit dem Photometer Eppendorf. Die arteriellen und venösen Sauerstoffspannungen wurden polarographisch nach Eschweiler mit der Elektrode von Thews bestimmt. Den Kohlensäurepartialdruck sowie pH, Standard-Bicarbonat und Basenüberschuß untersuchten wir mit der Mikro-Methode von Astrup und Verwendung des Nomogramms von Sigaard-Andersen.

Zur *Prämedikation* erhielten die Versuchspersonen 0,5 mg Atropin intravenös. 5 min später wurden 1,5 mg/kg Ketamine intravenös in genau 30 sec injiziert. Mit dieser Technik erreichten wir eine Narkosedauer von durchschnittlich 8,5 min.

Die Versuchsanordnung in ihrem zeitlichen Ablauf wird auf Abb. 1 dargestellt.

pO_2	pO_2	pO_2
Astrup	Astrup	Astrup
Blutzucker		Blutzucker
Transaminasen		Transaminasen
pränarkotisch	Narkose	postnarkotisch

Abb. 1

Ergebnisse

Das Verhalten der *Blutgase* wird auf Abb. 2 graphisch dargestellt. Eine signi-fikante Änderung der ermittelten Werte während und nach der Narkose gegenüber den pränarkotischen Ausgangswerten war nicht zu beobachten.

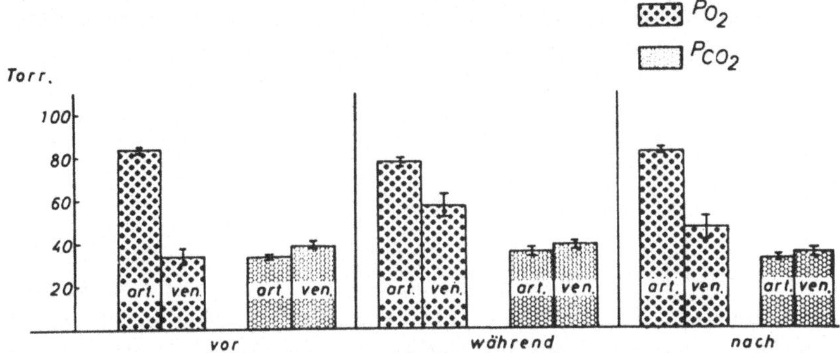

Abb. 2. pO_2 und pCO_2 unter dem Einfluß von 1,5 mg/kg Ketamine i.v. ($n = 10$)

Ebenso traten auch im Säure-Basen-Haushalt während und nach der Narkose mit Ketamine keine Änderungen auf (Abb. 3).

	Vor	Während	Nach	
pH	7,41	7,39	7,42	PH
	$s\bar{x} = \pm 0,006$	$s\bar{x} = \pm 0,007$	$s\bar{x} = \pm 0,012$	
B_E	−1,84	−2,36	−2,02	B_E
	$s\bar{x} = \pm 0,370$	$s\bar{x} = \pm 0,278$	$s\bar{x} = \pm 0,319$	
St_B	22,47	22,05	22,30	St_B
	$s\bar{x} = \pm 0,268$	$s\bar{x} = \pm 0,226$	$s\bar{x} = \pm 0,237$	

Abb. 3. Die Säure-Basenbalance unter dem Einfluß von 1,5 mg/kg Ketamine i.v.
($n = 10$)

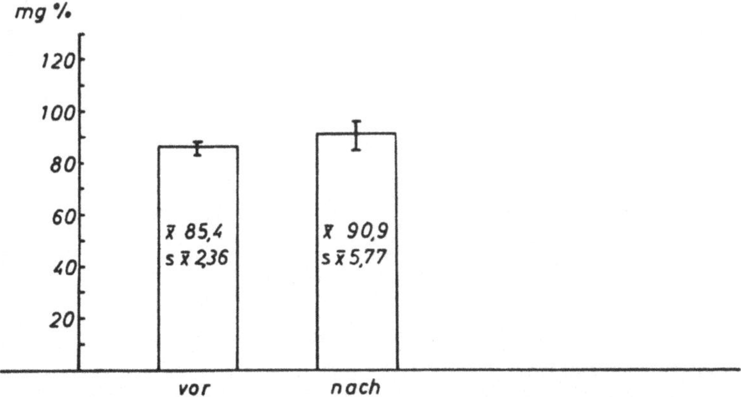

Abb. 4. Der Blutzucker unter dem Einfluß von 1,5 mg/kg Ketamine i.v. ($n = 10$)

9*

Die Steigerung von Blutdruck und Pulsfrequenz unter dem Einfluß von Ketamine ließ daran denken, daß es zu einer vermehrten Katecholaminausschüttung kommt. Diese wäre u. U. mit einer Erhöhung des Blutzuckerspiegels verbunden. Wie die Ergebnisse der Abb. 4 zeigen, bleibt aber der Blutzuckerspiegel vor und unmittelbar nach der Narkose unverändert.

Um einen bestehenden Leberschaden bei den Probanden auszuschließen, wurden vor der Narkose die Serum-Transaminasen bestimmt und die Werte nach der Narkose überprüft. Wie zu erwarten war, fanden sich keine Unterschiede.

Summary

In 10 volonteers (male, and female-age: 23–30 years) investigations were performed on the behaviour of the acid-base-balance, blood gases, blood sugar, and GOT so well as GPT before, during and after anesthesia with Ketamine (1.5 mg./kg. intravenously). No significant changes of the measured parameters could be observed.

Blutgasanalysen während Ketamine-Narkose unter Berücksichtigung von Prämedikation und Nachinjektionen

Von I. Podlesch

Aus der Anaesthesieabteilung der Universität Düsseldorf
(Direktor: Prof. Dr. M. Zindler)

Wir glauben, daß das Anwendungsgebiet von Ketamine vorwiegend in der pädiatrischen Anaesthesie liegt. Weil Kinder häufig ängstlich und unkooperativ sind, schien es interessant, die Wirkung von Ketamine auf die Atmung mit und ohne Prämedikation zu vergleichen. Die vorliegenden Untersuchungen wurden bei Atmung von Zimmerluft durchgeführt.

Abb. 1 zeigt pneumotachographisch gemessene Atemminutenvolumina nach 1–2 mg Ketamine/kg intravenös. Die Abnahme des Atemminutenvolumens in der 2. und 3. min post injectionem erfolgte durch Abnahme von Atemzugvolumen und Atemfrequenz.

Kinder zeigten eine geringere Beeinträchtigung des Atemminutenvolumens als Erwachsene.

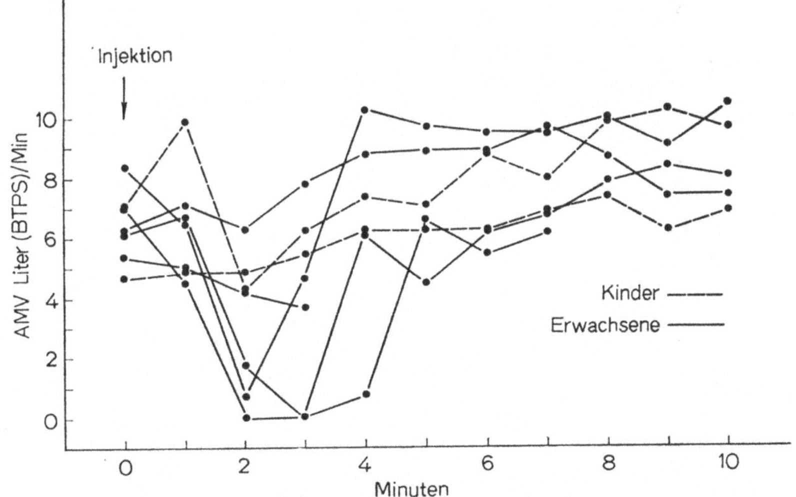

Abb. 1. Verhalten der Atemminutenvolumina nach Ketamine-Injektion und Atropinprämedikation

Abb. 2 zeigt Werte von Probanden mit einer Prämedikation in der Dosierung von 1 mg Atosil/kg, 1–2 mg Dolantin/kg und 0,01 mg Atropin/ kg, die ungefähr 45 min vor der Narkose verabreicht wurde. Auch bei diesem Versuch wird die Atmung der Kinder bis auf eine Ausnahme weniger stark beeinflußt als die der Erwachsenen.

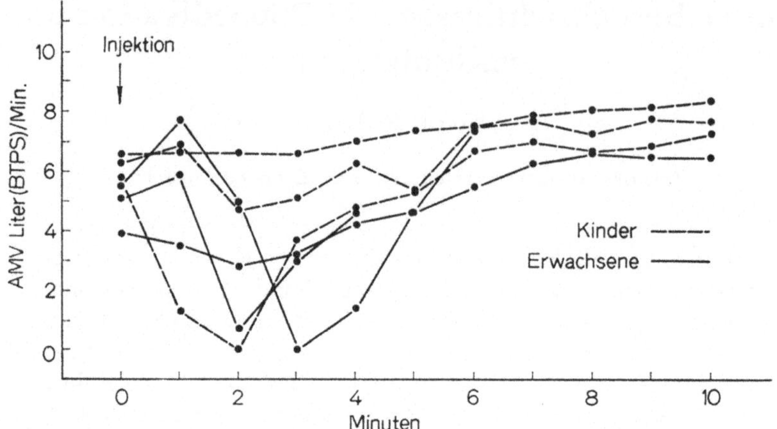

Abb. 2. Verhalten der Atemminutenvolumina nach Ketamine-Injektion und Promethazin-Pethidin-Prämedikation

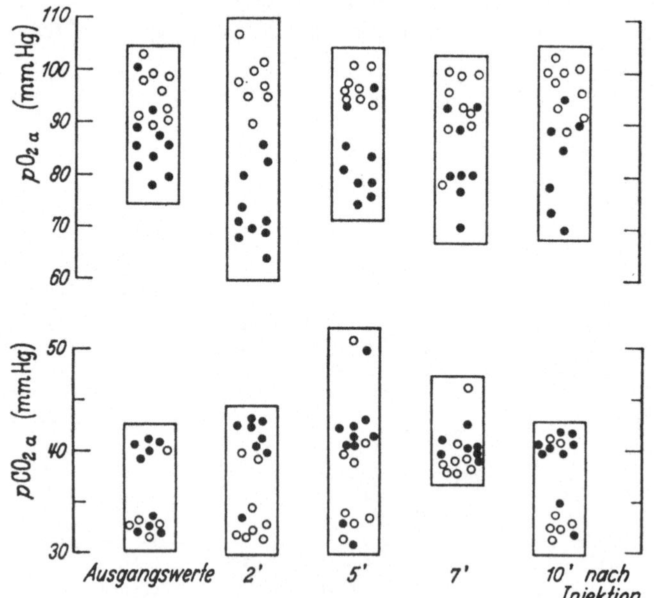

Abb. 3. ○ Patienten ohne Opiat-Prämedikation, ● Patient mit Atosil-Dolantin Prämedikation

Wir haben (Abb. 3) arterielle Sauerstoffdruckwerte und Kohlensäuredruckwerte zwischen Kindern mit und ohne Prämedikation verglichen. Die prämedizierten Patienten ließen eine stärkere Ketamine-Wirkung auf die Atmung erkennen. In der 2. min nach Ketamine-Injektion kam es zu einem Abfall des Sauerstoffdruckes. Für die gemessenen Werte ließ sich eine Sauerstoffsättigung von ungefähr 90% errechnen. Die Kohlensäuredruckwerte sind bis auf 2 Ausnahmen im Bereich der Norm geblieben.

Die Wirkung von Ketamine auf die Atmung ist unter unseren Versuchsbedingungen kurzzeitig. Da wir bei einzelnen Kindern mit Atosil-Dolantin-Atropin-Prämedikation nach der Narkose-Einleitung mit Ketamine eine Cyanose beobachtet haben, empfehlen wir die Bereitstellung einer Vorrichtung zur künstlichen Beatmung. Die Veränderungen von Blutgasen und Atemvolumina durch Nachinjektionen von 0,5–1 mg/kg Ketamine zur Verlängerung der Narkose unterschieden sich nicht von den berichteten Änderungen nach Erstinjektionen.

Diskussion

Kurka: Frau PODLESCH, wie lange haben Sie injiziert?

Frau **Podlesch:** Wir haben 1–2 mg/kg bei Kindern in 20 sec und bei Erwachsenen in 30–60 sec injiziert.

Corssen: Darf ich fragen, ob Sie bei Prämedikation mit einem Narkoticum eine Verlängerung der Aufwachphase beobachtet haben im Vergleich zu Patienten, die ohne Narkotikum vorbereitet wurden?

Frau **Podlesch:** Wir sahen eine Verlängerung der Aufwachphase um ungefähr eine Stunde. Wir registrierten, nach welcher Zeit die Kinder wieder ansprechbar waren, und diese Zeit war etwa 1 Std länger, wenn die Kinder ein Narkoticum erhalten hatten.

Corssen: Das deckt sich mit unseren Untersuchungen. Seit ungefähr 2 Jahren benutzen wir nur Scopolamin für die Prämedikation und haben nun Ergebnisse, die nachweisen, daß wir damit die Aufwachphase um ungefähr 50% verlängern.

Stöcker: Man hat den Eindruck, daß die Atmung sehr unregelmäßig wird. Herr LANGREHR hat heute morgen einige spirographische Registrierungen gezeigt, bei denen die Volumina zum Teil sehr deutlich und für längere Zeit ansteigen und zwischendurch abfallen. Auch ist die Atemmittellage etwas zur Inspirationsseite hin verschoben. Insgesamt sahen die Kurven, die Herr LANGREHR demonstrierte, fast so ähnlich aus wie pneumotachographische Volumenmessungen unter Dehydrobenzperidol. Es ist also die Frage, inwieweit diese respiratorischen Veränderungen gleichen Ursprungs sind.

Corssen: Ich möchte Frau Dr. PODLESCH fragen, ob sie Fälle beobachtet hat, bei denen eine echte Überdosierung erfolgte, und was geschah dann mit der Atmung?

Frau **Podlesch:** Von vielen Erscheinungen, die auftreten, weiß man nicht, ob sie auf eine echte Überdosierung zurückzuführen sind. Wir haben nach intramuskulären Injektionen bei Säuglingen gelegentlich Überstreckungen der Gliedmaßen und Opisthotonus gesehen. Ich weiß nicht, ob man diese Symptome als Folge einer Überdosierung bezeichnen kann. Ich hatte den Eindruck, daß bei diesen Kindern die Analgesie sehr tief war. Ich glaube, daß man nach sehr hoher Dosierung eine starke Atemdepression mit 2–3 min oder länger anhaltender Apnoe erzeugen kann.

Corssen: Das ist sehr interessant, daß Sie sich nicht festlegen wollen. Wir haben das auch vorgezogen. Auch wir beobachteten einige Opisthotonusfälle bei Kindern, die stets jünger als 1 Jahr waren. Dr. DILLON aus Los Angeles konnte ähnliche Beobachtungen machen.

Dillon: I have studied a little bit on the problem of children with heart disease. We used Ketamine for producing anesthesia in very small children for studying heart-defects. In a couple of slides I can demonstrate, that pCO_2, pH and pO_2 are really very little spread and none of these values are out of line. The pCO_2 increased a little, when the children come under the effects of Ketamine, and as they react, the pCO_2 goes down. We find this a very satisfactory way of keeping these children quiet for cardiac catheterisation. Well, some examinations, which are performed, lasted 4–5 h, and we have not enough agents to keep these children adequately anesthesized. Some of the dosages, which I'm not discussing now, have exceeded 1000 mgs over the duration of the procedure. So, the base success has not changed. We feel here in patients with a heart disease – and some of these children have had indeed failures –, some of them have only been one week old. We had no reason to feel prejediced to hurt these children in any way.

None of these values exceed values, which are known to exist in patients who are asleep normally without any effect of any drug whatever. I think, when we discuss this kind of problem, we should compare arterial values of blood on patients who are asleep without any drug effect because pCO_2 goes up, pO_2 goes down and saturation is down in patients who are asleep normally, at least values are not significantly different than those.

Langrehr: Die Antwort auf die eben gestellte Frage bezüglich der Dosisabhängigkeit und der eventuell auftretenden Atemdepression möchte ich so formulieren: Ich glaube, daß man in Dosisbereichen zwischen 1,5 bis 5 mg/kg intravenös keinen wesentlich dosisabhängigen Verlauf der Atmung beobachten kann. Bei einer geringeren Dosis kann ebenso einmal eine Apnoe auftreten wie bei einer höheren Dosis. Man hat nicht den Eindruck, daß hier eine Dosisabhängigkeit vorliegt. Weiterhin hat man auch nicht den Eindruck, daß die Atmung von der Injektionsgeschwindigkeit abhängig ist. Sie können also durch noch so langsame Injektion z. B. bei einem alten Menschen eine etwas längere Apnoe nicht vermeiden. Die typische Atemform und -frequenz ist also unabhängig von Dosis und Injektionsgeschwindigkeit.

Corssen: Wir hatten kürzlich einem 3 Monate alten Kind für einen ophthalmologischen Eingriff eine Dosis von 5 mg/lb und dann eine weitere Dosis von 2,5 mg/lb intramuskulär verabreicht. 15–20 min später trat ein sehr starker Opisthotonus auf, der etwa 1 Std anhielt und dann allmählich abklang. Dasselbe Kind kam 1 Woche später zu einer 2. ophthalmologischen Operation. Diesmal gaben wir 2 mg/lb intravenös, im Vergleich zu der intramuskulären Dosis also erheblich weniger. Es trat kein Opisthotonus auf. Dr. DILLON berichtete kürzlich, daß bei Kleinkindern unter einem Jahr erheblich häufiger sog. „purpose-movements" auftreten und unter Umständen die Durchführung des chirurgischen Eingriffes stören können. Dr. DILLON ist der Ansicht, daß man bei diesen Kleinstkindern u. U. die Verwendung von Ketamine vermeiden sollte. Unsere Erfahrung ist nicht ganz so profunde. Wir haben bei einer ganzen Reihe von Kleinkindern unseres Krankengutes – besonders bei Pneumoencephalographien – solche Bewegungen gesehen. Wir helfen uns, indem wir die Arme an die Oberschenkel mit Pflaster ankleben. Dr. DILLON, would you like to say something about purpose movements or extrapyramidal activity in these small infants?

Dillon: Well, we also have a very large pediatric neurologic service and we do an average of 2 or 3 pneumoencephalograms a day. We now use Ketamine as an agent of choice and obviously most of these children, because they have a pneumoencephalogram, have some neurological deficits. Our experience is: the more the deficit, the more the purpose movements. If we have a very small child e.g. one or two weeks old, don't ask me why they do this thing, but they do. These children have a very marked tendency to purpose movements. It seems that at about a year of age the tendency for this type of movement in this type of patients can be reduced unless the patient is of a very high level of neurological insufficiency and then the purpose movements continue and are a bit of a nuisance. But they seem to be related actually to the central nervous system integrity. The higher the integrity the less the tendency for movement.

Zindler: These patients with cardiac cateterization: were they breathing room air?

Dillon: Yes, room air.

Zindler: But they had arterial pO_2-values until 110. This must be a very good air!

Dillon: Not all patients had these high values. Others with heart desease have 60, and this is a very low value.

Dangel: Wir hatten einen Fall von Überdosierung bei einem ganz kleinen Kind, das versehentlich statt 8 mg/kg 40 mg/kg intramuskulär erhalten hatte und nun erstaunlicherweise einen völlig normalen Verlauf unter dieser Anaesthesie hatte. Weder die Atmung noch der Kreislauf waren gestört. Das Kind hat lediglich länger geschlafen als wir es sonst gewohnt sind. Wir haben weder einen Opisthotonus noch anderen besondere Bewegungen des Kindes bemerkt. Das steht im Gegensatz zu den Beobachtungen bei vielen anderen Kindern, besonders Kleinkindern, bei denen eine Pneumoencephalographie durchgeführt werden soll. Hier sehen wir häufig athetotische Bewegungen, die oft so stark sind, daß der Versuch, die Pneumoencephalographie durchzuführen, abgebrochen werden muß. Ich werde morgen auf diese Dinge noch näher eingehen. Wir haben vor allem den Eindruck, daß es weniger die Dosierung ist als der cerebrale Zustand des Patienten vor der Anaesthesie. Je mehr diese Kinder motorisch gestört sind, desto eher kommt es zu diesen Bewegungen, die, wenn sie schon vorhanden waren, sicher nicht durch die Anaesthesie unterdrückt werden.

Corssen: Wir können das nur unterstreichen. Dr. DILLON hat auch bereits angedeutet, daß Kinder für Pneumoencephalographien und ähnliche Eingriffe mit Ketamine anaesthesiert werden können. Auch wir haben festgestellt, daß die Anzahl der Patienten, die dann mit „purpose-movements" reagieren, erheblich höher ist. Als Zeichen einer echten Überdosierung, wie wir sie bei einem Kind mit 25 mg/lb intramuskulär gesehen haben und in einigen anderen Fällen mit relativ hoher intravenöser Dosierung, ist eine eigentümliche Atmungsart. Der Patient inhaliert tief und hält die Luft für mehrere Sekunden an, um anschließend einige oberflächliche Atembewegungen zu machen. In diesen Fällen ist die einzige Art der Behandlungsform natürlich die Gabe von Sauerstoff.

Das Verhalten der vestibulären Erregbarkeit nach Kurznarkose mit Ketamine

Von **F. Nagel**

Aus der Hals-Nasen-Ohrenklinik der Universität Mainz
(Direktor: Prof. Dr. W. KLEY)

Ein Kurznarkoticum ist unter anderem dadurch definiert, daß nach dem Wiedererwachen relativ schnell die Straßenverkehrstüchtigkeit erreicht wird. Die bequeme Anwendbarkeit von Kurznarkotica verbunden mit einem geringen Apparateaufwand und die allgemeine Tendenz der Patienten, schmerzhafte Eingriffe möglichst im Schlaf vornehmen zu lassen, machen dieses Narkoseverfahren bei Arzt und Patient gleichermaßen beliebt. Es ist daher verständlich, daß die pharmazeutische Industrie bestrebt ist, immer bessere und ungefährlichere Narkosemittel zu entwickeln. Der Arzt aber, der an einem ambulanten Patienten eine Narkose durchgeführt hat, trägt ein hohes Maß an Verantwortung bezüglich der Frage, wann dieser Patient ohne Schaden zu erleiden aus seiner Obhut entlassen werden kann, denn unsere Verkehrssituation verlangt nicht nur vom Autofahrer, sondern auch vom Fußgänger eine absolute Straßenverkehrstüchtigkeit.

Der Begriff der Straßenverkehrstüchtigkeit ist aber von komplexer Natur und an eine Reihe psycho-physischer Leistungen gebunden, so daß es nicht möglich ist, mit einem einzigen Testverfahren eine Beantwortung der sich stellenden Fragen zu finden. Es wurden daher verschiedene Methoden entwickelt, die die einzelnen Leistungen erforschen. Unter ihnen hat sich die Testmethode mit Prüfung des optisch-vestibulären Systems als brauchbar erwiesen, denn gerade sie läßt in Kombination mit den bewährten psycho-physischen Leistungstests eine relativ sichere Aussage bezüglich der Straßenverkehrstüchtigkeit zu.

Die Wirkung von Narkosemitteln auf den Vestibularapparat war schon oft Gegenstand von Untersuchungen und seit langem ist bekannt, daß in der postnarkotischen Phase oder nach dem Genuß einer entsprechenden Menge Alkohol ein sogenannter regelmäßiger Blickrichtungsnystagmus auftritt, d. h. beim Blick nach rechts oder links tritt ein horizontaler Rucknystagmus nach der Seite auf, in die gerade geblickt wird.

Dieser toxisch bedingte Blickrichtungsnystagmus muß unterschieden werden von den normalen Einstellrucken bei der Blickführung zur Seite, die transitorisch sind sowie von dem sogenannten physiologischen Endstellungsnystagmus, der beim extremen Seitenblick auftritt und nach NYLEN bei etwa 60% aller vestibulär Gesunden gefunden werden kann. Diese drei Nystagmusformen können für den Ungeübten Anlaß zur Verwechslung geben, wodurch die Aussagekraft des Blickrichtungsnystagmus wesentlich eingeschränkt wird.

Eine andere Nystagmusform, der optokinetische Nystagmus oder Eisenbahnnystagmus ist reflektorisch optisch bedingt. Er tritt auf, wenn schnell vorüberziehende Gegenstände fixiert werden. Die Augen folgen dem fixierten Gegenstand und schnellen dann zur Mittellinie zurück. Werden diese Augenzuckungen graphisch registriert, so erhält man ein typisches Kurvenbild. Die optokinetischen Reaktionen hängen aber stark von der Aufmerksamkeit des Untersuchten ab und deshalb tritt bei Intoxikationen zum Beispiel eine Verminderung dieser Folgebewegungen auf, wodurch sich das Diagramm verändert.

Seit MONTANDON eine Prüfung der Drehreizschwelle entwickelt hat, wissen wir, daß die Schwelle von extravestibulären „Faktoren", besonders empfindlich aber von Ermüdung beeinflußt wird. Die Bestimmung der Drehreizschwelle, die auf einem Drehstuhl durchgeführt wird, der eine gleichmäßige Beschleunigung zuläßt, beruht auf der Tatsache, daß ein perrotatorischer Nystagmus nur während einer Beschleunigung oder Verzögerung auftritt, nicht hingegen aber bei konstanter Drehgeschwindigkeit. Als Drehreizschwelle bezeichnet man die Drehbeschleunigung, die gerade eben einen perrotatorischen Nystagmus auszulösen vermag.

HAAS hat das Verhalten der Drehreizschwelle bei verschiedenen Narkosemitteln untersucht und dabei diese Methode als besonders brauchbar gefunden.

Im Rahmen unserer Untersuchungen haben wir die Frage geprüft, wie sich das optisch-vestibuläre System nach Narkose mit Ketamine verhält. Unser Interesse galt dabei dem Blickrichtungsnystagmus, der Optokinetik und dem Verhalten der Drehreizschwelle. Außerdem war es interessant zu erfahren, wie die Probanden selbst ihre Straßenverkehrstüchtigkeit in Relationen zu den gefundenen Untersuchungsergebnissen einschätzten.

Methode

Unsere Experimente wurden an insgesamt 10 (5 männlichen und 5 weiblichen) Personen im Alter zwischen 23 und 30 Jahren (Durchschnittsalter 26 Jahre) durchgeführt. Für die Versuche wurden nur gesunde Personen verwendet, wobei ganz besonderes Augenmerk einem intakten Vestibular- und Hörorgan geschenkt wurde. Personen mit pathologischen Vestibulogrammen oder Hörfehlern (z. B. pathologische Audiogramme) schieden für die Versuche aus. Zur Bestimmung der Drehreizschwelle stand uns ein elektronisch gesteuerter Drehstuhl nach TÖNNIES zur Verfügung.

Der eigentlichen Narkoseuntersuchung ging am Vortage neben anderen Testverfahren die Prüfung auf Endstellungs- und Blickrichtungsnystagmus sowie der Optokinetik und die Bestimmung der Drehreizschwelle voraus. Am Narkosetag wurde die Drehreizschwelle pränarkotisch noch einmal als sogenannte Tagesdrehreizschwelle bestimmt.

Nachdem den Probanden 1,5 mg/kg Körpergewicht Ketamine innerhalb 30 sec injiziert wurde, erfolgte nach dem Wiedererwachen neben anderen psychophysischen Leistungstests die Prüfungen auf Blickrichtungsnystagmus, die Optokinetik sowie die Bestimmung der Drehreizschwelle. Die Untersuchungen wurden in zeitlich genau festgelegten Abständen solange wiederholt, bis die pränarkotischen Ausgangswerte wieder erreicht waren.

Ergebnisse

Eine zusammenfassende Darstellung der Ergebnisse gibt Abb. 1. Die gefundenen Untersuchungsergebnisse zeigen, daß der Blickrichtungsnystagmus im Mittel 103 min nach erfolgter Injektion nicht mehr nachweisbar war. Er war als erster aller durchgeführter Testverfahren zur Norm zurückgekehrt.

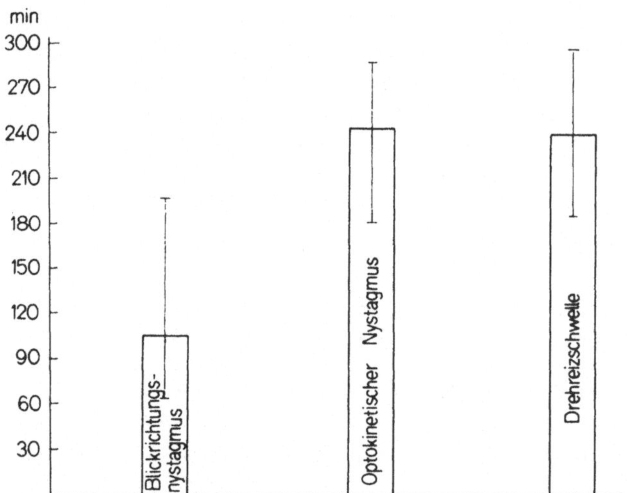

Abb. 1. Normalisierungszeiten optisch-vestibulärer Reaktionen nach Narkose mit Ketamine. Die Streuung ist durch I kenntlich gemacht

Der optokinetische Nystagmus beanspruchte im Durchschnitt 242 min bis das Ausgangskurvenbild wieder erreicht war und die Drehreizschwelle erforderte im Mittel 238 min bis der pränarkotische Wert wiedererlangt war.

Die meisten Probanden glaubten auf Grund ihres Befindens, daß sie durchschnittlich 70 min *vor* Normalisierung der letzten Testergebnisse, wieder straßenverkehrstüchtig seien.

Diskussion

Die Feststellung von JUST sowie KLEIN, daß Patienten nach Erlöschen des „Endstellungsnystagmus" (gemeint ist Blickrichtungsnystagmus) ohne Bedenken allein nach Hause entlassen werden können, ist auf Grund unserer Ergebnisse für die Ketaminenarkose nicht zutreffend.

Auch der optokinetische Nystagmus ist kein sicheres Zeichen der Ernüchterung, denn 5 Probanden, also die Hälfte, wiesen schon ein normales optokinetisches Nystagmogramm auf, obwohl die Ausgangswerte der psycho-physischen Leistungstests noch nicht wieder erreicht waren.

Im Durchschnitt hatte die Drehreizschwelle lt. der statistischen Ausrechnung früher als die Optokinetik ihren pränarkotischen Wert wieder erreicht. Dies kommt aber dadurch zustande, daß bei 2 der Probanden die Ausgangsdrehreizschwelle nicht wieder gefunden wurde, und die Versuche wegen physiologischer Übermüdung abgebrochen wurden. Diese fehlenden Werte konnten für die Ermittlung der Durchschnittszeiten nicht berücksichtigt werden, so daß bei der Angabe von Durchschnittszeiten das Wiedererlangen der Normalzeiten bei der Optokinetik länger erscheint, obwohl im konkreten Falle die Normalisierungszeiten für die Drehreizschwelle alle höher liegen als beim optokinetischen Nystagmus. Die verlängerte Erholung der Drehreizschwelle nach Alkoholgenuß wurde von FORSTER als eine zentrale Intoxikation gedeutet. HAAS hat diese These auf Grund seiner Untersuchungsergebnisse mit Narkosemitteln ebenfalls vertreten und auch wir glauben, daß die temporär heraufgesetzte Drehreizschwelle nach Narkose mit Ketamine in der gleichen Ursache zu suchen ist.

Wir sind bei unseren Untersuchungen zu der Überzeugung gekommen, daß die Drehreizschwelle ein brauchbarer und empfindlicher Test bei unserer Versuchsanordnung gewesen ist. Wir halten sowohl die Optokinetik als auch die Beurteilung des Blickrichtungsnystagmus bezüglich der Frage der Ernüchterung und der Straßenverkehrstanglichkeit nach Narkose mit Ketamine weniger geeignet.

Summary

In 10 male, and female volonteers (age 23–30 years) the behaviour of optico-kinetic and sight line nystagmus as well as rotatory stimulus threshold of the vestibular apparatus were tested after awakening of anesthesia with 1.5 mg./kg. Ketamine intravenously. The tests were continued until the preanesthetically ascertained norms were reached. The obtained values show, that acting the duration of the applicated dosis of Ketamine is long. Ketamine is not an short acting anesthetic.

Optico-kinetic and sight line nystagmus are methods which are not convenient for testing the recovery time after anesthesia with Ketamine.

Literatur

Aschan, G., M. Bergstedt u. a.: Positionalnystagmus in man during and after alcohol intoxication. Quart. J. Stud. Alcohol **17**, 381 (1956).

Bender, M. B., and F. H. O. Brien: The influence of barbiturate on various forms of nystagmus. Amer. J. Ophthal. **29**, 1541 (1946).

Bergström, O., and H. Koch: The effect of chlorpromazine on the vestibular function. Acta oto-laryng. (Stockh.) **46**, 484 (1956).

Binker, E.: Vergleichende Untersuchungen über die Straßenverkehrstauglichkeit nach Thiopental- und Methohexital-Kurznarkosen. Schweiz. med. Wschr. **91**, 1285 (1961).

Blomberg, L. H.: Evipan-Nystagmus and inequality in labyrinthine sensitivity. Acta oto-laryng. (Stockh.) **47**, 283 (1957).

— The significance of so-called "end position nystagmus" and its relation to nystagmus produced by evipan. Acta psychiat. scand. **33**, 138 (1958).

Decher, H.: Vestibularis-Feindiagnostik mittels Nystagmographie. Theoretische und klinische Medizin in Einzeldarstellungen Band 28. Heidelberg: Dr. Alfred Hüthig Verlag 1965.

Ey, W.: Störungen des oculo-vestibulären Systems bei alkoholisierten Personen. Dtsch. ophthal. Ges. 1964, 349.

Forster, B.: Elektronystagmographische Untersuchungen über den Drehbeschleunigungsnystagmus nach Alkoholgaben. Dtsch. Z. ges. gerichtl. Med. **47**, 282 (1958).

Flügel, F., u. D. Soyka: Über den Einfluß von Neuroleptika und Schlafmittel auf das optisch-vestibuläre System. Nervenarzt **34**, 506 (1963).

Frenzel, H.: Spontan- und Provokationsnystagmus als Krankheitssymptom. Berlin-Göttingen-Heidelberg: Springer 1955.

Frey, R.: Über die Verkehrstüchtigkeit eines Menschen nach Applikation von Hypnotika und Narkotika in der ambulanten Praxis. Therapiewoche **12**, 345 (1962).

Gutman, J., F. Bergmann, and M. Chaimovitz: The mechanisme of nystagmus induced by anaesthetics. Exp. Neurol. **9**, 175 (1964).

Haas, E.: Die Beeinflussung optisch-vestibulärer Reaktionen durch Kurznarkotika. Arch. Ohr.-, Nas.- u. Kehlk.Heilk. **182**, 569 (1963).

Jatho, K.: Die Wirkung der Alkoholintoxikation auf den Vestibularapparat unter besonderer Berücksichtigung der Störung der vestibulär oculo-motorischen Regelfunktionen. I. Kritische Betrachtung und Deutung nystagmischer Phänomene. Z. Laryng. Rhinol. **44**, 1 (1965).

— II. Ergebnisse experimenteller Untersuchungen. Z. Laryng. Rhinol. **44**, 104 (1965).

Just, O.: Die Anaesthesie beim ambulanten Kranken. Langenbecks Arch. klin. Chir. **289**, 101 (1958).

Kapp, W.: Straßenfähigkeit nach ambulanten Narkosen in der Zahn- und Kieferheilkunde. Dtsch. zahnärztl. Z. **21**, 1244 (1966).

Kornhuber, H.: Physiologie und Klinik des zentralvestibulären Systems. HNO-Heilkunde. Kurzgefaßtes Handbuch in 3 Bänden. Bd. III/Teil 3: Seite 2150. Stuttgart: Thieme Verlag 1966.

Klein, R.: Verkehrstüchtigkeit und Kurznarkotika. Dtsch. Z. ges. gerichtl. Med. **49**, 187 (1959).

Kreuscher, H., u. R. Frey: Die Verkehrstüchtigkeit unter der Mitwirkung von Anaesthetica, Hypnotica, Analgetica und Ataractica. Arzneimittel-Forsch. **12**, 1056 (1962).

MITTERMAIER, R.: Die experimentellen Gleichgewichtsprüfungen. HNO-Heilkunde. Ein kurzgefaßtes Handbuch in 3 Bänden. Band III/Teil 1, Seite 581. Stuttgart: Thieme Verlag 1965.

MONTANDON, A.: A new technique for vestibular examination. Acta oto-laryng. (Stockh.) 44, 594 (1954).

NYLEN, C. O.: zitiert bei STENGER i: HNO-Heilkunde. Ein kurzgefaßtes Handbuch in 3 Bänden, Band III/Teil 1, Seite 554. Stuttgart: Thieme Verlag 1965.

ROSSBERG, G., u. H. H. STENGER: Klinik der peripheren Vestibularisstörungen. HNO-Heilkunde. Ein kurzgefaßtes Handbuch in 3 Bänden, Band III/Teil 3, Seite 1697. Stuttgart: Thieme Verlag 1966.

SCHÜLE, H.: Die intravenöse Kurznarkose in der Kieferchirurgie; experimentelle Untersuchungen und klinische Erfahrungen. Dtsch. zahnärztl. Z. 21, 1225 (1966).

TRINCKER, D.: HNO-Heilkunde. Ein kurzgefaßtes Handbuch in 3 Bänden, Band III/Teil 1, Seite 311. Stuttgart: Thieme Verlag 1966.

Ein Leistungsvergleich nach Ketamine und Methohexital

Von **A. Doenicke, J. Kugler, M. Emmert, M. Laub** und **H. Kleinert***

Aus der anaesthesiologischen Abteilung (Leiter: Priv.-Doz. Dr. A. Doenicke) der Chirurgischen Poliklinik (Dir.: Prof. Dr. F. Holle) und der Neurophysiologischen Abteilung (Leiter: Priv.-Doz. Dr. J. Kugler) der Nervenklinik der Universität München (komm. Dir.: Prof. Dr. M. Kaess)

I. Problem

Seit 1961 führen wir laufend Untersuchungen über Hirnfunktion und Anaesthesie im Hinblick auf die Verkehrsfähigkeit von Kranken und Gesunden nach Narkosen durch. Im Rahmen dieser Untersuchungen haben wir zuletzt 1966–1968 diese Methode auch zum Untersuchen der Nachwirkungen von CI-581 benützt. Es sollten die Nachwirkungen dieses neuen Narkosemittels mit der eines bekannten Präparates verglichen werden; wir benützten dazu Methohexital.

II. Methode

12 freiwillige, gesunde Versuchspersonen im Alter von 22 bis 30 Jahren mußten sich jeweils zu 2 Narkosen zur Verfügung stellen. Bei 6 Personen wurde zuerst eine Methohexital-Narkose und ca. 14 Tage später eine CI-581-Narkose durchgeführt, bei den restlichen 6 Personen erfolgten die Narkosen in umgekehrter Reihenfolge. Den Versuchspersonen war nicht bekannt, welche Narkose sie erhielten. Die Dosis von 2 mg/kg des CI-581 wurde durchschnittlich in $1^1/_2$ min, die des Methohexital in 30 sec injiziert. Als Prämedikation erhielten die Versuchspersonen nur 0,5 mg Atropin.

Zum Erfassen der Leistung nach Narkotika, Psychopharmaka und Analgetika hat sich in zahlreichen Untersuchungen zu verkehrsmedizinischen Problemen die nachfolgend dargestellte psychodiagnostische Testkombination bewährt. Selbstverständlich kann man auch mit anderen Untersuchungen die Leistung messen. Die von uns bevorzugte Kombination ergänzte jedoch besonders günstig die subjektiven Äußerungen der Versuchspersonen, die gezielten Fragen und die EEG-Untersuchung. Die Testuntersuchungen dauerten durchschnittlich 40 min, ihre Reihenfolge wurde unverändert beibehalten.

---

* Die Arbeit wurde mit Unterstützung der Deutschen Forschungsgemeinschaft durchgeführt.

Folgende Testmethoden wurden angewendet:

1. Der *Labyrinth-Test* benutzt drei, in Umfang und Schwierigkeitsgrad sich steigernde Labyrinthe in quadratischer Form. Die Versuchspersonen mußten versuchen, vom Zentrum aus in möglichst kurzer Zeit den Weg nach außen zu finden; eingeschlagene Irrwege werden mit Fehlerpunkten bewertet.

2. Beim *Zähltest* schreibt die Versuchsperson die natürliche Zahlenreihe von 1000 ab rückwärts bis zur Zahl 975 auf. Als zusätzliche Bedingung wird die Zahlenreihe von links nach rechts und in Fünfer-Kolonnen gestaffelt, in der Weise, daß die Zahl 995 wieder unter der Zahl 1000 steht.

3. Der *Reaktionstest nach Mierke* stellt mit Hilfe eines Gerätes zur Aufgabe, aufleuchtende Zeichen und Farben richtig zu beantworten. Ein wesentliches Moment stellt dabei die getrennte Anordnung der aufleuchtenden Lampen (als Impulsgeber) von den Antworttasten dar. Das Programm, d. h. die Zusammenstellung der Zeichen und Formen, ist in bestimmten Grenzen wählbar, ebenso mittels eines Stufenreglers, der Rhythmus der nacheinander aufleuchtenden Zeichen- und Farbimpulse. Nicht oder falsch beantwortete Impulse werden von einem Zählwerk als Fehler notiert. Dabei muß festgestellt werden, daß die Möglichkeit der Beantwortung eines Impulses so lange gegeben ist, bis ein neues Zeichen (oder Farbe) aufleuchtet. Wird diese durch den Stufenregler bestimmte Zeitspanne für die Beantwortung nicht genutzt, gilt der Impuls als nicht beantwortet.

4. Beim *Track-Tracer-Test* muß die Versuchsperson auf einer Tafel eine vorgezeichnete Schlangenlinie mit einem Stift nachfahren, und zwar in möglichst kurzer Zeit. Beim Verlassen der Schlangenlinie kommt der Stift mit Kontaktpunkten in Berührung. Dies wird auf elektrischem Wege als Fehler automatisch registriert.

5. Im *Konzentrationsleistungs-Test nach Düker* muß die Versuchsperson einfache Rechenaufgaben im Kopf lösen: von je 2 zusammengehörenden Additionsaufgaben (bestehend aus: 3 Summanden, jeder absolut kleiner als 10, mit unterschiedlichen Vorzeichen) ist jeweils die Summe zu bilden; die Ergebnisse müssen im Kopf behalten werden, um dann zwischen beiden die Differenz zu bestimmen und diese als Ergebnis in ein dafür bestimmtes Kästchen einzutragen. Dieser Rechenvorgang wiederholt sich in jeder Aufgabe (= ein Additionspaar). Bei unseren Untersuchungen mußten innerhalb 30 min möglichst viele Aufgaben gelöst werden.

Mit Hilfe dieser Tests wurden im wesentlichen folgende Formen der Leistungs- und Konzentrationsfähigkeit geprüft:

1. Konzentrationsfähigkeit bei allen Tests, besonders bei Test V

2. sensomotorische Koordination   bei Test IV

3. Kombinationsgabe   bei Test I und V

4. logisches Denken   bei Test I und V

5. Situationsüberblick   bei Test I und II

6. abstraktes Vorstellungsvermögen   bei Test II und V

7. Reaktionsfähigkeit (= richtiges Schalten) und
Reaktionsschnelligkeit (= schnelles Schalten)   bei Test III

10*

III. Ergebnisse

Die zeitlichen Beziehungen (Abb. 1) d. h. die Dauer der Bewußtseinsänderung, wie sie bei dieser Beobachtungsserie festgestellt wurden, deckten
sich mit den aus dem EEG ermittelten Zeiten (Mittelwerte von 12 Versuchspersonen). Von Injektionsbeginn bis zum Eintritt des Bewußtseinsverlustes
(Erlöschen der Ansprechbarkeit), gingen nach CI-581 ebenso wie nach
Methohexital ca. 45 sec, d. h. bei CI-581 trat der Bewußtseinsverlust noch
während der $1^{1}/_{2}$ min dauernden Injektion ein. Bis zum Wiedereintreten der
Ansprechbarkeit war die Zeit nach CI-581 mit $14^{1}/_{2}$ min doppelt so lange
wie nach Methohexital und bis zum Einsetzen der Reorientierung mit
24 min 3mal so lange wie nach Methohexital.

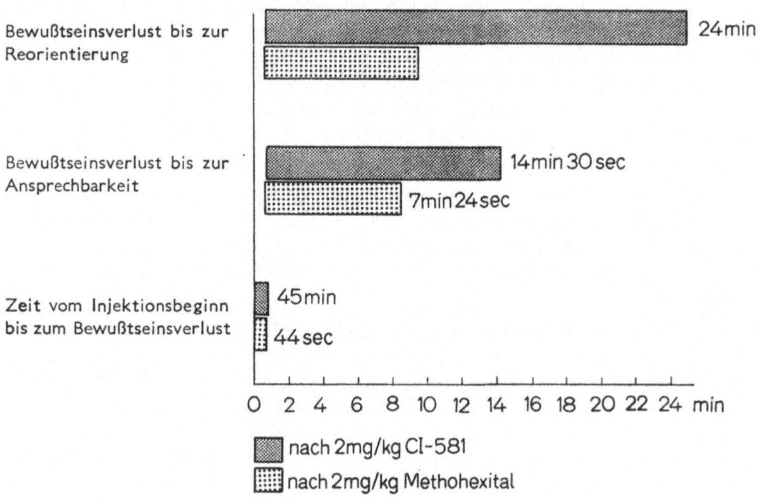

Abb. 1. Dauer der Bewußtseinsänderung. Mittelwerte von 12 Versuchspersonen

Ergänzend wurde zum Beurteilen der vegetativen Funktionen die Pulsfrequenz (Abb. 2) palpatorisch gezählt und zeigte im Gesamtverlauf gute
Übereinstimmung mit den aus dem EKG der EEG-Kurven errechneten
Werten. Der Anstieg der Pulsfrequenz in den ersten 10 min nach CI-581 ist
größer als nach Methohexital, die Rückkehr zum Ausgangsverhalten erfolgt
nach CI-581 später als nach Methohexital.

Unregelmäßige Myokloni waren bei 2 von 12 Versuchspersonen in den
ersten Minuten der Narkose an den proximalen Bereichen der oberen
Extremitäten und am Schultergürtel erkennbar (nach Methohexital war es
bei einer Versuchsperson in der 5. min nach Injektionsbeginn zu rhythmischen, klonischen Zuckungen der Extremitäten gekommen).

Mimische, gestikulatorische Spontanbewegungen oder Automatismen konnten wir bei einigen Untersuchten vor der 24. min beobachten. Einige Versuchspersonen zeigten einen ängstlichen, andere einen zufriedenen Gesichtsausdruck. Es kam aber auch teils zu koordinierten Bewegungen und Affektäußerungen, die offenbar mit visuellen oder anderen sensorischen, traumhaften Erlebnissen in Zusammenhang standen. So versuchten einige Versuchspersonen mit dem Fuß in die Luft zu schlagen oder Arme zu heben. Später wurden Flug- und Schwebeträume berichtet; eine Versuchsperson stand auf, um aus dem Fenster zu springen, in der Annahme fliegen zu können. Einige Versuchspersonen schrien laut, wobei Angstäußerungen erkennbar waren.

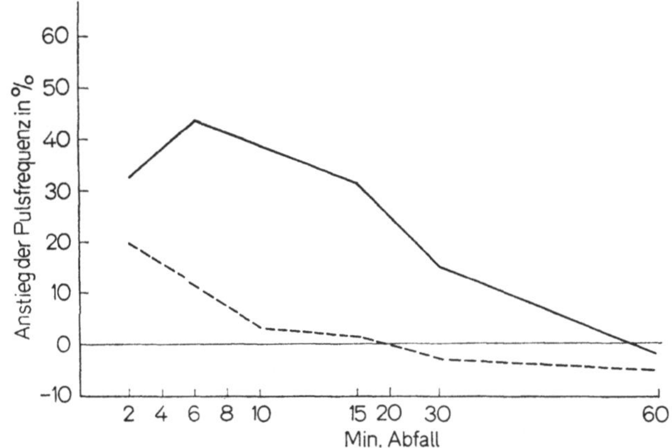

Abb. 2. Pulsfrequenz. Mittelwerte von 12 Versuchspersonen

Einer der Verfasser hat sich selber beiden Narkoseformen unterzogen und schildert das subjektive Erleben nach Injektion von CI-581 wie folgt:

„Bei den ersten subjektiven Erlebnissen glaubte ich mich in einem komplizierten Röhrensystem zu befinden, das mich an eine Ölraffinerie erinnerte. Eine treibende Kraft schoß mich durch die bunten, gelegentlich abgewinkelten Rohre. Ich wunderte mich über das Zustandekommen dieser seltsamen Umstände und glaubte von Verwandten verhext worden zu sein. Mir schien dies nun ein ewiges Schicksal zu sein, worüber ich sehr traurig wurde.

Einige Zeit später konnte ich zuerst akustische Eindrücke aus der Umgebung wahrnehmen, die zuvor fehlten. Die Stimmen der im Raum anwesenden Personen klangen fern, aber trotzdem laut und schallend. Dabei konnte ich zwar die Laute hören, aber nicht verstehen. Ich glaubte, daß es sich um die Stimmen von Verwandten handle, die mich verhext hätten.

Im weiteren Verlauf konnte ich visuelle Eindrücke wahrnehmen. Der Raum erschien mir dämmrig-neblig. In der entfernten Lichtung einer Röhre erschien der Kopf eines Kollegen. Nun verstand ich einige Worte und begann zu antworten. Meine Sprache erschien mir selber lallend und dröhnend. Zwischendurch wiederholte sich die Vorstellung verhext zu sein. Später ist mir gesagt worden, daß ich eigenartige Laute ausgestoßen habe. Meine Zunge erschien mir überaus groß, aber sehr leicht zu sein. Auch in den Extremitäten spürte ich eine auffallende Leichtigkeit.

Kurz vor dem Erwachen konnte ich wieder verstehen, was in der Umgebung gesprochen wurde und sah die Umwelt wieder, wenn auch stark verschwommen und sich ständig im Kreise drehend. Allerdings fühlte ich mich noch sehr schwach und es war mir übel.''

Zu diesen Äußerungen sind die während der EEG-Ableitung notierten Beobachtungen aufschlußreich:

Zeit/min	subjektiv	objektiv
0.–3.		Augen auf, starrer Blick
4.–6.		Injektionsende, Schmatzen, streckt die Zunge weit heraus, bewegt die Hände
7.–9.		streckt die Zunge heraus, lautes Brummen, Grimassieren
10.–12.		bewegt sich, Husten, Brüllen
13.–15.		lautes Brüllen, Hilferufe
16.–18.	„was ist los"	lautes Brüllen, hebt den Kopf
19.–21.	„es ist komisch – wo bin ich"	schreien
22.–24.	„ich sehe mich als Schwartenmagen", „mit Ihnen spreche ich nicht mehr", „dies ist unmöglich", „es ist eine andere Welt"	brüllen, starke körperliche Unruhe
25.–27.		brüllen, bewegt Arme kreisend
28.–30.	„was mache ich mit", „ich bin verrückt", „ich habe Hunger"	brüllen
31.–33.		körperliche Unruhe
34.–36.	„es dreht sich alles"	winkt mit der Hand
37.–39.		allgemeine Unruhe
40.–42.	„ich könnte micht totlachen"	streckt die Zunge heraus, schreit
43.–45.		starkes Atmen, Brüllen
46.–48.		dreht den Kopf hin und her
49.–51.		streckt die Zunge heraus, brüllt.
52.–54.	„ich sah Pastellfarben – braun, orange, es ist alles in Fluß"	häufige Bewegungen
55.–57.	„ich sah Menschen in anderen Dimensionen, es war wie ein Kandinsky-Gemälde"	häufige Bewegungen
58.–60.	„man fühlte sich so verlassen"	häufige Bewegungen
61.–63.		häufige Bewegungen
64.–66.	„mein Mund ist pelzig"	unruhig

(Fortsetzung von Seite 150)

Zeit/min	subjektiv	objektiv
67.–69.		häufige Bewegungen
70.–72.		häufige Bewegungen
73.–75.	„ich sehe schlecht, es ist alles verschwommen"	häufige Bewegungen
76.–78.	„akustisches Empfinden hatte ich nicht. Ich war in einem System drinnen, man fließt im Großen und Ganzen, die Menschen waren verzerrte Typen, ich habe mich nicht sprechen gehört"	
79.–81.	„es waren Striche, die ineinanderflossen, ich flog davon und sah Leute"	häufige Bewegungen
82.–84.		häufige Bewegungen
85.–87.		häufige Bewegungen
88.–90.	„es strömt auf einem ein und selbst ist man passiv"	häufige Bewegungen
91.–93.		Beruhigung
94.–96.		liegt ruhig
97.–99.		liegt ruhig
100.–102.		liegt ruhig
103.–105.		liegt ruhig
106.–108.		liegt ruhig
109.–111.		liegt ruhig
112.–114.		liegt ruhig
115.–117.		liegt ruhig
118.–120.		liegt ruhig

Insgesamt überwogen bei allen Versuchspersonen in den traumhaften Perioden irreale Vorstellungen mit Bewegungserlebnissen und Farbeindrücke (Tab. 1 und 2). Taktile, akustische und schmerzhafte Reize waren in dieser Periode unwirksam. Anschließend bestanden in der Regel Phasen mit flüchtiger Depersonalisation, Derealisation und Körperschemastörungen bis zu 60 min. Von diesem Zeitpunkt an vermochten die Versuchspersonen mit Selbstbezogenheit und Selbstkritik zu berichten, daß sie geträumt hätten. Doch berichteten fast alle über wechselnde Übelkeit, Schwindel und Sehstörungen bis zu 2 Std. Bei 5 Versuchspersonen trat in dieser Periode *Erbrechen* auf (Tab. 3).

Bei der unter anderen Bedingung mit elektroenzephalographischer Kontrolle beobachteten Gruppe von Versuchspersonen wurde auf Trauminhalte aus den unvermittelbar protokollierten verbalen Äußerungen geschlossen und zugleich bestehende Verhaltensweisen notiert (Tab. 2)

Tabelle 1. *Traumerlebnis nach Injektion von CI-581*

Versuchsperson Nr.	Trauminhalt	Farbeindrücke	Bewegungsphänomene	Traum war angenehm unangenehm indifferent
1	„Ich war auf einem Berg und sollte dort in eine Schublade gelegt werden; dabei wechselte ich auf verschiedene Höhenstufen. Ich fühlte mich dann selber als Schublade."	rot, grün	geradlinige Fortbewegung	indifferent
2	„Ich war in einem farbigen Traumstaat; dort fühlte ich mich als Amöbe."	blau	keine	angenehm
3	„Ich war eine bunte Harlekin-Figur. In einem großen Gebäude wechselte ich ruckartig von Etage zu Etage; die Etagen hatten jeweils verschiedene Farben."	grün, keine genauere Erinnerung	keine Erinnerung	indifferent
4	„Ich war eine farbige geometrische Gliederpuppe, die sich im leeren Raum bewegte."	rot, orange	geradlinige Fortbewegung	angenehm
5	„Ich schwebte mit großer Geschwindigkeit durchs Weltall; dabei traf ich auf Marsmenschen, die mich weitergeleitet haben."	rot, rosa	geradlinige Fortbewegung	angenehm
6	„Ich schwebte im unbegrenzten, farbigen Raum. Ich fragte mich selber: bin ich dazu verdammt, hier zu bleiben?"	rot, gelb	schwebende Bewegungen	angenehm
7	„Ich drehte mich auf einer Kreistangente im unendlichen Raum. Ich versuchte höher zu kommen; ein Mann half mir."	rot, orange	Rotationsbewegung	angenehm
8	„Ich sah viele weiße, schloßähnliche Krankenhäuser an mir vorüberziehen; auch Ärzte und Schwestern zogen vorbei."	weiß, blau	Rotationsbewegung	indifferent
9	„Ich bewegte mich in einer sand- oder plastikartigen Masse. Die Bahn konnte ich nicht selber bestimmen."	rot, grün	keine genauere Erinnerung	indifferent

Tabelle 1 (Fortsetzung)

Versuchs-person Nr.	Trauminhalt	Farb-eindrücke	Bewegungs-phänomene	Traum war angenehm unangenehm indifferent
10	„Ich sah Fadenmännchen, die sich drehten; ich drehte mich mit ihnen."	rot, grün	Rotations-bewegung	angenehm
11	„Ich war in einem großen, weißen Saal mit vielen Menschen; ich fühlte mich wie völlig in Schaum-gummi eingehüllt"	weiß, grau	keine Er-innerung	indifferent
12	„Ich sehe lauter geometri-sche Figuren; ich drehe mich mit ihnen."	blau, grün	Rotations-bewegung	unangenehm

Tabelle 2

Versuchs-person Nr.	Traumhafte Erlebnisse	Farb-eindrücke	Traum war unangenehm indifferent	Besonderheiten
1	„Ich sah Marsmen-schen und fuhr auf der Achterbahn."	weiß, grau	unangenehm	Körperschema-störungen
2	„Ich hatte Angst vor dem Nichts, alles war eckig."		unangenehm	Körperschema- und Sprach-störungen
3	„Ich sah kantige Köpfe, ich war Ja-mes Bond."	blau	indifferent	Körperschema-störungen, Dys- und Parästhe-sien
4	„Ich glaubte fliegen zu können und war festgebunden."	keine	unangenehm	Körperschema-störungen, Parästhesien
5	„Ich sah ein Badezim-mer und schwbte über einer Wendel-treppe auf und ab."	weiß, rosa	indifferent	Körperschema-störungen, Dys- und Parästhe-sien
6	„Ich fühlte mich in einer anderen Welt."	rot	indifferent	keine
7	„Ich sah alle Varian-ten von rot, ich drehte mich in den Farben."	rot, blau	indifferent	Körperschema-störungen, Dys-ästhesien
8	„Ich war in ein Hör-spiel verwickelt", „ich habe wie ein Kind die Welt ent-deckt."	rosa, rot, blau, orange	angenehm	Dys- und Par-ästhesien

Tabelle 2 (Fortsetzung)

Versuchs-person Nr.	Traumhafte Erlebnisse	Farb-eindrücke	Traum war unangenehm indifferent	Besonderheiten
9	„Ich spielte Fußball", „es war alles neutral, endlos, zeitlos."	keine	indifferent	Körperschema-störungen, Dys-ästhesien
10	„Ich sah runde Dinge, die sich ineinander-schoben."	weiß, blau	angenehm	keine
11	„Ich war in einem Röhrensystem und wurde bedroht", „ich sah Menschen in anderen Dimen-sionen."	braun orange	unangenehm	Parästhesien
12	„Ich flog zwischen Hochhäuser, und durch Fenster."	weiß, hellblau	indifferent	Körperschema-störungen Parästhesien

Bei diesen Versuchspersonen handelt es sich um spontane Äußerungen während der EEG-Ableitung.

Tabelle 3. *Erbrechen und Übelkeit im Anschluß an das Erwachen aus der Narkose mit CI-581*

Versuchs-person Nr.	Erbrechen post injectionem 1 h	2 h	3 h	4 h	Übelkeit post injectionem 1 h	2 h	3 h	4 h	Ist Vp. 1 h post injectionem aufgestanden ja / nein
1	++	++	−	−	+	++	−	−	nein
2	−	−	−	−	++	++	+	−	ja
3	−	+	−	−	−	−	−	−	ja
4	−	−	−	−	++	+	−	−	nein
5	−	−	−	−	++	+	+	−	ja
6	++	+	−	−	++	++	−	−	ja
7	++	+	−	−	++	++	−	−	ja
8	+	−	−	−	++	++	−	−	nein
9	+	−	−	−	+	+	−	−	nein
10	−	−	−	−	−	−	−	−	ja
11	−	−	−	−	−	−	−	−	ja
12	−	−	−	−	+	−	−	−	ja

Zeichenerklärung: ++ Erscheinungen stark oder mehrmals, + Erscheinungen gering oder flüchtig, − Erscheinungen fehlen.

Nachträglich über das *subjektive Erleben* befragt, äußerten 5 von 12 Versuchspersonen, daß sie den Beginn der CI-581-Injektion „angenehm" empfanden, 7 bezeichneten ihn als indifferent. Über das Erwachen und die Traumperiode äußerten 4 von 12 Versuchspersonen, daß sie angenehm,

2 daß sie unangenehm und 6 daß sie indifferent gewesen sei. Dagegen fanden nach Methohexital 11 von denselben 12 Versuchspersonen sowohl den Beginn der Narkose als auch das Erwachen daraus angenehm.

Die 1 Std nach Injektionsbeginn durchgeführten *psycho-experimentellen* Testuntersuchungen (Abb. 3) zeigten nach CI-581 eine Leistungseinbuße von 70%, nach Methohexital, das kürzer wirkte eine solche von ca. 20%. Im späteren Verlauf, 2, 4 und 8 Std nach der Narkose erfolgte der langsame Angleich an das Ausgangsverhalten, bei CI-581 langsamer als bei Methohexital.

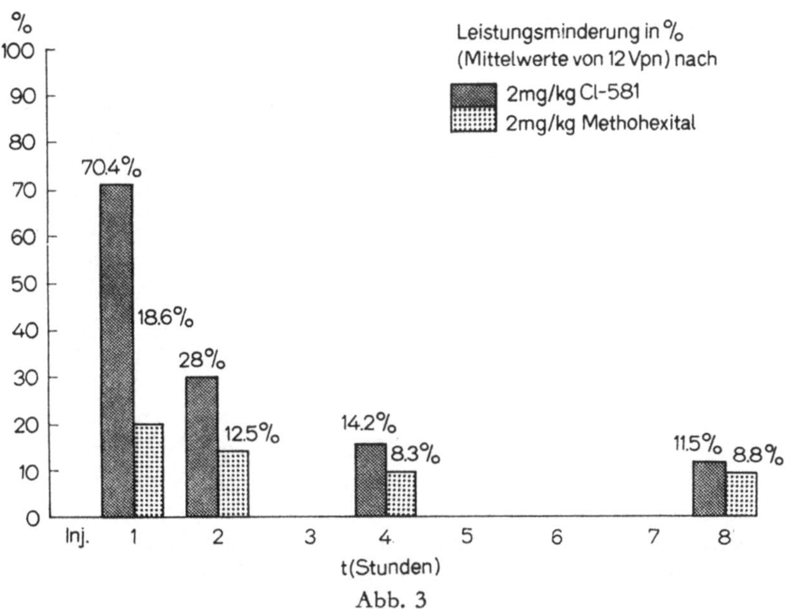

Abb. 3

Mit einer gleichen Versuchsanordnung hatten wir früher nach sog. Einschlafdosen von Thiobarbituraten Werte festgestellt, die zum Vergleich dienen können: 1 Std nach Injektionsbeginn war das Prüfen der Leistungsminderung mit dieser Testkombination unmöglich, weil die Versuchspersonen noch nicht reaktionsfähig waren. 2 Std nach Injektionsbeginn betrug die Leistungsminderung noch 40%, lag bei 4 Std über den Werten von CI-581 und nach 8 Std bei 20%.

Summary

Ketamine is not an short acting anesthetic. The experimentally investigated minimization of the psycho-physic abilities has a prolonged recovery time. The recovery period lies between those after Methohexital and Thiopental.

Untersuchungen über die psycho-physische Leistungsfähigkeit nach Ketamine

Von **H. Kreuscher, S. Fuchs** und **F. Bornemann**

Aus dem Institut für Anaesthesiologie der Universität Mainz
(Direktor: Prof. Dr. R. Frey)

Die relativ kurze Narkosedauer mancher intravenöser Narkosemittel wie beispielsweise der Thiobarbiturate führte zur Einbürgerung von Begriffen wie *kurz-* oder *ultrakurzwirkende* Mittel. Diese besondere Qualitätsbezeichnung hatte die Annahme zur Folge, daß solche Mittel besonders für die Anwendung bei ambulanten Patienten geeignet seien.

Die Bezeichnung „ultrakurz" ist aber für die Thiobarbiturate insofern irreführend, als nach der Wiedererlangung des Bewußtseins noch lange Zeit Einschränkungen der psycho-physischen Leistungsfähigkeit bestehen, die gerade für den ambulanten Patienten erheblich physische und auch juristische Konsequenzen haben.

Bei der Prüfung eines neuen Narkosemittels interessieren daher auch seine Eigenschaften bezüglich des Verhältnisses der Narkosedauer zur Dauer des sog. „hang-over" – also derjenigen Beeinträchtigung psychophysischer Leistungen, die eine Voraussetzung für die volle Eigenverantwortlichkeit als Verkehrsteilnehmer im weitesten Sinne ist.

Besonders strenge Maßstäbe sind dabei für die Beurteilung der *Straßenverkehrstüchtigkeit bzw. Fahrtüchtigkeit* anzulegen.

Auch dem Ketamine ging der Ruf „kurzwirkend" voraus. Unsere klinischen Beobachtungen ließen jedoch Zweifel an der Richtigkeit dieser Qualitätsbezeichnung aufkommen.

Wir haben darum mit einer bereits bei früheren vergleichenden Untersuchungen mit Thiopental, Methohexital und Propanidid bewährten Testkombination die Dauer der Beeinträchtigung bestimmter psycho-physischer Leistungen nach Anwendung von Ketamine geprüft.

Methodik

Die Versuchsanordnung, durch die die psycho-physische Leistungsfähigkeit nach Ketamine beurteilt werden sollte, bestand aus folgenden Tests:

1. Fallstab-Test. Hierbei muß der Proband einen plötzlich fallenden Stab ergreifen. Der Fallbeginn wurde elektromagnetisch ausgelöst und akustisch markiert. Nach der Formel $s = 1/2 \cdot b \cdot t^2$ läßt sich aus der Fallhöhe die Reaktionszeit bestimmen.

2. Konzentrations-Leistung-Test (Düker). Auf einem vorgeschriebenen Testbogen löst die Versuchsperson 30 min lang Rechenaufgaben, die ein besonderes Maß an Konzentration und Aufmerksamkeit erfordern. Dieser Test wurde, da er viel Zeit erfordert, als Kontrollversuch an das Ende der Versuchsreihe gestellt. Um die Konzentrationsleistung in kürzerer Zeit prüfen zu können, wurden die Aufgaben des Dükerschen Tests 4 min lang als Diapositive an eine Wand projiziert. Die Geschwindigkeit der Diafolge konnte der Proband selbst bestimmen.

3. Tachistoskop-Test. Hierbei werden 5 zweistellige Zahlen, hell auf dunklem Grund, 1 sec lang an eine Wand projiziert. Es sollen möglichst viele Zahlen erkannt und anschließend aus dem Gedächtnis niedergeschrieben werden.

Die einzelnen Kriterien, die durch diese Testkombination beurteilt werden, sind:

Fallstabtest:	1. Sensomotorische Reaktion
	2. Aufmerksamkeit
	3. Motorische Koordination
K-L-T Düker:	1. Konzentration
	2. Arbeitstempo
	3. Ermüdbarkeit
Tachistoskoptest:	1. Auffassungsvermögen
	2. Erinnerungsvermögen
	3. Aufmerksamkeit
	4. Blendempfindlichkeit
	5. Akkomodation

Die Untersuchungen wurden an 10 gesunden männlichen und weiblichen Versuchspersonen im Alter zwischen 23 und 30 Jahren durchgeführt. Am Vortage wurden die Tests geübt, um einen unkontrollierbaren Leistungszuwachs durch Training auszuschalten.

Vor dem Versuch wurden die Ausgangswerte bestimmt und anschließend, nach Prämedikation mit 0,5 mg Atropin, 1,5 mg/kg Ketamine intravenös injiziert.

Sobald es der physische Zustand des Probanden erlaubte, d. h. im Durchschnitt 76 min nach der Ketamine-Injektion, wurden die Tests in der Reihenfolge ihrer geübten Kombination so lange wiederholt, bis die pränarkotisch ermittelten Leistungswerte wieder erreicht waren.

Ergebnisse

Bei Beginn der postnarkotischen Prüfung wurden bei allen Tests erhebliche Leistungsminderungen verzeichnet (Abb. 1–3). Die zusammenfassende Beurteilung der ermittelten Werte ergibt (Abb. 4), daß die pränarkotisch ermittelten Ausgangswerte für

sensomotorische Reaktion
Aufmerksamkeit und
motorische Koordination

durchschnittlich nach 225 min wieder erreicht wurden. Die Streuung der Einzelergebnisse lag zwischen 165 und 250 min. Herabgesetzte Konzentration bestand noch 197 min nach der Ketamine-Injektion bei einer Streuung zwischen 150 und 240 min.

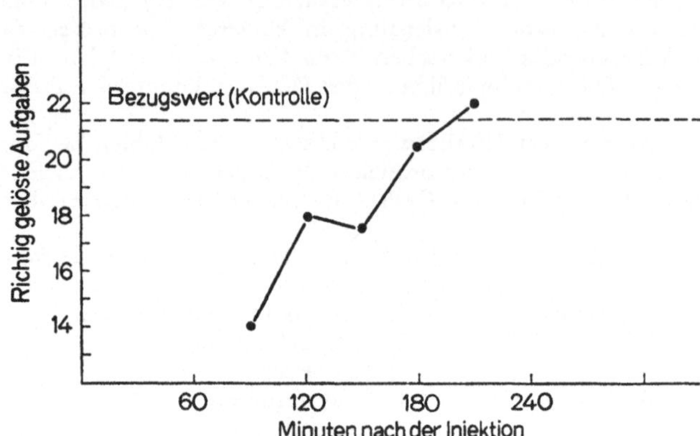

Abb. 1. Dükerscher Konzentrations-Leistungs-Test: Graphische Darstellung der Mittelwerte

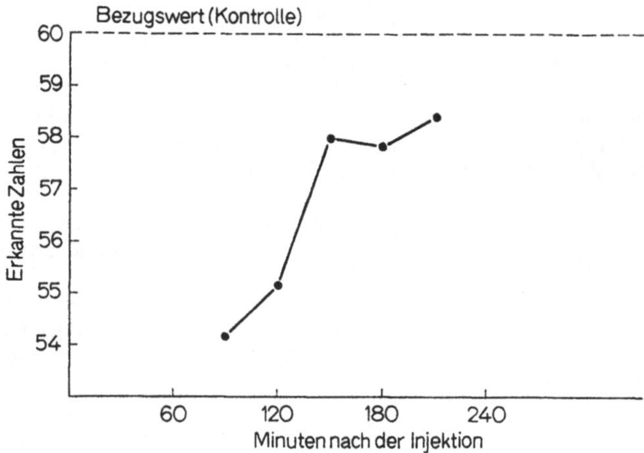

Abb. 2. Tachistoskop-Test: Graphische Darstellung der postnarkotischen Mittelwerte

Einschränkungen des Auffassungsvermögens
                 Erinnerungsvermögens
                 der Aufmerksamkeit
                 der Blendempfindlichkeit und
                 der Akkomodation

bestanden im Durchschnitt 208 min nach der Ketamine-Injektion. Die Einzelergebnisse lagen zwischen 160 und 240 min.

Der Konzentrations-Leistungs-Test (DÜKER) zeigte nach dieser Zeit in keinem Falle auffällige Ermüdungserscheinungen nach längerer Konzentrationsleistung.

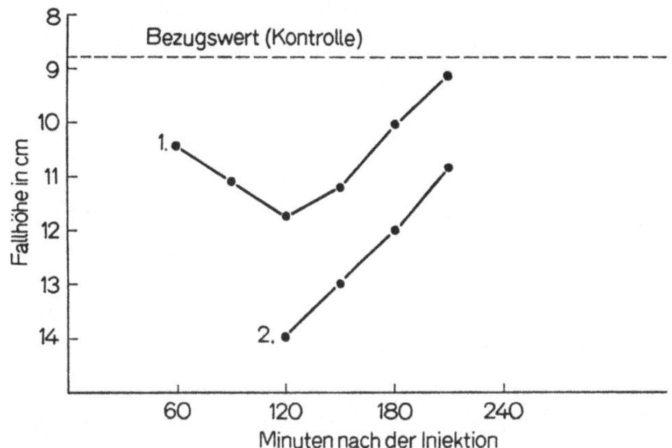

Abb. 3. Fallstab-Test: Die obere Kurve (1) gibt die Mittelwerte der Versuchspersonen 1–7, die untere Kurve (2) die Mittelwerte der Versuchspersonen 8–10 wieder

Psycho-physische Leistungsgruppe	Dauer der postnarkotischen Leistungsminderung
Auffassungsvermögen Erinnerungsvermögen Aufmerksamkeit Blendempfindlichkeit Akkomodation	
Konzentration	
Sensomotorische Reaktion Aufmerksamkeit Motorische Koordination	
	60 120 180 240 300
	Minuten nach der Jnjektion

Abb. 4. Graphische Darstellung der durchschnittlichen postnarkotischen Minderung der psycho-physischen Leistungen nach 1,5 mg/kg Ketamine intravenös

Schlußfolgerung

Die Ergebnisse unserer Untersuchungen zeigen, daß nach 1,5 mg/kg Ketamine i.v. bei einer durchschnittlichen Narkosedauer von 8 min erst 4 Std nach der Injektion von Ketamine diejenigen Funktionen wieder normalisiert sind, die eine Mindestvoraussetzung für die eigenverantwortliche Teilnahme am Straßenverkehr sind.

Wie die Untersuchungen von NAGEL zeigen, muß auch zu dieser Zeit noch mit erheblichen Störungen des Vestibularapparates gerechnet werden, die eine Straßenverkehrstauglichkeit ausschließen. Andererseits konnten wir feststellen, daß unsere Versuchspersonen nach durchschnittlich 90 min in einem Zustand waren, der die Entlassung mit einer verantwortlichen Begleitperson erlaubt hätte.

Unter den Bedingungen unserer Versuchsanordnung konnten wir feststellen, daß sich Ketamine bezüglich der Dauer einer postnarkotischen Minderung der psycho-physischen Leistungsfähigkeit ähnlich verhält wie Thiopental. Seine Eignung für ambulante Patienten muß darum einschränkend beurteilt werden.

Summary

In 10 male and female volunteers (mean age 26 years) the effect of 1.5 mg./kg. Ketamine on some psycho-physical efficiencies was tested. Sensomotoric reaction, motoric coordination and alertness was decreased 225 min after the injection. The ability for concentration was decreased 127 min, the powers of comprehension and recollection so well as sensitivity against blinding, and the ability for accomodation were decreased for 208 min. The ability for coordination of eye-movements was disturbed for 245 min after injection. The duration of the influence on psycho-physic efficiencies after Ketamine-anaesthesia is comparable to those of Thiopental. The term "short acting" anaesthesic would not be justified for Ketamine.

Traumähnliche Erlebnisse bei Kurznarkosen mit Ketamine, Thiopental und Propanidid

Von **K. Rumpf, J. Dudeck, H. Teuteberg, W. Münchhoff** und **H. Nolte**

Aus der Nervenklinik (Kommissar. Direktor: Prof. Dr. K.-H. Schiffer), dem Institut für Anaesthesiologie (Direktor: Prof. Dr. R. Frey) und dem Institut für Medizinische Dokumentation und Statistik (Direktor: Prof. Dr. S. Koller) der Universität Mainz

In klinischen Erfahrungsberichten über Ketaminenarkosen wurden bereits mehrfach Traumerlebnisse und eigenartige Phänomene während der Aufwachphase erwähnt [1, 2]. Es erschien daher angebracht, anläßlich einer vergleichenden Untersuchung von Kurznarkosen mit Thiopental, Propanidid und Ketamine an den beteiligten Versuchspersonen systematisch eine Befragung vorzunehmen nach derartigen Erlebnissen während der Narkose und während der anschließenden Aufwachphase. Über die medizinischen Daten dieser Vergleichsuntersuchung berichten Nolte u. Mitarb. an anderer Stelle; dort sind auch die genauen Einzelheiten von Versuchsplan und Versuchsablauf angeführt.

Methode

Die *Versuchsgruppe* bestand aus 18 unausgelesenen, gesunden Versuchspersonen (Vpn), 9 männlichen und 9 weiblichen, im Alter von 19 bis 29 Jahren. Überwiegend handelte es sich um Studenten verschiedener Fachrichtungen (15 Vpn). Von daher darf begründet angenommen werden, daß die Gruppe einen überdurchschnittlichen Intelligenz- und Differenzierungsgrad aufwies. Für die Verbalisierung der in Frage stehenden psychischen Phänomene war dies zweifellos ein Vorteil; ob es möglicherweise auch für die Häufigkeit ihres Auftretens eine Rolle spielte, darüber lassen sich gesicherte Aussagen nicht machen.

An allen Vpn wurde am Tag vor dem ersten Narkoseversuch eine orientierende psychologische Untersuchung mittels einfacher geeichter Fragebogentests vorgenommen. Zur Anwendung kamen die beiden Eysenckschen Fragebogen MMQ (Maudsley Medical Questionnaire) und MPI (Maudsley Personality Inventory). Die Gruppenmittelwerte für die „neurotischen Tendenzen" lagen dabei mit 7,6 im MMQ und mit 17,2 im MPI jeweils im mittleren Normbereich, ebenso auch der Mittelwert für die Extraversionstendenz im MPI (29). Den genannten Testresultaten zufolge war die Gruppe als hinreichend psychisch normal anzusehen.

Die *Versuchsanordnung* war derart, daß jede Vp in unterschiedlicher, statistisch permutierter Reihenfolge jedes der drei Narkotica erhielt, und zwar in den Dosierungen: 4 mg/kg Thiopental, 7 mg/kg Propanidid, 2 mg/kg Ketamine. Der Abstand zwischen zwei Kurznarkosen einer Vp betrug mindestens 6 Tage.

Nach dem Aufwachen und 60 min nach Injektion wurde jede Vp nach Inhalt und Art evtl. aufgetretener traumartiger oder anderer ungewöhnlicher Erlebnisse befragt; wurden solche angegeben, so wurde die Vp 24 Std nach dem Versuch nochmals darüber befragt. Die Doppelblindmethode war dabei gesichert, die Vp und der Befragende wußten nicht, welches Mittel im akuten Versuch gegeben worden war.

Ergebnisse

Die *Ergebnisse* hinsichtlich der Häufigkeit des Auftretens von Narkoseträumen zeigt Tab. 1. Bei unserer Versuchsanordnung fand sich demnach ein deutliches Überwiegen traumartiger Phänomene bei Ketaminenarkosen.

Tabelle 1. *Traumerlebnis in Kurznarkose bei je 18 Vpn*

Nach Thiopental	0 Vp
Nach Propanidid	1 Vp
Nach Ketamine	18 Vpn

Von der *Eigenart* dieser „*Ketamine-Träume*" soll im folgenden die Rede sein. Sie werden überwiegend als „utopisch "(8mal) und „phantastisch" (3mal) gekennzeichnet; „irreal" oder „rätselhaft" sind weitere typische Bezeichnungen. Lediglich 1 Versuchsperson fand das im Traum Erlebte ganz normal und unauffällig.

Das Narkoseerleben bezeichneten 6 Versuchspersonen unserer Gruppe als angenehm, 8 Versuchspersonen als unangenehm, die restlichen 4 Versuchspersonen als neutral (s. Tab. 2). Die lustbetonte Qualität des Erlebens ging dabei in keinem Falle soweit, daß deshalb eine Wiederholung des Versuches gewünscht wurde. Die Traumszenen werden meist ausgesprochen farbig erlebt (14 gegen 4 Versuchspersonen), wobei ein dominierendes Rot am häufigsten angegeben wird.

Tabelle 2. *Kennzeichnung des Narkoseerlebens nach Ketamine (18 Vpn)*

Angenehm	6 Vpn
Unangenehm	8 Vpn
Neutral	4 Vpn

Veränderungen im Zeiterleben, wie sie 11 Versuchspersonen angeben, sind in Tab. 3 dargestellt.

Tabelle 3. *Zeiterleben im Ketamine-Traum (18 Vpn)*

Außerhalb jeder Zeit	7 Vpn
Zeit geht schneller	2 Vpn
Zeit geht langsamer	2 Vpn
Zeit unauffällig	7 Vpn

Das Erleben des Raumes geben 5 Versuchspersonen als verändert an; bei 4 von ihnen spielten die Traumszenen in einem unbegrenzten, endlosen Raum, der jedoch nicht der Weltraum gewesen sei. Vom Weltraum berichtete in unserer Serie lediglich 1 Versuchsperson; sie flog mit einer Rakete auf Besuch zu benachbarten Planeten.

Verfolgt oder bedrängt fühlten sich im Traum 2 der 18 Versuchspersonen. Bei 4 Versuchspersonen wird die Thematik von Tod oder Gestorbensein erwähnt.

Die Angaben unserer Versuchspersonen über ihre Gestimmtheit im Narkosetraum sind in Tab. 4 zusammengestellt.

Tabelle 4. *Stimmungslage im Ketamine-Traum (18 Vpn)*

Heiter, beschwingt	3 Vpn
Herabgestimmt, besorgt	8 Vpn
Ohne Besonderheit	7 Vpn

Sehr häufig treten in den Träumen Bewegungserlebnisse unterschiedlicher Intensität auf. 15 Versuchspersonen sprechen von einem gleichzeitigen Kreisen und Fallen wie auf einer Achterbahn, oder von sausender Fahrt in der Horizontalen, vom Kreisen wie auf einem Karussell oder schließlich auch von einem ruhigen Schweben im Raum.

Bemerkenswert ist, daß nur ein Drittel der Gruppe (6 Versuchspersonen) angibt, während des Träumens die Szenen ganz unbezweifelt für real gehalten zu haben. 12 Versuchspersonen sprechen hingegen davon, daß sie zumindest zeitweise auch im Traum unter dem Eindruck standen, das Erlebte könne doch nicht ganz wirklich sein. Bei gut der Hälfte der *Trauminhalte* (10 Versuchspersonen) läßt sich ein naheliegender persönlicher oder situativer Bezug zum Träumer erkennen. So erlebt eine Versuchsperson im Narkosetraum die Autofahrt zusammen mit ihrem Verlobten noch einmal, die wenige Stunden zuvor stattgefunden hatte. Die Studentin mit dem bereits erwähnten Raketenflug-Traum hatte kurz vorher in der Zeitung den Bericht über den neuesten Raketenstart in den USA gelesen. Eine andere Studentin sieht im Traum – es war gerade in der Vorweihnachtszeit – den Weihnachtsmann mit seinem Gefolge vom Himmel herabkommen. Eine weitere Versuchsperson erlebt sich zu dieser Zeit auf einem riesigen rotierenden Adventskranz sitzend. 3 Versuchspersonen erleben im Narkosetraum, daß irgend ein „Versuch" mit ihnen unternommen werden soll. 4 Versuchspersonen geben an, der Traum habe sie an den letzten James-Bond-Film erinnert.

Einige typische Beispiele noch für andere Trauminhalte: eine Versuchs, person fühlt sich durch ein System langer, farbiger Röhren hindurchgeschleudert; eine andere schwebt in einem unendlichen Raum auf große rote Bogen zu. Eine dritte erlebt sich auf einem Tisch liegend und sieht zu-

11*

wie sie sich bis auf einen Punkt auflöst in lauter Fäden, die dann kunstvolle geometrische Gebilde darstellen.

Insgesamt war aus dem näheren Umgang mit unseren Versuchspersonen der deutliche Eindruck zu gewinnen, daß durchaus Zusammenhänge anzunehmen sind zwischen Persönlichkeitseigenart sowie intrapsychischer Situation einer Versuchsperson und der Besonderheit ihres Narkoseerlebens. So neigten ausgeglichene, syntone und affektiv stabile Versuchspersonen offensichtlich mehr zu ruhigen, „friedlichen" und eher angenehmen Traum- und Aufwacherlebnissen, wohingegen bei unausgeglichenen, affektiv gespannt wirkenden und konfliktbelasteten Versuchspersonen eine Tendenz zu mehr „dramatischen", bedrohlichen und dementsprechend eher negativ getönten Erlebnissen zu beobachten war.

Das von Hemmer [3] bei potenzierter Narkose beschriebene besondere Traummotiv eines Überwältigtwerdens von fremdartiger Wirklichkeit, gegen die man sich nicht wehren kann, wird auch von unseren Versuchspersonen vielfach angegeben.

Die *Aufwachphase* verläuft bei Ketamine deutlich protrahiert. Es vergehen im Regelfall 30–60 min vom Narkosebeginn an, ehe der Proband konstant wieder bei völlig klarem Bewußtsein ist, in 3 Fällen dauerte es bis 75 min, in einem Fall rund 90 min. Gut 80% der Versuchspersonen (15) geben einen wellenförmigen Verlauf dieser Phase an mit zeitweiligem Zurücksinken in schlafnahe Bereiche, wobei 9 Versuchspersonen eine Fortsetzung ihres Narkosetraums angeben. Das *Übergangsstadium* zwischen narkotischer Schlafverfassung und Wachbewußtsein wird von der Mehrzahl unserer Versuchspersonen (14 von 18) als unangenehm empfunden. In dieser hypnoiden Grenzverfassung fehlen dem Probanden augenscheinlich noch die adäquaten Orientierungsmaßstäbe zur Gestaltung des Wahrnehmungsfeldes und zum Erfassen der realen Umweltsituation. Er ist daher während dieser Zeit besonders leicht irritierbar und offenbar auch in gewisser Weise disponiert zu abnormen Reaktions- und Erlebensweisen. Aus diesem Grund sollten Stimulationen jeder Art in diesem Stadium unterbleiben, da sie die genannten Reaktionen zu provozieren geeignet sind. Es ist durchaus möglich, daß auch die mit unserer Versuchsanordnung unvermeidlich verbundene Stimulation (wie die regelmäßige Analgesieprüfung und Befragung) hier einiges Zusätzliche provoziert hat.

Unmittelbar nach dem Erwachen ist die Sprache noch lallend und undeutlich artikuliert, vielfach werden zunächst nur wenige Worte oder Redewendungen perseverierend wiederholt.

Eine der ersten Äußerungen ist meist, man komme sich so beschwipst vor wie von einem starken Rausch. Es folgen dann Klagen über verschwommenes Sehen, bisweilen auch Doppeltsehen und über die Schwere der Glieder. Von Schwindelgefühlen und von einem Schwanken der Umgebung ist ebenfalls häufig die Rede.

Die Hälfte der Versuchspersonen (9) berichtet von Wahrnehmungs-
anomalien wie Veränderungen der optischen Größenverhältnisse und
Verzerrungen der Perspektive, sowie darüber, daß Personen und Gegenstände der Umgebung ihnen eigentümlich fremd und unwirklich er-
schienen.

6 Versuchspersonen, ein Drittel der Gruppe, erleben den eigenen
Körper als verändert, entstellt oder entfremdet. Hierher gehören Äußerungen wie: Kopf und Extremitäten seien jetzt ganz eckig und kantig, man
fühle sich wie gestaucht und in die Breite gegangen, die Finger seien ganz
dünn wie Spinnen geworden und ähnliches mehr.

In 2 Fällen werden Sinnestäuschungen der Körperfühlssphäre angegeben: ein Student glaubt mittels der angelegten EKG-Schnüre elektrisiert zu
werden, und eine Studentin hatte das Gefühl, ihr Körper werde ausein-
andergezerrt wie auf einer mittelalterlichen Streckfolter.

Eine passagere Situationsverkennung in der Aufwachphase war bei
Versuchsperson 7 zu beobachten: wegen des vermeintlichen Schwankens
der Umgebung glaubte sie sich in einer fliegenden Weltraumkapsel zu
befinden; das leise Surren des EKG-Schreibers hielt sie dabei für das Flug-
geräusch.

Ebenfalls zu einer vorübergehenden Situationsverkennung kam es bei
Versuchsperson 15, sie glaubte, zur weiteren Behandlung auf eine andere
Station verlegt worden zu sein. Hierbei spielte ein abnormes Bedeutungs-
erleben für sie eine Rolle: sie hatte an ihrem Arm einen Blutstropfen gesehen, der vom Entfernen der Injektionskanüle herrührte und das hatte bei ihr
zu der Vorstellung geführt, der Versuch sei schiefgegangen, sie sei nun
schwer verletzt behandlungsbedürftig.

In ähnlicher Weise bestand bei Versuchsperson 17 zeitweilig die Vorstellung, der Versuch sei bei ihm mißlungen, die Ärzte stünden jetzt ratlos
um ihn herum, da er für sein Leben eine geistige Störung davon zurück-
behalten werde.

Wie bereits erwähnt, gibt die Hälfte unserer Gruppe (9 Versuchspersonen) während der Aufwachphase hypnagoge visuelle Erlebnisse an im
Sinne einer Fortsetzung ihres Narkosetraums, zumeist bei geschlossenen
Augen. Formal wird man hier – in der Terminologie der deutschen Psychopathologie – am ehesten von pseudohalluzinatorischem Erleben zu reden
haben, da der leibhaftige Realitäts- und Wahrnehmungscharakter der echten
Halluzinationen diesem Erleben weitgehend fehlt.

Es bleibt festzustellen, daß die Versuchspersonen sich ohne Ausnahme
von den genannten Erlebnissen distanzieren, sobald sie anhaltend die volle
Bewußtseinsklarheit wiedererlangt haben und der Prozeß der Reorientierung abgeschlossen ist.

Die Befragung 24 Std nach dem Versuch ergab in keinem Falle zusätzlich erinnerte Erlebnisse; das Gesamterleben wird dagegen jetzt besser

geordnet und zusammenhängender dargestellt. Nach dem Urteil vieler Versuchspersonen sei das Narkoseerleben in der Rückerinnerung noch am ehesten einem eindrücklichen Schlaftraum zu vergleichen.

Zusammenfassung

Anläßlich einer vergleichenden Untersuchung von Kurznarkosen mit Thiopental, Propanidid und Ketamine an 18 gesunden Versuchspersonen wurde das Auftreten traumartiger Phänomene bei den Narkosen registriert.

Im Rahmen unserer Versuchsanordnung ergab sich dabei ein deutliches Überwiegen von Narkoseträumen nach Ketamine (Thiopental:Propanidid: Ketamine = 0:1:18). Einzelne Qualitäten der Ketamine-Träume und Beispiele ihrer Inhalte werden dargestellt, anschließend wird von abnormen Erlebnissen während der Aufwachphase berichtet. Von jeglicher Stimulation in dieser Phase wird abgeraten, da sich die Versuchsperson darin meist in besonders labiler psychischer Verfassung befinden. Ein psychodynamischer Zusammenhang zwischen Persönlichkeitseigenart und Besonderheiten des Narkoseerlebens wird in vielen Fällen als wahrscheinlich angenommen. Den Gesamtversuch überdauernde abnorme psychische Phänomene sind in keinem Falle beobachtet worden. Die Versuchspersonen distanzierten sich ausnahmslos von ihren Erlebnissen, sobald sie die volle Bewußtseinsklarheit wiedererlangt hatten.

Summary

The occurrence of dreamlike phenomena during anaesthesia with Thiopentone, Propanidid and Ketamine was studied in 18 healthy volunteers.

Dreams occurred significantly predominant in Ketamine-anaesthesia (Thiopentone:Propanidid:Ketamine = 0:1:18).

Some qualities and contents of these dreams are described. The abnormal experiences during the phase of awakening from Ketamine-anaesthesia prohibit stimulation at this stage. A psychodynamic correlation between personality and peculary of the experiences in anaesthesia seems probable. There were no abnormal psychic phenomena lasting longer than the experiment.

All volunteers renounced their experiences when fully awake.

Literatur

1. DOMINO, E. F., et al.: Human pharmacology of CI-581. Fed. Proc. **24**, 268 (1965).
2. — — Pharmacologic effects of CI-581. Clin. Pharmacol. Ther. **6**, 279 (1965).
3. HEMMER, R.: Beobachtungen über psychische Veränderungen unter potenzierter Narkose. Zbl. Neurochir. **13**, 360 (1953).
4. JASPERS, K.: Allgemeine Psychopathologie. 6. Aufl. Berlin-Göttingen-Heidelberg: Springer 1953.
5. LEUNER, H.: Die experimentelle Psychose. Berlin-Göttingen-Heidelberg: Springer 1962.

Psychische und vestibuläre Effekte von Ketamine

Von **A. Benke** und **W. Unger**

Aus der II. Chir. Abt. der Krankenanstalt Rudolfstiftung, Wien
(Vorstand: Prof. Dr. P. Kyrle)

Wir haben CI-581 für 96 Narkosen bei Erwachsenen verwendet. Eine psychotische Symptomatologie haben wir bei 27 Fällen beobachtet. Es handelte sich dabei um postnarkotisch auftretende Symptome psychopathologischer Natur, die zum Großteil in der Zeitspanne zwischen Ansprechbarkeit und vollständiger Orientierung auftraten, oft nur durch mehr oder weniger intensive Exploration aufgedeckt werden konnten und nach Eintritt der vollständigen Orientierung bis auf eine Ausnahme wieder zurückgingen. Es blieb nur eine unangenehme Erinnerung. Bei der einen Ausnahme handelte es sich um ein stundenlang anhaltendes stupuröses Zustandsbild, das sich schließlich aber ebenfalls restlos zurückbildete. Wir haben entsprechend der Häufigkeit verschiedener Symptome 4 Gruppen gebildet:

1. Perseverationssymptome: 11mal
2. Depersonalisationserlebnisse: 10mal
3. Unruhe (als Ausdruck von Angst): 13mal
4. In dieser Gruppe werden diejenigen Phänomene zusammengefaßt, die sich nicht zwanglos in die Gruppen 1–3 einordnen lassen:

retrograde Amnesie	2mal	Halluzinationen	2mal
Logorrhoe	1mal	Artikulationsstörungen	1mal
lautes Schreien (Enthemmung)	4mal	Stupor	1mal

Zum Teil traten bei einem Patienten Symptome von zwei oder mehr Gruppen auf, so waren z. B. Perseverations- und Depersonalisationssymptome 3mal bei ein und demselben Patienten zu beobachten, Unruhe, Depersonalisation und Logorrhoe bei einem Patienten usw.

Nun einige erklärende Worte und charakteristische Beispiele zu den einzelnen Gruppen:

1. Zur Perseveration. Sie wird psychiatrisch zu den „formalen Denkstörungen" gezählt, also zu jenen Störungen, zu denen z. B. auch die Sperrung, Umständlichkeit, Denkhemmung, Ideenflucht, Zerfahrenheit etc. gehört. Die Perseveration ist ein Kernsymptom der Cerebralsklerose und der epileptischen Wesensveränderung – eine Großhirnstörung, deren leitendes Symptom das Haftenbleiben an einem Gedankengang, das zähflüssige, träge und einfallsarme Denken ist. Die Patienten fragen unaufhörlich immer wieder dasselbe: Bin ich schon operiert? Ist schon alles vorbei? Wo bin ich? etc.

2. Zur Depersonalisation. Dabei handelt es sich um Entfremdungserlebnisse des eigenen Seelenlebens, des Körpers oder einzelner Körperteile. Sie gehört zu den subjektiven Persönlichkeitsstörungen, d. h. zu den Störungen des Ichbewußtseins. Das eigene Ich oder einzelne Körperteile erscheinen fremd, irreal. Depersonalisationserlebnisse kommen in klassischer Form bei der Schizophrenie, ferner bei der endogenen Depression, der Psychopathie und physiologisch im Zustand der hochgradigen Ermüdung vor. Wir hörten z. B.: Die Hände gehören nicht mir; ich kann mich nicht rühren; ich habe ein eigentümliches Gefühl in den Armen und Beinen; mein Mund ist geschwollen, fremd, gehört nicht mir; etc.

3. Zur Unruhe (als Ausdruck der Angst). Sie wurde von uns 13 mal beobachtet. Ist an sich kein rein psychiatrisches Symptom, sondern bildet den Übergang zu physiologischen Reaktionen. Angst kommt nun bei diversen Psychosen gehäuft vor und bildet oft ein Kernsymptom (Schizophrenie, Depression etc.).

Bei genauerer Analyse zeigt sich, daß die Angst bei unseren Fällen meist mit Träumen, Depersonalisationserlebnissen, Logorrhoe, Übelkeit, Erbrechen, Schwindel, lautem Schreien als Zeichen der Enthemmung, einer weinerlichen Stimmungslage – die Patientin verlangt ihr Kind – gekoppelt war.

4. Sammelgruppe. 2 mal sahen wir *Halluzinationen*; Einer sieht Besucher (Verwandte) mit übergroßen Köpfen – Makropsien, wie man sie auch bei occipitalen Herden findet; eine Patientin glaubt, ein Schnellzug kommt auf sie zu und nimmt sie mit – also eher ein Zeitrafferphänomen.

Logorrhoe – ein Enthemmungsphänomen – wurde einmal beobachtet; stundenlang dauernder Stupor – ein Hemmungsphänomen – trat ebenfalls 1 mal auf; lautes *Schreien am Ende der Operation* – wieder ein Enthemmungsphänomen – beobachteten wir 4 mal; es war 2 mal mit einem Traum – Schwesterntanz in der Feuerhalle, Kampf mit einem Hund mit anschließendem Tod, gekoppelt; 2 mal konnten wir keine „Gründe" für das Gebrüll am Ende der Operation erheben.

Sowohl in Gruppe 3 als auch in Gruppe 4 mußten wir jeweils auf *Träume* verweisen. An sich stellt der Traum einen Schutzmechanismus der Psyche gegenüber einer Störung des normalen Schlafes dar. Uns wurde 7 mal von Träumen berichtet. Die Träume waren zum Teil angenehm, meistens jedoch unangenehm, z. T. indifferenter Natur, 2 mal sexuell gefärbt. 1 Patient träumte indifferent vom Operieren; einer träumte vom „perversen Pflege-personal im Saal;" einer von kleinen Figuren, die ihm drohten – also Mikropsien, wie man sie auch beim Delirium tremens beobachten kann –; einer träumte von einer Feuerhalle, in der die Schwestern als Flammen um ihn herumtanzten – also ein Traum im Sinne eines phantastischen Deliriums, wie wir es z. B. bei der Epilepsie finden –; einer hat einen Kampf mit einem Hund zu bestehen, unterliegt und stirbt; einer hatte einen sexuell gefärbten Traum und einer träumte schließlich angenehm von seiner Familie ohne Details angeben zu können.

Zusammenfassend kann man sagen, daß psychopathologische Phänomene der verschiedensten Natur durch das Präparat erzeugt werden können. Wir haben völlig konträre Symptome wie Angst – Euphorie (angenehme Träume), Hemmung und Enthemmung (Stupor einerseits – Logorrhoe und lautes Schreien andererseits), Makropsien und Mikropsien (kleine Figuren auf der einen Seite und übergroße Köpfe auf der anderen Seite), phantastische und triviale deliriumähnliche Zustände (Schwesterntanz in der Feuerhalle und Figuren, die den Patienten bedrohen).

Wir glauben nicht, daß diese Symptome durch das verwendete Succinylcholinchlorid oder durch das gleichzeitig verabreichte Lachgas verursacht wurden.

Vestibuläre Symptome. Störungen im Bereich des VIII. Hirnnervs führen subjektiv zu Schwindel, objektiv zu Gleichgewichtsstörungen, Schwanken beim Stehen, Abweichungen von der eingeschlagenen Richtung beim Gehen (besonders beim Augenschluß), Vorbeizeigen beim BARANY-schen Zeigeversuch und zu Nystagmus. Da es sich bei uns um Patienten unmittelbar nach einer Narkose handelte, haben wir uns auf die subjektive Angabe des Schwindelgefühls und des „Brechreizes" sowie auf die objektive Feststellung des Nystagmus und Erbrechens beschränkt. Zur Abgrenzung des „oculären Schwindels" gegenüber dem echten, vestibulären Drehschwindel begnügten wir uns mit den Angaben der Patienten hinsichtlich aufgetretener Sehstörungen wie Doppelbilder, verschwommenes Sehen etc. Wir beobachteten:

Schwindel	59mal
Nystagmus	15mal
Sehstörungen	65mal
Brechreiz	40mal
Erbrechen	17mal

Sehstörungen gekoppelt mit Schwindel waren in 54 Fällen zu beobachten. Wir hatten also bei den 15 Fällen mit Nystagmus zweifellos einen echten Drehschwindel durch Irritation des vestibulären Systems vorliegen, da es sich um keinen blickparetischen Nystagmus handelte. Die restlichen Angaben hinsichtlich des Symptoms „Schwindel" müssen aber auf die häufigen Sehstörungen bezogen und als „oculärer Schwindel" als Folge von latenten Augenmuskellähmungen gedeutet werden.

Diskussion

Langrehr: Die Problematik dieses Stoffes könnte bequem einen Tag füllen. Ich möchte nur eine einzige Bemerkung zu den Phänomenen, welche sich in der Zeit vom 1. verbalen Kontakt bis zur völligen Orientierung in Raum, Körper und Zeit abspielen, machen. Diese Zeit ist von Nachschlafintervallen unterbrochen. Auch Konvergenzstörungen sind stark ausgeprägt. Ehe man Terminologien wie „klein"- und „groß"-Sehen verwendet, muß man natürlich die Konvergenzstörung ausschließen. Der ganze Körper bietet ein Gefühl als ob man eine „Lokalanaesthesie" des gesamten Körpers hätte. Weil der analgetische Effekt diesen ersten verbalen Kontaktmoment überdauert, sind Bemerkungen wie „wo sind meine Hände", „wo ist mein Mund", „ich habe ein Gefühl wie Schaum und Pappe" als Versuch des Patienten zu deuten, sein völlig irritiertes Körpergefühl zu interpretieren. Ehe man psychiatrische Formulierungen wie „Verfremdung" oder ähnliches für diese Erscheinungen verwendet, muß man berücksichtigen, daß hier eine ganz außerordentlich tiefgreifende Störung der normalen Afferenzen auf den Menschen vorliegt. Berücksichtigen Sie dazu bitte auch, daß der Patient im Gegensatz zu allen anderen mir bekannten Narkoseformen ein erinnerungsfähiges Rest- oder Kleinerlebnis bei dieser Narkose hat. Wenn Sie ihn dann in der Aufwachzeit mit Untersuchungen irritieren oder den Afferenzeinstrom, so wie es schon für das Sernyl früher gemacht wurde, sehr stark werden lassen, dann beobachten Sie bei diesen Patienten die merkwürdigsten Effekte. Es liegen also eine Reihe von tatsächlichen Vorgängen vor, die eine große Zahl der Antworten, die auf Befragungen gegeben werden, zwanglos erklären. Interessant sind für mich eigentlich nur solche Patienten, die Tage oder doch viele Stunden später noch kleine oder große Köpfe sehen. Ich weiß nicht, ob es sich dann um ein psychiatrisches Phänomen handelt.

Wir haben in unseren 1300 Fällen solche Phänomene nicht gesehen, allerdings sind wir keine Psychiater. Gibt es Berichte über echte Halluziantionen, über echte psychiatrische Phänomene?

Kugler: Vom psychiatrischen Standpunkt aus wird man sich außerordentlich hüten, den Terminus „Halluzinationen" oder irgend ein anderes psychiatrisches Phänomen mit diesen Dingen zu verbinden. Herr NOLTE hat vollkommen recht gehabt, wenn er sich darauf beschränkte zu sagen: „Wir haben es mit pseudohalluzinatorischen, periodischen Erscheinungen zu tun, die eng gekoppelt sind mit all dem, was wir an funktionellen Abläufen finden."

Es gibt zwar gewisse Dinge wie Metamorphopsie oder Heteropsie, – diese haben mit der Konvergenz nichts mehr zu tun –. Das sind aber für mich Phänomene, die aus echten mnestischen Residuen stammen und durch Enthemmung aktiviert werden.

Das ist genau dasselbe wie die Anosognosie und die Körper-Schema-Störung, die bei der parietalen Funktionsstörung eintritt und die der nach der Narkose Erwachende nunmehr erlebt als Phänomen wie „durch Röhren kriechen", „ins All geschossen sein" oder „irgendwo schweben". Das alles ist nur erklärbar im Zusammenhang mit der Abnahme der peripheren Afferenzen, die in erster Linie die taktilen, propriozeptiven und akustischen Systeme betreffen. Die Leute brüllen, und man sieht eine verminderte Leistung der Schallwahrnehmung. Was sie visuell tun, weiß ich nicht. Das konnten wir nicht prüfen. Es ist aber anzunehmen, daß auch hier einige vertiginöse und vestibuläre Störungen damit verbunden sind; teils als Abnahme der Erregbarkeitsschwelle, teils aber auch als Enthemmung und Aktivationssymptome, die in zentralen Regionen aktiviert sein müssen.

Corssen: Wir haben schon sehr früh aufgrund unserer Untersuchungen an Gefangenen ähnliche Symptome beschrieben und waren uns darüber klar, daß die Droge psychotrope Effekte hat. Wir haben deshalb Patienten im Erwachsenenalter vorher genau untersucht, bevor wir CI-581 gegeben haben. Seit etwa $1^1/_2$ Jahren haben wir in Michigan überhaupt keine richtigen halluzinatorischen oder ähnliche psychotische Zustände mehr gesehen, weil wir vermieden haben, die Droge Patienten zu geben, von denen wir wissen, daß sie eine Tendenz zu solchen psychotischen Symptomen haben. Mit anderen Worten, wir haben seit dieser Zeit Ketamine auf die pädiatrische Anaesthesie beschränkt. Hierbei haben wir das Alter von 14 Jahren als die Grenze angenommen, von der ab wir sehr vorsichtig sind, Ketamine anzuwenden. Nur in der Behandlung der schwerverbrannten Patienten haben wir Ausnahmen gemacht und konnten merkwürdigerweise sehr wenig oder gar nichts in bezug auf psychotische Zustände bei Erwachsenen sehen. Dr. Domino glaubt, daß das mit der Verminderung der Afferenz bei diesen Patienten zusammenhängt, denn es handelt sich um bis zu 85% drittgradig Verbrannte. Diese Patienten haben erhebliche Einbußen in der Möglichkeit, afferente Impulse aufzunehmen. Wir haben bei über 1000 Kindern in den letzten $1^1/_2$ Jahren nur dreimal eine sehr kurz dauernde halluzinatorische Reaktion festgestellt und sind mit diesem Ergebnis natürlich sehr zufrieden. Ich möchte noch eine Mitteilung erwähnen, die mir Dr. Ronald Stephen in Dallas/Texas vor etwa 14 Tagen machte: 2 seiner Assistenten hatten LSD genommen um die psychotischen Reaktionen auf diese Droge an sich selbst zu studieren. Später ließen sich dieselben Assistenten 1 mg/lb CI-581 intravenös spritzen. Es war dann sehr interessant, daß die halluzinatorischen oder pseudo-halluzinatorischen Zustände, die beide Assistenten mit LSD erlebten, nach CI-581 nicht auftraten, daß aber

frühzeitige Stimulationen nach CI-581 in beiden Fällen einen Psychose-
ähnlichen Zustand auslösen konnten, die aber nichts mit dem von LSD
ausgelösten Zustand zu tun hatten. Ich weise auf das Ergebnis dieses Selbst-
versuches besonders deshalb hin, weil ein sehr bekannter amerikanischer
Anaesthesiologe kürzlich in der „Medical World News" eine Zusammen-
fassung der Forschungsergebnisse des Jahres 1967 gegeben hat und hierbei
leider ausführte, daß die Untersuchungen mit CI-581 daran erinnern, daß
wir im Zeitalter des LSD leben und wahrscheinlich hier irgendwelche
Zusammenhänge bestehen.

Allgemeine Erfahrungen mit Ketamine als Einleitungsnarkotikum

Von **C. Zegveld**

Anaesthesiol. Abt., Centraal Ziekenhuis Alkmaar, Niederlande

Ketamine haben wir ausschließlich zur Einleitung von Narkosen, d. h. durch einmalige Injektion angewendet. Die Ketamine-Dosis betrug stets 100 mg unabhängig vom Körpergewicht des Patienten. Die Injektionsgeschwindigkeit wurde möglichst konstant gehalten. Demzufolge lagen die Dosierungen zwischen 0,68 und 2 mg/kg/min. Mit dieser Versuchsanordnung wurden 75 Patienten untersucht. Es wurden Kurettagen und große Abdominaleingriffe durchgeführt. Die Zeitdauer des Eingriffe war daher verschieden und lag zwischen 5 und 97 min.

Nach der intravenösen Ketamine-Injektion, die man mit der Verabreichung einer Einschlafdosis eines Barbiturates vergleichen könnte, wurde die Narkose in gewohnter Weise fortgesetzt und kein weiteres Adjuvans verabreicht. Wie immer dienten Blutdruck, Puls, Atmung, Hauttemperatur und Schweißabsonderung als Kriterien für die Beurteilung der Narkosetiefe.

Folgende Wirkungen des Ketamine wurden beurteilt:

Analgesie
muskelerschlaffende Wirkung
neurovegetative Stabilisierung
Herabsetzung der respiratorischen Leistung

Weiterhin wurde das Zusammenwirken von Ketamine mit:

Analgetica
Anaesthetica und
Muskelrelaxantien

sowie etwaige Nebenwirkungen und mögliche Inkompatibilitäten beobachtet.

Die ausschließlich durch Ketamine bedingte *Schlafdauer* konnten wir nicht ermitteln, weil sofort nach der Einleitungsphase immer ein Lachgas-Sauerstoff-Gemisch verabreicht wurde.

Ob die *Prämedikation* auf die Wirkung des Ketamines einen Einfluß ausübt, hat sich aus diesen Versuchen nicht ergeben. Im Vergleich mit anderen Narkoseeinleitungen hat sich jedoch keine einzige zusätzliche

Schwierigkeit ergeben, die darauf hindeuten könnte, daß die übliche Prämedikation zu hoch oder zu niedrig dosiert war und daß sie anders zusammengesetzt sein sollte.

Es hat sich herausgestellt, daß – mit einigen Ausnahmen – die optimale Dosierung bei 1,5 mg/kg liegt. Diese Menge wurde in 1 min verabreicht. Bei dieser Dosierung tritt die *Analgesie* schon nach durchschnittlich 40 sec ein, d. h. also, wenn 1 mg/kg verabreicht wurde.

Der *Schlaf* tritt durchschnittlich nach 45 sec ein, also beinahe gleichzeitig mit der völligen Analgesie.

Die erreichte Analgesie ist ausgezeichnet; während der ersten 15–20 min werden afferente Schmerzreize offenbar überhaupt nicht mehr zentral wahrgenommen. Reaktionen auf den operativen Eingriff fehlen in fast allen Fällen sowohl motorisch als auch vegetativ vollkommen. Deshalb ist es merkwürdig, daß die Lidschluß- und Larynxreflexe bestehen bleiben. Dagegen fehlt der Hustenreflex, wenn der Patient ohne Verabreichung von Relaxantien endotracheal intubiert wird, was meist sehr gut möglich ist.

Diese Eigenschaften lassen vermuten, daß Ketamine offenbar bestimmte Thalamus-Regionen oder aber die afferente Reizleitung des Trigeminus erst in höherer Dosierung beeinflußt. Dadurch unterscheidet sich die Einleitung mit Ketamine deutlich von der Einleitung mit einem Barbiturat.

Weiterhin wurden folgende Unterschiede zu anderen Narkosemitteln beobachtet: Der auffallendste ist wohl die starke und sehr rasch nach der Einleitung mit Ketamine eintretende *Blutdrucksteigerung*. Die Blutdruckerhöhung bleibt 5–20 min bestehen um danach ganz allmählich zu normalen Werten zurückzukehren. Unter dem Einfluß von Halothan erfolgt diese Senkung schneller, oft bis zu Werten, die unter dem Ausgangsniveau liegen. Die gleiche plötzliche Steigerung zeigt auch die *Pulsfrequenz*. Die Wiederkehr zu normalen Werten erfolgt schneller als es beim Blutdruck der Fall ist. Diese plötzliche Steigerung der Pulsfrequenz und des Blutdruckes ist nicht Ausdruck einer vegetativen Reaktion auf Schmerzreize, denn sie findet auch statt, wenn noch nicht operiert wird und selbst, wenn noch nicht endotracheal intubiert worden ist. Ein Nachteil der Blutdrucksteigerung ist die erschwerte Blutstillung im Operationsfeld. Die Normalisierung des Blutdruckes und der Pulsfrequenz erfolgt in der Regel gleichzeitig mit dem Ende der Analgesie. Zu dieser Zeit ist die Verabreichung eines Analgeticums oft notwendig.

Hinsichtlich der *Atmung* ist der Unterschied zur Einleitung mit Barbituraten deutlich, indem eine Atemdepression nicht zu beobachten ist. Gelegentlich kommt während einer sehr kurzen Periode eine vorübergehende Bradypnoe vor.

In unserer Beobachtungsreihe wurden einige Appendektomien ohne Relaxantien durchgeführt. Bei Operationen, die üblicherweise eine Curarisierung erfordern, wurden geringere Curaremengen verwendet als bei herkömmlichen Anaesthesieverfahren. Das gleiche gilt für die Dosierung von Analgetica. Trotz ausreichender Muskelerschlaffung und Analgesie war eine endotracheale Intubation nicht notwendig. Ebenso war das Einlegen eines Guedel-Tubus nicht erforderlich, da die Muskulatur der Zunge und des Mundbodens einen Tonus beibehält, der zur Sicherung freier Atemwege ausreicht. Auch die ausreichende Ventilation ist bei dieser geringen Curarisierung immer gesichert. so daß die Erhaltung der spontanen Atmung zur Routine dieser Narkosetechnik gehört.

Neurovegetative Reaktionen wie Schwitzen und plötzliche Änderungen der Pulsfrequenz, des Blutdrucks und der peripheren Durchblutung sind bei einer guten Technik ebenso selten wie bei anderen Methoden, so daß in dieser Hinsicht keine Gegenindikation von Ketamine festgestellt werden konnte.

Es ist uns nicht bekannt, ob es Medikamente gibt, die mit Ketamine nicht vereinbar sind.

Während der Aufwachphase befinden sich die Patienten oft in einem merkwürdigen Zustand, der bereits wiederholt beschrieben wurde. Dieser subpsychotische Zustand tritt nicht auf, wenn die Kombinationsnarkose relativ lange Zeit gedauert hat. In diesen Fällen kann die Aufwachphase verlängert sein und läuft dann ohne psychische Nebenerscheinungen ab. Hieraus könnte man schließen, daß Ketamine für die psychischen Nebenwirkungen verantwortlich ist. Die Metaboliten dieses Mittels können in einem späteren Stadium wenigstens im psychogenen Bereich keine Wirkung mehr entfalten.

Der schnelle Abbau und die rasche Inaktivierung des Ketamines sind aus dem baldigen Erwachen nach einer Operation von langer Dauer erkennbar. Hat der Eingriff hingegen nur kurze gedauert, so werden, von dem Zeitpunkt der Injektion an gerechnet, dennoch immer 20–30 min vergehen, ehe der Patient wieder ansprechbar ist. Eine völlige zeitliche und örtliche Orientierung und eine adäquate Reaktion erfordern manchmal einige Stunden.

Oft kommt zwischen dem Aufwachen und der Reorientierung eine Phase vor, während der dem Patienten kurzfristig übel ist und er sich manchmal ein wenig erbricht.

Es ist auffallend, daß die Analgesie postoperativ derart gut ist, daß im größeren Teil unserer Fälle ein Analgeticum überhaupt nicht oder nur sehr spät nach dem Eingriff gegeben werden mußte. Dies ist ein sehr überzeugender Unterschied zu anderen Narkoseformen.

Zusammenfassung

Wir können feststellen, daß Ketamine als Einleitungsnarkoticum ebenso brauchbar ist wie jedes andere von uns dafür verwendete Narkosemittel. Die Analgesie ist so ausgezeichnet, daß wir glauben, daß gerade auf diesem Gebiet weitere Untersuchungen gerechtfertigt sind.

Some Clinical Considerations about the Use of Ketamine

By **L. Lecron**

C. G. T. R. Montignies-Le-Tilleul, Belgien

We used Ketamine in not more than 150 patients. In the following we present our small experiences using this drugs in different techniques.

Ketamine is not a short acting anesthetic like methohexital or propanidid, as well by the duration of the anesthesia, particular of the intramuscular application, as by the recovery time.

Indications for the use of Ketamine are extremely wide. The product has no antagonism to other drugs. Particular adventages of Ketamine we found in the following indications:

1. Induction of anesthesia in children may be done without danger by intramuscular injection. In these cases no respiratory depression occurs. The psychic trauma may be avoided, mainly in childhood, when preoperatively preparations are running in unfamiliar surroundings.

The dose of 20 mg/10 lbs gives an excellent induction of a halothane-anesthesia. The intramuscular method with advised doses has only indications for interventions longer than 30 min, because the recovery time is prolonged although without danger of cardio-respiratory depression.

2. In addition of local and regional anesthesia reduced doses, either intravenously or intramusculary, according to the time required for the operation, give the patient a state of comfortable analgesia.

3. In general anesthesia in adults, we combined Ketamine with neuroleptanalgesia: for short interventions we used small doses of fentanyl and droperidol. In addition we gave Ketamine. During a 30-min-period for laparotomie we needed 4 ml Thalamonal and 60–70 mg of Ketamine intravenously. After endotracheal intubation of the curarisized patients anesthesia was maintained by spontanous inhalation of nitrous-oxyde-oxygen.

For anesthesia lasting longer than 1 h, 7–8 ml Thalamonal and 40 mg of Ketamine intravenously are convenient. There seems to be an interesting pharmacological synergia: neuroleptanalgesia has a moderate effect on the tachycardia and bloodpressure-rise caused by Ketamine. We used reduced doses of both, Thalamonal and Ketamine. Ketamine eliminates, besides other things, the trouble in particular patients by consciousness during the operation.

We did not observe hallucinations in our patients. Nevertheless, we restrict the use of Ketamine on drinkers. There we noted in some cases a state of agitation and excitation, which required medication with Valium in 3 cases.

We observed 1 case with tachycardia (frequency 200/min.) in a 6 years old child during surgery of an inguinal hernia. Not any particular reason was found; the tachycardia stopped spontaneously.

As mentioned above Ketamine is, according to our short experience an anesthetic of choice. The particular adventages are the absence of respiratory and cardiovascular depression.

It would be of high interest to determine the blood-pressure-rise and tachycardia effected by these drugs. Intrinsic factors or mechanisms which have an adrenergic stimulatory effect could be the reason of these unconvenient side-effects.

Die Ketamine und Barbiturate.
Vergleichende klinische Beobachtungen

Von **P. Kurka**

Aus der II. chirurg. Abteilung des Wilhelminenspitals, Wien
(Vorstand: Doz. Dr. K. Holub)

Um zwei Narkosemittel klinisch miteinander vergleichen zu können, erscheint es vorteilhaft, wenn man diese Narkosemittel bei derselben Operation erprobt. Besonders die Appendektomie als Routineoperation ist bei gleichen Voraussetzungen dazu geeignet. Nach Anlegen einer Gordh-Nadel wurde das Narkoticum, also Thiopentobarbital oder das Phencyclidinepräparat CI-581, intravenös gespritzt. Schon von diesem Augenblick an kann man einen deutlichen Unterschied zwischen der Wirkung dieser beiden Präparate beobachten. Während die mit dem Thiobarbiturat narkotisierten Patienten ruhig und ohne Excitationserscheinungen einschlafen und die Atmung allmählich abzuflachen beginnt, beobachten wir bei der Narkose mit CI-581 sehr bald eine gewisse Erstarrung des Gesichtes des Patienten und das baldige Auftreten eines mehr oder minder ausgeprägten Nystagmus. Bei der von uns verwendeten Dosierung, nämlich 2 mg pro Kilogramm Körpergewicht, war bei relativ langsamer Injektion der Gesamtmenge in etwa 2 min nur sehr selten eine echte Atemdepression zu beobachten. Schon in diesem Stadium also sind die wesentlichen Unterschiede zwischen den beiden Narkosemitteln deutlich zu erkennen. Bei der Barbituratnarkose Lähmung und das Fehlen zentraler Erregungssymptome, bei der Anaesthesie mit CI-581 Symptome, die der Neuroleptanalgesie ähneln. Dieser grundsätzliche Unterschied ist auch während der ganzen Operation zu beobachten. Bei der dissoziativen Anaesthesie mit CI-581 bleibt der Tonus der quergestreiften Muskulatur nicht nur erhalten, er scheint auch zeitweilig erhöht. Während bei der Barbituratanaesthesie ein stärkerer Muskeltonus sowie das Bewegen von Händen und Füßen als Symptome einer zu flachen Anaesthesie angesehen werden können, kann man im Toleranzstadium der Dissoziationsnarkose nicht selten Muskelzuckungen an den Extremitäten, motorische Unruhe und auch Kopfbewegungen beobachten. Auch in ihrer Wirkung auf das vegetative Nervensystem unterscheiden sich die beiden erwähnten Narkotica grundsätzlich. Während den Thiobarbituraten eine Erregbarkeit des parasympathischen Nervensystems nachgewiesen wurde, schließen mehrere Autoren aus der zu beobachtenden Puls- und Blutdrucksteigerung nach CI-581 auf eine sympathicomimetische Nebenwirkung dieses Präparates. Sofort nach Beginn der Injektion von CI-581 kommt es zu einer Blutdrucksteigerung, die bei unseren jugendlichen Patienten je nach Ausgangslage etwa 20 mmHg betragen hat. Parallel dazu ist ein leichtes Ansteigen der Pulsfrequenz sowie eine Blässe des Gesichtes auf Grund der peripheren Konstriktion der Gefäße zu beobachten. Das Maximum der Steigerung von Blutdruck und Pulsfrequenz ist nach etwa 5 min erreicht und nach etwa 20–30 min sind diese Symptome wieder abgeklungen. Will man eine entsprechende Narkosetiefe für die Zeit der Appendektomie aufrecht erhalten, ist man gezwungen, in bestimmten Zeitabständen kleinere Barbituratmengen nachzuinjizieren, um den durch Abbau und Abflutung gesunkenen Barbituratspiegel im Blut aufrecht zu erhalten. Hingegen war es nur einmal nötig, die von uns gegebene Einleitungsdosis von 2 mg CI-581 pro Kilogramm Körpergewicht durch eine Nachinjektion zu ergänzen.

Selbstverständlich unterscheiden sich die beiden Narkosemittel auch in der Aufwachphase grundsätzlich voneinander. Das Erwachen aus der Barbituratnarkose ist im allgemeinen ruhig. Nach kurzen Narkosen ist der Patient rasch ansprechbar. Erbrechen wird selten beobachtet, jedoch sind jugendliche Patienten in der Aufwachphase manchmal recht unruhig. Das geradezu plötzliche Einsetzen des Toleranzstadiums bei Injektion von CI-581 verleitet dazu, dieses Mittel als Kurznarkoticum anzusehen. Dies ist jedoch nicht der Fall. Das Erwachen geht langsam vor sich und bis zur völligen Orientiertheit des Patienten vergehen oft 60–90 min. Es ist sehr zu empfehlen, den Patienten nach der Operation nicht durch Fragen oder Manipulationen zu stören. Denn in der Aufwachphase kommt es bei der dissoziativen Anaesthesie nicht selten zu psychischen Reaktionen der Patienten. Oft wurde von unseren Patienten angegeben, daß sie viel geträumt hätten. Über die Art der Träume kann meist keine Auskunft gegeben werden, selten wurde „Schönes" oder „Schlechtes" geträumt. Häufig werden immer wieder dieselben Worte oder Sätze wiederholt. Motorische Unruhe, Halluzinationen und postoperatives Erbrechen sind selten. Man gewinnt also den Eindruck, daß in der Aufwachphase die mit Thiobarbiturat narkotisierten Patienten dem Anaesthesisten weniger Kopfzerbrechen machen als die mit Ketamine narkotisierten. Es darf bei dieser Gelegenheit nicht unerwähnt bleiben, daß CI-581 eine wesentlich stärkere postoperative Analgesie als die Thiobarbiturate erzeugt.

Zusammenfassung

Es kann festgestellt werden, daß die Anaesthesie mit CI-581 der Barbituratnarkose durch ihre geringere Toxizität und größere therapeutische

Breite sowie der stärkeren postoperativen Analgesie überlegen ist. Auch die
sympathicomimetische Wirkung ist, wenn es sich nicht um hypertone
Patienten handelt, ein Vorteil. Hingegen ist CI-581 kein Kurznarkoticum
und es ist auch für eine Anwendung bei ambulanten und älteren Patienten
nicht zu empfehlen. Die psychomimetischen Komplikationen in der Aufwachphase können durch geeignete Maßnahmen im Aufwachraum auf ein
Minimum reduziert werden.

Diskussion

Frau **Podlesch**: Ich möchte noch etwas zur Kombination von Ketamine mit anderen Narkosemitteln sagen. Wir haben nach der Einleitung mit Ketamine Halothan gegeben und bei einem Patienten einen sehr starken Blutdruckabfall beobachtet. Ich vermute, daß das unruhige Blutdruckverhalten durch eine endothorakale Stimulation entweder des Vagus oder des Sympathicus zustandekommt. Unter 0,5–1% Halothan im Einatemgemisch sehen wir gelegentlich Blutdruckabfälle bis auf 60 mmHg. Ich würde jedenfalls mit einer Halothannarkose nach Einleitung mit Ketamine vorsichtig sein.

N. N.: Ich wollte fragen, ob Erfahrungen vorliegen über das Zusammenwirken von Ketamine mit vorher gegebenen Medikamenten. Ich denke hierbei an Reserpin oder Phenothiazinderivate.

Langrehr: Wir haben bei etwa der Hälfte unserer Fälle vor der Ketamine-Anwendung eine Prämedikation mit Thalamonal und Bellafolin oder mit Pethidin und Bellafolin gegeben. Wir hatten hierbei den Eindruck, daß außer einer naturgemäßen Verlängerung der Anaesthesiezeit und deutlichen Veränderung der Blutgaswerte nach Vorgabe von Dolantin sonst keine unerwünschten Neben- oder Gegenwirkungen solcher Substanzen festzustellen sind. Das gilt zumindest für Thalamonal, Dolantin und Bellafolin sowie Lachgas und Fluothane.

A. The Utilization of Ketamine as an Agent of Induction Combined with Neuroleptanalgesia

By **G. Szappanyos, M. Gemperle** and **G. Gemperle**

Département d'Anesthêsiologie des Cliniques Universitaires, Hopital Cantonal de Genève

The continuous search to facilitate and ameliorate the induction phase of general anesthesia led us to try the Ketamin (CI-581) for its proved positive properties, with almost no undesirable effect on the respiratory and cardiovascular system.

Its brief, limited duration of action, the maintenance of the pharyngeal reflexes and muscle tone not requiring the support of the jaw, were all in its favour in our selection to use it as an induction agent with different types of intravenous or inhalational agents.

The positive effects of the drug upon the cardiovascular system with almost no alterations of the respiratory function made it sound like close to the ideal agent for induction.

A strict comparison of new compounds with those already in use is essential. To be widely acceptable as an intravenous anesthetic, this drug will have a difficult task ahead of it. It has to show an obvious advantage over already accepted drugs and its desirable effects must outweigh its less desirable side effects.

What are the characteristics of a good agent for the induction of general anesthesia?

1. Fast, pleasant, short hypnotic action with analgesia.
2. No depressing effect on the respiratory or cardiovascular system.
3. No undesirable side effects such as laryngo and bronchospastic action, excitatory phase, cough, vomiting, hiccough, tissue irritation if given i.v., i.m. or rectally.
4. No contraindication.

Many agents have been used, mostly by the intravenous route, but inhalational agents were preferred in many well indicated cases, not to mention the rectal administration of different drugs in mainly pediatric anesthesia.

Reviewing the literature about the intravenous induction agents, one finds a great number of chemically related or unrelated agents. The intravenous barbiturates have almost entirely taken over this field chiefly for their rapid, pleasant action and ease of control.

They are all hypnotic agents without analgesic properties and they even increase sensitivity to pain. At the expense of the markedly depressed respiration and cardiovascular system, one could achieve a pleasant induction for the patient with considerable spastic side effects on the coronary system of the anesthesiologist. I would just remind you of Sir ROBERT MACINTOSH's remark that "it is fatally easy to give Pentothal", and the many thousands of uneventful administrations may only emphasize the skill and judgment of the administrator rather than the safety of the drug. Existing compounds, even if they are widely accepted, do not meet all our requirements, and the search for anesthetics not showing the undesirable drawbacks is continuously on.

The clinical trials of the new non-barbituric group showed distinct advantages such as no respiratory depressant effect, enhanced cardiovascular activity, analgesia, etc. Its shortcomings, such as high incidence of thrombophlebitis and weak analgesic action, led to its oblivion after initial enthusiasm. The inhalation induction technique has many distinct advantages over the intravenous route and is widely used on account of its easy controllability and reversibility. It is rather unpleasant to the patient and this fact, at least in our institution where it was a standard induction technique in conjunction with Neuroleptanalgesia, led us to try a more comfortable way of induction.

The widely accepted classical induction of Neuroleptanalgesia consists of the injection of 10–25 mg. Dehydrobenzperidol i.v. followed by induction with a mixture of 3:1 Nitrous Oxyde-Oxygen usually lasting 3 to 5 min, at the end of which the respiration must be assisted or even controlled. The analgetic compound, Fentanyl, in 0.2–0.4 mg. is injected after the induction and followed by intubation under Succinylcholin (1 mg./kg.) relaxation. Maintenance of surgical anesthesia is carried out with small (0.05–0.1 mg.) repeated doses of Fentanyl and a mixture of 3:1–1:1 Nitrous Oxyde-Oxygen with controlled respiration.

The expected cardiovascular effects of Droperidol, the decrease in the arterial pressure (both systolic and diastolic) with marked diminution of the peripheral resistance (vasodilation) due to its adrenergic blocking action, are well known.

The induction with Nitrous Oxyde-Oxygen seems ideal from the pharmacological point of view because it does not potentiate these actions, but it is slow and has a rather unpleasant excitatory phase, especially in younger patients. They experience vivid, nightmarish dreams and usually recall even the intubation. The continuous search to ameliorate the technique incited us to use different intravenous agents among which Epontol was found to be the most desirable. But in geriatric anesthesia and in emergency situations, even this induction technique was not satisfactory and we tried the CI-581 in these cases, later extending its indication.

The technique of induction was modified from the standard and two different methods were used to benefit from the actions of the CI-581 in conjunction with the neuroleptic agent.

45 cases were done, divided into two groups. In the first group, 30 cases above the age of 55 were included and selected to undergo different surgical interventions. The majority of these cases was considered as either emergency or poor risk.

The technique used was as described below:

Premedication:

> 1 hour prior to the induction, intramuscularly
> — 1–2 ml. Thalamonal
>> (2,5 –5   mg Dehydrobenzperidol
>> 0,05–0,1 mg Fentanyl)
> — 0,5 mg Atropine.

Induction of NLA:

1. Blood pressure and pulse control.
2. Intravenous infusion of either:
   10% Rheomacrodex (100–200 ml.)
    5% Glucose-levulose
   10% Glucose (200–400 ml.)
3. Injection of 10–25 mg. Dehydrobenzperidol i.v.
4. Oxygenation for 3–5 min during which frequent blood pressure and pulse controls were carried out.
5. Slow injection (60–100 sec) of 2 mg./kg. CI-581 i.v.
6. Intubation under Succinylcholine relaxation (1 mg./kg.).
7. Continuous controlled ventilation but with Nitrous Oxyde-Oxygen in 3:1 mixture.
8. Injection (after an average of 5 min) of Fentanyl 0.2–0.4 mg. i.v.

Maintenance of NLA:

1. Controlled respiration with Nitrous Oxyde-Oxygen 3:1 or 1:1 mixture.
2. Utilization of a relaxing agent as needed (Alloferin, Curare, Succinylcholine drip).

In the second series of 15 patients, between the ages of 18 and 55 and considered as good risks, the technique was modified or, rather, the agents were injected in a different order.

Premedication:

Unchanged.

Induction of NLA:

1. Blood pressure and pulse control.
2. Intravenous infusion of the already mentioned solutions.
3. Oxygenation for 3 min.
4. Slow injection (60–100 sec) of 2 mg./kg. CI-581.
5. Continuous oxygenation (spon. resp.).
6. Intubation (about 45–60 sec after the injection of CI-581) under Succinylcholine relaxation (1 mg./kg.).
7. Injection of 10–25 mg. Dehydrobenzperidol i.v., immediately followed by
8. Injection of Fentanyl 0.2–0.4 mg. i.v.
9. Controlled respiration with Nitrous Oxyde-Oxygen 3:1 mixture.

Maintenance of NLA:

Unchanged.

Discussion

We recommend the first technique for it seemed more advantageous from both its pharmacological and its clinical safety point of view. In both techniques we emphasized the infusion of intravenous fluids prior to the induction in order to compensate for the relative hypovolemia, due to the α blocking, peripheral resistance decreasing action of the Droperidol (similar, but most likely central, effect of CI-581).

The initial injection of the Droperidol, with a waiting period of 3–5 min, not only allowed us to see the primary effect of its action but also provided us with sufficient time for maximal oxygenation, thus increasing the margin of safety in poor risk patients. The induction with CI-581, with no observable respiratory depressant effect, also counteracted the bradycardic effect of Droperidol and increased the blood pressure, which was usually 10–15 percent below the original reading after the injection of Droperidol.

The tachycardia and increase of blood pressure was proportional and entirely related to the speed of injection of the CI-581. The further advantage was that the pharyngeal reflexes were fully maintained (danger of aspiration minimized), and there was no laryngeal obstruction due to the muscular relaxation of the jaw and pharyngeal muscles with the tongue obstructing the glottis. The analgetic effect of the drug was a welcome feature and, on electrocardiographic tracings during the induction and intubation, we could not see arrythmias that were described with other intravenous agents. There was no prolonging effect on the action of the

Succinylcholine. The emergence of the anesthesia was smooth and dreams or hallucinations were not observed. Post anesthetic, drug-induced psychic disturbances were not seen in our series. Patients questioned never recalled unpleasantness of the induction nor ever noticed the introduction of the endotracheal tube.

In several emergency cases, in which the stomach was full (blood or foodstuff), we have seen neither vomiting nor regurgitation during the effect of CI-581, but the intubation technique was also modified. Instead of using one full dose of Succinylcholine injection, we used the Succinylcholine drip method to avoid fasciculation and occasional vomiting due to the contraction of the abdominal muscle and diaphragm.

The second technique of induction does not offer advantages and we do not advise it for the following reasons:

1. Although it provides us with seemingly maximal safety by not having the Droperidol injected prior to the intubation (the way we proceed when we use Epontol induction), it can mask the initial effect of Droperidol, and one cannot dose it individually as one can with a patient awake. If required for safety measures we give the Droperidol in small, divided doses.

2. The tachycardia and elevation of blood pressure are also more pronounced, even with slow injection of CI-581, than with the other method.

Arrythmias, vomiting during induction and intubation were not observed in this series either. The use of multiple agents in the induction and during the maintenance of the surgical anesthesia is a controversial subject and needs careful, controlled, honest evaluation. By combining agents we not only try to significantly reduce the amount of each agent used, but also to exploit the advantageous properties of each drug if used separately. The induction stage, which is one of the most critical phases of the anesthesia – just like the take-off or landing of a modern jet airplane – does not only have to be safe, but also must be acceptable and pleasant to the patient. We believe that the described technique fulfills these requirements and in certain cases will add to the safety of the induction. Our aim is not to proclaim this new drug as the "most" and "only", but to place it in its proper place in our armamentarium. We would like to emphasize that the disastrous results which can follow the administration of any kind of agent are mainly due to faults in judgment, to careless evaluation of patients and to the improper selection of many of our otherwise very valuable drugs.

Zusammenfassung

Auf der Suche nach einem komfortablen Einleitungsanaestheticum für die Neuroleptanalgesie (NLA) verwendeten die Autoren Ketamine wegen seiner geringen Nebenwirkungen auf die respiratorischen und kardiovasculären Systeme. Nach Gabe von 10–25 mg Dehydrobenzperidol i.v. erhielten die Patienten 2 mg/kg Ketamine i.v. Danach wurde die NLA in üblicher Weise mit Fentanyl (0,2–0,4 mg i.v.) und Muskelrelaxantien sowie einem N_2O-Gemisch unterhalten. Der besondere Vorteil dieser Methode liegt in dem stabileren Kreislaufverhalten während der Einleitungsphase der NLA.

B. The Utilization of Ketamine as an Adjunct with Spinal and Epidural Analgesia

By **G. Szappanyos, M. Gemperle** and **G. Gemperle**

Département d'Anesthésiologie des Cliniques Universitaires, Hopital Cantonal de Genève

Spinal and, to a lesser degree, epidural anesthesia has experienced more wawes of popularity and unpopularity than any other method. One of the chief reasons was the fear of the lumbar puncture which was due to either the patient's dreadful recollection of a previous unpleasant personal experience or just a hearsay evidence from a well-informed drinking partner in the neighbourhood bar. The usual first question asked after the convincing, comforting, reassuring words from the visiting anesthesist is: "Will I be awake during the operation?" "To be or not to be?" This is the question which we ask ourselves, for to give rather large doses of an intravenous adjunct to those regional techniques would nullify their advantages over other general anesthetic methods. On the other hand, to perform a block could be a spectacular technical achievement with a continuously moving patient, not speaking of the necessity of the stand-by "psycho-anesthesist" – to use GEORGE P. PITKIN's expression, "to maintain the patients on the table and distract their minds from the frightening unknown."

To ensure safety and comfort of the patient during spinal or epidural anesthesia, one has to use an agent of supplementation which has the following characteristics:

1. rapid analgetic and hypnotic activity with brief duration (important in the induction phase to assess accurately the success of the block);
2. no appreciable effect on the respiration;
3. no undesirable action on the cardiovascular system;
4. maintenance of the pharyngeal and laryngeal reflex activity;
5. maintenance of the normal muscle tone above the extent of the block;
6. possible abolition of the visceral traction reflexes (such as nausea, vomiting, hiccough, bradycardia);
7. good tissue tolerance given i.v.;
8. doses could be repeated if required.

Most of the agents used fall short of these requirements; therefore, based on the promising clinical and experimental evidences, we tried the CI-581 as an induction and supplementation agent with local techniques. The pharmacological details of said drug were given in another paper; therefore, omitting unnecessary repetition, we describe our technique. The total number of cases was 50, equally divided between the two techniques.

Drugs Used

For the spinal anesthesia, either Pontocaine 1% (Winthrop) or LAC 43 1% (Marcain-A.B. Bofors) was used and mixed by the anesthesist, with Dextrose 10% to adapt it to different specific conditions. The epidural blocks were performed with Marcaine-Adrenalin 0.5% (A.B. Bofors).

Premedication

Either 25–50 mg. Meperidine
with 0.5 mg. Atropine
or only 0.5 mg. Atropine.

Induction

1. blood pressure – pulse control;
2. intravenous infusion of either
   10% Rheomacrodex,
    5% Glucose-Levulose or
   10% Glucose (if there was no contraindication to their use) in the quantity of 10 percent in ml. of the patient's estimated blood volume;
3. lateral decubitus positioning of the patient;
4. injection i.v. 1–2 mg./kg. CI-581 with blood pressure, pulse control;
5. performance, 30–60 sec after the injection of the CI-581, of the block;
6. assessment of the extent of the block, usually 3–5 min following the spinal and 15 min after the epidural block.

Discussion

Reviewing the literature one finds that in approximately one-third of the cases of fatal spinal anesthesia, the block was supplemented with some kind of intravenous or inhalational agent. In many instances, the injudicious use of a supplementary agent was in a direct cause/effect relationship with the ensuing cardiovascular collapse or respiratory failure. In spite of the dangers involved, several mostly intravenously administered drugs are used. The CI-581 was tried in our institution and found not only to be satisfactory, but also to have the least side effect.

Although it is not a hypnotic, it creates a peculiar type of state of mind, especially if given in small doses (1 mg./kg.), with complete amnesia. The protective reflexes are fully maintained, as well as the muscle tone. It is an important feature of the drug since the lateral decubitus position favors laryngeal obstruction in patients having, for instance, Sodium Pentothal injection.

The transient increase in blood pressure and pulse rate is variable and also negligible due not only to the slow injection of the product but also to the small quantity used. The basic psychic disposition of the patients was more the determining factor in the selection of the dosage than was the premedication. The analgesic effect of the 1 mg./kg. was sufficient. The recovery time after 1 mg./kg. was 5 to 7 min and sometimes, even during the analgesic effect, patients were able to cooperate but still had total amnesia. With the 2 mg./kg. dose patients were in total catalepsy and cooperation could not be obtained. With these doses neither the respiratory rate nor the depth was altered. The recovery was smooth, but patients had dreams which were not unpleasant and did not cause anxiety. Only two patients, in the geriatric group, experienced frightening dreams. The maintenance, or rather supplementation with CI-581, of the blocks was required only in those cases in which the surgical manipulation extended beyond the planned procedure, and the block anatomically was not sufficient. We had three cases diagnosed as acute appendicitis in the geriatric group which were actually 2 acute cholecystitis and 1 mesenterial thrombosis. The manipulation of the bowels caused distress, nausea and retching. The immediate i.v. injection of 3 mg./kg. relieved the symptoms in spite of the CI-581 being apparently inefficient in protecting against visceral pain. This relatively large dose of CI-581 administered during an effective spinal block caused moderate tachycardia and increased blood pressure, but the evaluation was not valid because the manipulation and retching had the same effect on the patient.

The wellknown and disturbing extrapyramidal movements seen during light barbituric anesthesia were not observed in adults with the CI-581.

The present clinical experiences are not sufficient to vindicate the absolute superiority of the CI-581 compared to other well accepted and perhaps better understood intravenous agents. However, one has to admit its distinct advantages and utilize it in well selected cases. The unchallenged popularity of the intravenous barbiturics comes mainly from the patient's enthusiastic remarks and not from the employing anesthesists. Unfortunately, in today's sophisticated age and society, we get to a point where patients will dictate and select the agent of their choice. We know that the barbiturate nucleus is characterized by certain disadvantageous effects which cannot be modified by altering its side chains; therefore, we believe that new intravenous compounds are needed and we welcome among us our newest fascinating product, the CI-581. A strict comparison with the already existing drugs is necessary and contradictory findings will be useful, provided that the experiments are carried out under the same working conditions.

Zusammenfassung

Die experimentellen Untersuchungen bei Tier und Mensch zeigen eindeutig die positiven Effekte von Ketamine auf das kardiovasculäre System, seine potente analgetische Wirkung und die fehlende Depression der laryngealen und pharyngealen Schutzreflexe. Aus diesem Grunde hat sich Ketamine zur Einleitung und Unterstützung einer Spinal- oder Epiduralanaesthesie bewährt.

Bibliography

1. Barron, D. W., and J. W. Dundee: The recently introduced rapidly-acting barbiturates; a review and critical appraisal in relation to thio-pentone. Brit. J. Anaesth. **33**, 81 (1961).
2. Bourreau, J.: Premiers essais cliniques d'un anesthésique intraveineux d'action ultra-courte, le G 29505. Anesth. et Analg. **16**, 869 (1958).
3. Burstein, C. L., F. J. Lo Pinto, and W. Newman: Electrocardiographic studies during endotracheal intubation. I. Effects during usual routine techniques. Anesthesiology **11**, 224 (1950).
4. G. Woloshin, and W. Newman: Electrocardiographic studies during endotracheal intubation. II. Effects during general anesthesia with IV procaine. Anesthesiology **11**, 299 (1950).
5. Chen, G.: Evaluation of phencyclidine-type cataleptic activity. Arch. int. Pharmacodyn. **157**, 193 (1965).
6. —, at al.: The neuropharmacology of 2-(o-chlorophenyl)-2-methylamino-cyclohexanone hydrochloride. J. Pharmacol. exp. Ther. **152**, 332 (1966).
7. —, D. McCarthy, and C. R. Ensor: Studies on the cardiovascular effect of 2-(o-chlorophenyl)-2-methylamino-cyclohexanone. HCl (CI-581) in laboratory animals. Memo of January 12, 1966 to Dr. Bratton.
8. Corssen, G., and E. F. Domino: Dissociative anesthesia: further pharmacologic studies and first clinical experience with the phencyclidine derivative CI-581. Anest. Analg. **45**, 29 (1966).
9. — — Dissociative anesthesia: further pharmacologic studies and first clinical experience with the phencyclidine derivative CI-581. Anest. Analg. **45**, 29 (1966).
10. Domino, E. F., et al.: Human pharmacology of CI-581, a new intravenous agent chemically related to phencyclidine. (Abstract 771) Fed. Proc. **24**, 268 (1965).
11. — — Pharmacologic effects of CI-581, a new dissociative anesthetic, in man. Clin. Pharmacol. Ther. **6**, 279 (1965).

12. Dundee, J. W.: Intravenous Anesthesia. I. A. C.; Little, Boston: Brown and Company, vol. 2/4 (1964).
13. —, and D. W. Barron: The barbiturates. Brit. J. Anaesth. **34**, 240 (1962).
14. Edwards, G., et al.: Deaths associated with anesthesia. Anaesthesia **11**, 194 (1956).
15. Feurstein, V.: Das intravene Narkoticum G 29505: vorläufiger klinischer Bericht. Anaesthesist **6**, 177 (1957).
16. Frey, R. u. K. J. Herrmann: Ein intravenöses Kurznarkoticum aus der Gruppe der Phenoxyessigsäureamid (G 29505) Tierversuche, Selbstversuche und erste klinische Erfahrungen. Anaesthesist **6**, 170 (1957).
17. Gruber, C. M.: The effects of anesthetic doses of sodium thiopentobarbitol, sodium thio-ethamyl, and pentothal sodium upon the respiratory system, the heart and blood pressure in experimental animals. J. Pharmacol. exp. Ther. **60**, 143 (1937).
18. Henschel, W. F. u. O. Just: Zur Anwendung des neuartigen intravenösen Kurznarcoticums G 29505 (Phenoxyessigsäureamid-Verbindung) bei poliklinischen Eingriffen. Anaesthesist **6**, 174 (1957).
19. Horton, H.: Electrocardiographic findings during laryngoscopy and endotracheal intubation. Brit. J. Anaesth. **27**, 326 (1955).
20. Huguenard, P.: Emploi clinique du G 29505. Anesth. et Analg. **16**, 952 (1959).
21. Jacoby et al.: Cardiac arrhythmias: effect of vagal stimulation and hypoxia, Anesthesiology **16**, 1004 (1955).
22. Johnson, S. R.: The effect of some anaesthetic agents on the circulation in man. Acta chir. scand. Suppl. **158** (1951).
23. Kaump, D. H.: Preclinical toxicological studies on CL-369 (CI-581). Memo of December 10, 1963 to Dr. Bratton.
24. — N. D. A. toxicological studies on CL-369 (CI-581); Acute toxicity in dogs. Memo of January 5, 1965 to Dr. Bratton.
25. — Local tolerance studies on CI-581 following intraarterial injection in rats and dogs. Memo of January 20, 1967 to Dr. Bratton.
26. Kern, E.: La N, N-diéthylamide de l'acide 2-méthoxy-4-allylphénoxyacétique (G 29505) -pharmacologie. Anesth. et Analg. **16**, 942 (1959).
27. King, C. H., and C. R. Steshen: A new intravenous or intramuscular anesthetic. Anesthesiology **28**, 258 (1967).
28. Kreuscher, H., and H. Gauch: (The effect of phencyclidine derivative Ketamine (CI-581) on the human cardiovascular system). (Ger) Anaesthesist **16**, 229 (1967).
29. Natof, H. E., and M. S. Sadove: Cardiovascular collapse in the operating room. Philadelphia and Montreal: J. B. Lippincott Company 1958.
30. Payne, J. P., and D. A. Wright: Observations on the pharmacology of a eugenol derivative, G 29505. Brit. J. Anaesth. **34**, 368 (1962).
31. Raffan, A. W.: Reflex cardiac arrest under anesthesia. Anaesthesia **9**, 116 (1954).
32. Rosner, S., W. Newman, and C. L. Burstein: Electrocardiographic studies during endotracheal intubation. VI. Effects during anesthesia with thiopental sodium combined with muscle relaxant. Anesthesiology **14**, 591 (1953).
33. Swerdlow, M.: A new intravenous anesthetic – G. 29 505. Brit. J. Anaesth. **33**, 104 (1961).
34. Virtue, R. E., et al.: An anesthetic agent: 2-orthochloro-phenyl-2-methyl-amino cyclohexanone HCL (CI-581). Anesthesiology **28**, 823 (1967).
35. Wright, D. A., and J. P. Payne: A clinical study of intravenous anaesthesia with a eugenol derivative, G 29505. Brit. J. Anaesth. **34**, 379 (1962).

Vergleich zwischen Ketamine und Diazepam als Adjunkt zur Periduralanaesthesie

Von **J. Lassner**

Diazepam ist unter dem Namen Valium bekannt, und meine Bemerkungen gehen darauf hinaus, diesen Stoff mit verschiedenen anderen und insbesondere mit Ketamine als Adjunkt zur Peridualanaesthesie zu vergleichen. Herr Kollege SZAPPANYOS hat seine kritischen Bemerkungen hauptsächlich auf die Barbiturate gerichtet. Ich stimme mit ihm weitgehend überein. Tatsächlich halte ich die Barbiturate nicht als die bestgeeigneten Mittel als Adjunkt für eine Peridual- oder eine Spinalanaesthesie. Der Vergleich mit Ketamine wäre aber wahrscheinlich anders ausgefallen, wenn nicht nur die Barbiturate ins Auge gefaßt worden wären, sondern auch die anderen heute verfügbaren Mittel, insbesondere das Gamma-hydroxybutyrat, das Hemineurin und vor allem das Valium. Uns stand nur ein sehr beschränktes Quantum von Ketamine zur Verfügung. Ketamine ist in Frankreich nicht zugelassen, so daß eine Verwendung nur bei vorheriger Aussprache mit den Patienten möglich war. Wie ich später noch bemerken will, war meine persönliche Einstellung zu dem Mittel durch eine Selbsterfahrung auch so geworden, daß eine derartige Aussprache mit dem Patienten vor der Verwendung mir unbedingt notwendig erschien. Die Patienten, die Ketamine bekommen haben, müssen als Sonderfälle angesehen werden.

Während Ketamine sympathicotonisch wirkt und daher, ähnlich wie das Gamma-hydroxybutyrat den Blutdruck steigert, was bei der Spinal- und Peridualanaesthesie aber günstig ist, verstärkt das Diazem, wenn auch nur geringgradig, die Tendenz zum Blutdruckabfall. Die sogenannte analgetische Wirkung von Ketamine macht es möglich, die Lumbalpunktion durchzuführen, ohne daß der Patient reagiert, während nach Gabe einer Dosis von 8–12 mg Diazepam Abwehrbewegungen auch beim Anlegen der Hautquaddel auftreten, die erheblich stören können. Beide Substanzen beeinträchtigen die Atmung kaum. Trotz der erwähnten Vorteile, scheint mir das Risiko einer etwaigen psychischen Störung nach Ketamine die Anwendung dieser Substanz als Adjuvans nicht rätlich zu machen.

Diskussion

Langrehr: Dr. SZAPPANYOS, may I ask you about the behaviour of the heart rate in the combination of Ketamine and neurolept-analgesia?

Szappanyos: It depends upon the technique you use. If you use the first technique, which we recommend, then first of all we inject droperidol and afterwards Ketamine. In this case, you have the initial effect of droperidol. The hypertensive effect of Ketamine is in this case very minimal. Only in a few cases did we see an increase of blood pressure and pulse rate more than 10%. Using the second technique, that means primarely application of Ketamine, you will have tachycardia and rising blood pressure, and after application of droperidol the drop of the blood pressure and pulse rate is much sharper than in the first techique.

Kreuscher: Dr. SZAPPANYOS, I have two questions: I cannot recognize the adventage of the combination of drugs used to produce neurolept analgesia, and CI-581. The relatively clear conditions of the neurolept-analgesia will be confused by a compound with very pronounced action on the cardiovascular system on the one side, with a psychotropic action on the other.

And the second question: Dehydrobenzperidol is an alpha-blocking drug. Should that be the pharmacodynamic background of the lesser fall of blood pressure if you administer CI-581 following dehydrobenzperidol?

Szappanyos: To your first question: We start by giving an intravenous infusion prior to the injection of droperidol; we fill up the cardiovacular system with a large amount of fluid to compensate the relative hypovolemia caused by droperidol. That is one way to avoid the blood-pressure drop and certainly in poorest patients we do not start a neurolept analgesia having not that amount of liquid in the cardiovascular system. It was surprising to me, that with both, droperidol, which has an alpha-blocking action and causes vasodilatation in the periphery and CI-581, also causes vasodilataion and decrease of peripheral resistence. But droperidol has a peripheral action and CI-581 a central action. Now to the second question: all right, droperidol and CI-581 are psychomimetic acting drugs. But we use these combinations just for induction and we show you the length of the surgical interventions of our cases: It was always more than $1^1/_2$ hour. If the procedure lasts less than $1^1/_2$ hour, we do not use neuroleptics. In these cases we use a classical type of any kind of anesthesia e. g. with Halothane or Penthrane.

Corssen: I would like to ask Dr. LASSNER about the rationale behind comparing a sedative such as Valium with an agent like Ketamine, which is really not a sedative. Ketamine has profound analgetic action, which is why we are using it as a sole anaesthetic agent for a variety of surgical procedures. If you compare Ketamine with its rather mild sedative action with a very strong sedative such as Valium, I think, that is a very unusual attempt to compare two drugs, which have nothing to do with each other.

Lassner: The question certainly is to the point: The reason is that we have been not comparing two drugs for anesthesia but we have been looking for good adjuncts for peridural anesthesia. There is no need for an analgesic substance in peridural anesthesia, which procures anaesthesia in the field of operation. The question is, how to put a patient under peridural or spinal anesthesia in a state of rest, and I feel that drugs like Ketamine have little to offer for this specific purpose.

Kalff: Ich habe einige Fragen an Herrn LASSNER: In welcher Dosis verabreichen Sie Valium bei Peridural-Anaesthetsie? Welchen Einfluß hat Valium auf den Blutdruck bei Peridural-Anaesthesie? Und welchen Einfluß hat Ketamine bei der Periduralanaesthesie? Sind Sie in der Lage, durch Ketamine bei der Periduralanaesthesie einen Blutdruckabfall abzufangen?

Lassner: Die Dosierung als Beruhigungsmittel liegt beim Erwachsenen zwischen 10 und 15 mg. Der Einfluß des Mittels auf den Blutdruck bei dieser Dosierung ist sehr gering.

Wir haben diesem Mittel den Vorzug gegeben vor den meisten anderen, die wir ausprobiert hatten (z. B. Dehydrobenzperidol), da eben die Periduralanaesthesie einen Einfluß auf den Blutdruck ausübt und das Mittel, das verwendet wird, um Beruhigung oder den Schlaf herbeizuführen, diesen Blutdruckabfall nicht verstärken soll.

So hatte z. B. das Presuren, das wir seinerzeit versucht hatten, eine erhebliche Verstärkung des Blutdruckabfalles bei der Peridural-Anaesthesie mit sich gebracht, während das bei dem Valium nicht der Fall ist. Ich habe nicht genug Erfahrung mit dem Ketamine bei der Peridural-Anaesthesie, was den Blutdruck betrifft, um darüber Auskunft geben zu können; aber Herr SZAPPANYOS wird vielleicht antworten können.

Szappanyos: In dogs with open chest operation anesthetized with pentothale we saw a remarkable decrease of every motoric parameter. That is one reason, why we don't like to use Ketamine as an adjunct neither with neuroleptic nor as an induction agent nor with spinal or epidural anesthesia.

Die Anwendung von Ketamine vorwiegend in der Kinder- und Neurochirurgie

Von **B. Brunckhorst**, **K. Horatz** und **G. König**

Aus der Anästhesieabteilung des Universitäts-Krankenhauses Hamburg-Eppendorf
(Direktor: Prof. Dr. K. Horatz)

Einer der größten Gegner des Kinder behandelnden Arztes ist die Angst. Die Angst des Kindes vor dem Unbekannten, vor dem Schmerz. So trifft man gerade auf dem Gebiet der Anaesthesie immer wieder auf Bemühungen, die Narkose möglichst unbemerkt, möglichst spielerisch zu beginnen, wie z. B. jener Kollege, der das Narkosegemisch einem Teddybären entströmen ließ. In diesem Zusammenhang kam uns das intramuskulär zu injizierende CI-581 sehr gelegen, zumal wir im Laufe der Erprobung feststellten, daß man die Injektion mit dem in der Prämedikation üblichen Atropin zusammenfallen lassen kann. Eine halbe Stunde vorher gaben wir bei Kindern unter einem Jahr eine Rektiole Chloralhydrat, bei Kindern über einem Jahr 25–50 mg Phenothiazine per os. Bei einer Dosierung von 5–10 mg Ketamine i.m. pro Kilogramm Körpergewicht erreichten wir so eine Analgesie und Bewußtlosigkeit, die ausreichend war, diagnostische und kleinere chirurgische Eingriffe durchzuführen. So erwies sich das CI-581 als nahezu ideal für Luftencephalographien in der Neurochirurgie. Hierbei zeigt sich ein Bestehenbleiben des Muskeltonus als Vorteil, da das Kind beim Einführen der Punktionsnadel mit Unterstützung sitzen und die in den Lumbalkanal eingedrückte Luft sofort aufsteigen kann. Während der folgenden Röntgenaufnahmen läßt die Analgesie stetig nach und die längerdauernde Bewußtlosigkeit, die später einer Benommenheit weicht, gewährleistet aber noch ein völlig ruhiges Verhalten des Kindes. Sollte anschließend ein größerer chirurgischer Eingriff notwendig werden, ist ohne Bedenken eine erneute Narkose möglich, deren Einleitung von dem Kind widerstandslos hingenommen wird. Als Beispiel diene das Protokoll eines 5jährigen Kindes von 31 kg Gewicht.

Am 15. 12. 1967 wurde nach Gabe von 50 mg Phenothiazin per os um 8 Uhr die Narkose mit 150 mg CI-581 i.m. unter Zugabe von 0,4 mg Atropin eingeleitet. Um 8.10 Uhr zeigte das Kind bei der Lumbalpunktion keinen Schmerzreiz mehr und ließ die zahlreichen Röntgenaufnahmen bis 9.15 Uhr ruhig über sich ergehen. Da dieselben keine restlose Klärung des Krankheitsbildes brachten, entschloß man sich um 10.30 Uhr zur Anlegung eines Bohrloches mit Ventrikelpunktion und anschließender Ventrikulographie. Die Narkose wurde mit 30 mg CI-581 i. v. eingeleitet und nach 15 min mit 15 mg CI-581 i. v. um weitere 15 min verlängert.

Um 13.30 Uhr entschloß man sich nach beendeter Diagnostik zur Anlegung einer Torkildsen-Drainage. Hierzu leiteten wir bei dem noch sehr schläfrigen Kind die Narkose mit 30 mg CI-581 i. v. erneut ein unter Zugabe von 0,3 mg Atropin i. v. Anschließend intubierten wir das Kind unter Muskelrelaxierung und führten die Narkose mit einem Lachgas-Sauerstoff-Gemisch unter Zugabe von 0,5 Vol.-% Halothan weiter und gingen auf kontrollierte maschinelle Beatmung über.

Während der ganzen Narkosedauer zeigten sich nur minimale Blutdruckschwankungen, während die Pulsfrequenz infolge der wechselnden Narkosetiefe stärker schwankte. Das über mehrere Tage kontrollierte Blutbild, die Leberfunktionsproben und der Urinstatus zeigten keine nennenswerten Abweichungen von der Norm.

Dieses Beispiel läßt erkennen, daß sich das CI-581 sowohl als Mono-Anaestheticum eignet als auch zur Kombination mit den bisher üblichen Anaesthetika. Man kann also bei Kindern in jedem Falle die Narkose durch intramuskuläre Injektion von CI-581 beginnen, und zwar bei ängstlichen und kontaktarmen Kindern bereits auf Station in der für sie gewohnten Umgebung. Man kann es dann von der Art des chirurgischen Eingriffes abhängig machen, ob das CI-581 allein ausreicht, oder praktisch nur der Einleitung gedient hat und man die Narkose mit Lachgas-Sauerstoff unter Halothan-Zusatz fortführt, wobei hier zu erwähnen ist, daß man nach der eingangs beschriebenen CI-581-Einleitung mit wesentlich geringeren Halothan-Konzentrationen die gewünschte Narkosetiefe erzielt.

Wir führten in dieser Form 450 Narkosen mit CI-581 durch, und zwar 200 in der Chirurgie, 150 in der Neurochirurgie, je 50 in der Augenklinik und Kinderklinik. Hierbei zeigte sich das CI-581 als Monoanaestheticum bei kleinen chirurgischen Eingriffen als völlig ausreichend. Also z. B. bei

Punktionen, Incisionen, kleinen Wundversorgungen,
kurzfristig einzustellenden Frakturen,
Arteriographien,
Luftencephalographien sowie in der
Augenklinik bei Tonometrien,
         Funduskopien,
         Tränenwegsspülungen und
         einfachen Schieloperationen.

Bei allen anderen Operationen erwies sich CI-581 für die Einleitung zwar als vorzüglich, es mußte aber zur Weiterführung ein Lachgas-Sauerstoff-Halothan-Gemisch entweder über eine Maske oder einen Trachealkatheter zugeführt werden, um die entsprechende länger und gleichmäßig anhaltende Narkosetiefe zu erreichen. In der Neurochirurgie ist CI-581 als Monoanaestheticum auch bei etwas ausgedehnteren Eingriffen am Kopf zu verwenden, wenn bei schnellem Vorgehen des Operateurs rasch die wenig schmerzempfindliche Dura erreicht wird und man durch *wiederholte* Gaben von CI-581 intravenös nur eine Ruhigstellung des Kindes erzielen will. In jedem Falle ist es aber hierbei angezeigt, einen sicheren venösen Zugang zu haben, um eventuell auftretende Blutverluste ausgleichen zu können. Wir haben auf diese Weise 20 Revisionen des Ventrikelteils eines Pudenz-Ventiles durchgeführt sowie 25 epi- bzw. subdurale Hämatome ausgeräumt und waren nur in einem Falle gezwungen, die Operation kurz zu unterbrechen, um das unruhige Kind intubieren und mit einem Lachgas-Sauerstoff-Gemisch beatmen zu können. In keinem der Fälle kam es zu größeren Blutdruckschwankungen, wohl aber zur Steigerung der Pulsfrequenz um 10–30 Schläge pro Minute. Die Eigenatmung war in allen Fällen ausreichend, wobei zu erwähnen ist, daß wir in der Prämedikation alle atemdepressiv wirkenden Medikamente vermieden haben. Einen Eingriff möchte ich noch speziell erwähnen, für den das CI-581 als Monoanaestheticum prädestiniert erscheint:

Es handelt sich um *Saugbiopsien des Duodenums* bei Kindern und Kleinkindern. Hier ist die erhaltene Spontanatmung mit intakten Kehlkopfreflexen von besonderem Vorteil. Das Vorgehen bei dieser Untersuchung besteht im Einführen einer Sonde durch den Mund, die durch den Untersucher bis in den Magen und schließlich unter Röntgenkontrolle in das Duodenum vorgeschoben wird, an dessen Schleimhaut die Biopsie entnommen werden soll. Voraussetzungen für den Untersucher sind dabei der freie Zugang zur Mundhöhle, in der er die Sonde manövrieren kann, und das Fehlen von Würgereflexen, die das Einführen erschweren und zu Erbrechen führen können. Darüber hinaus ist das Erhaltensein des Schluckreflexes wünschenswert, was bei möglicherweise auftretendem Erbrechen die Aspirationsgefahr vermindert.

An unserer Kinderklinik wurden so in Gegenwart eines Anaesthesisten 20 Kinder im Alter von 2–7 Jahren untersucht. Diese Kinder blieben 6 Std vor dem Eingriff nüchtern, erhielten als Prämedikation eine altersentsprechende Atropin-Gabe von 0,1–0,5 mg subkutan sowie CI-581 intramuskulär, und zwar 5 mg pro Kilogramm Körpergewicht. Nach 3–5 min trat Bewußtlosigkeit bei erhaltener Spontanatmung ein. Bei dieser Dosierung ließ sich der Mund trotz des erhaltenen Tonus der Muskulatur leicht zum Einführen der Sonde öffnen. Unter Schluckbewegungen des Kindes ließ sich die Sonde mühelos in den Oesophagus und Magen vorschieben, ohne daß Würgereflexe oder Erbrechen aufgetreten wären. Selten vorgekommene versehentliche endotracheale Intubation wurde sofort durch Husten des Kindes als solche erkennbar. Ein solcher Husten konnte in einen kurzen Hustenanfall übergehen, einen Glottiskrampf haben wir nicht beobachten können. Bei fast allen Kindern wurde während der Untersuchung eine vermehrte Salivation beobachtet, wobei der Speichel entweder aus dem Munde floß oder geschluckt wurde. Bei der röntgenologisch beobachteten Passage der Sonde vom Magen über den Pylorus in das Duodenum erschien dem Untersucher die Passage verzögert zu sein. Dies ist vielleicht ein Nachteil, der aber durch den Vorzug einer entspannten Bauchmuskulatur wieder aufgewogen wird, so daß ein zusätzliches manuelles Dirigieren der Sonde von außen durch die Bauchdecke möglich ist. Abschließend läßt sich also sagen, daß sich das CI-581 vorzüglich für die Kindernarkose eignet, und zwar entweder als Einleitung bei großen chirurgischen Eingriffen oder als Monoanaestheticum bei diagnostischen und kleineren chirurgischen Eingriffen. Dies kann man um so mehr behaupten, als das CI-581 eine außerordentlich geringe Toxizität und eine sehr große therapeutische Breite besitzt.

Die von verschiedenen Anaesthesisten beschriebene atemdepressorische Wirkung des CI-581 konnten wir nicht feststellen unter der Voraussetzung, daß in der Prämedikation kein atemdepressorisch wirkendes Medikament verwendet wurde. Diese Feststellungen können wir durch zwei Fälle von Überdosierung untermauern, bei denen zwei Kinder im Alter von einem und anderthalb Jahren statt der üblichen 5 mg pro Kilogramm Körpergewicht 25 mg pro Kilogramm Körpergewicht erhielten, was einer Gesamtmenge von 250 mg CI-581 entspricht. Bei beiden Kindern verhielten sich Blutdruck und Pulskurve während der verlängerten Anaesthesiezeit nahezu konstant, die Eigenatmung war ausreichend, was durch den klinischen Befund und die arterielle Sauerstoffsättigung belegt wurde. Lediglich die Phase der Bewußtlosigkeit und späteren Benommenheit war stark verlängert. Die über mehrere Tage durchgeführten Laboruntersuchungen zeigten keinerlei pathologische Veränderungen.

Summary

In 450 children Ketamine was given for diagnostic procedures like spinal puncture, pneumoencephalogram, arteriographia and for small surgery like incisions, sutures or repositions of bone fractures. After premedication with atropine and phenothiazinederivatives Ketamine was applied in a dose range of 5–10 mg/kg intramusculary.

3–5 minutes after injection the children became unconscious without respiratory depression. It was possible to extend the duration of anesthesia either by maintenance with halothane and/or nitrous oxyde or by repeated injections of Ketamine. In 2 children, the extremely high doses of 25 mg/kg was tolerated without any changes in blood-pressure and pulse-rate.

Liver-functions and hematograms were not influenced by Ketamine in our patients.

Erfahrungen mit Ketamine bei Kindern

Von **Ilse Eckart**

Anästhesie-Abteilung des Städt. Rudolf-Virchow-Krankenhauses in Berlin
(Dir.: Chefärztin ILSE ECKART)

Patienten, Eingriffe und Prämedikation

Wir führten bei 150 Kindern Ketamine-Narkosen durch. Ihr Alter lag zwischen 5 Monaten und 12 Jahren und betrug im Durchschnitt $3^1/_2$ Jahre. Die Kinder wogen zwischen $3^1/_2$ und 61 kg, im Mittel 15,4 kg.

Tabelle 1. *Übersicht über 150 Operationen,*
bei denen Ketamine intravenös oder intramuskulär angewendet wurde

Eingriffe in der Mundhöhle	71
Zahnsanierungen	9
Operationen im Gesicht	18
Extremitätenoperationen, Frakturen	24
Phimosen-Operationen	15
Herniotomien, Orchidopexien	8
Appendektomien	5

Tab. 1 zeigt die in Ketamine-Narkose vorgenommenen Eingriffe. Über die Hälfte der Kinder waren Patienten der Kieferchirurgischen Abteilung, bei denen kleinere Eingriffe in der Mundhöhle und im Gesicht durchgeführt wurden. Dazu gehörten Lippenkorrekturen, Wundversorgungen, Fixierung von Platten durch Drahtnaht, Probeexcisionen, das Anlegen von Wasmundschienen und Sekundärnähte am Gaumen. Das Entfernen der Fäden nach Gaumenplastiken bei Spaltkindern wurde durch die Ketamine-Anaesthesie wesentlich erleichtert, ebenso Zahnsanierungen bei debilen Kindern. Frakturrepositionen und kleine chirurgische Eingriffe ließen sich ohne apparativen Aufwand durchführen.

Als Prämedikation erhielten 50 Kinder 20–40 min vor Narkosebeginn 0,01 mg/kg Körpergewicht Atropin intramuskulär injiziert. Bei 55 Kindern gaben wir zusätzlich Pethidin in einer Dosierung von 1 mg/kg Körpergewicht; in 45 Fällen wurde keine Prämedikation verabfolgt.

Narkosetechnik und Narkoseverlauf

Zu Beginn der Narkose erhielten 107 Kinder 3,0–7,5 mg/kg Körpergewicht Ketamine als 5%ige Lösung intramuskulär injiziert. Bei 43 Kindern wurden 1,5–2 mg/kg Körpergewicht Ketamine als 1%ige Lösung intravenös verabfolgt. Die mittlere Injektionsgeschwindigkeit betrug dabei 2 mg/sec.

Zur Verlängerung der Narkose wurden bei Bedarf Nachinjektionen vorgenommen und zwar in einer Dosierung von 1 mg/kg Körpergewicht intravenös. Auch die Kinder, bei denen die Narkoseeinleitung durch intramuskuläre Injektion erfolgte, erhielten die Nachinjektion intravenös verabreicht. Durch die bereits bestehende Narkose entfällt die Schwierigkeit der Venenpunktion beim Kleinkind. Außerdem kann durch die intravenöse Nachinjektion die Gesamtdosis des Narkotikums geringer gehalten werden, und durch den schnelleren Wirkungseintritt wird eine Störung oder Unterbrechung der Operation vermieden.

Bei intravenösen Injektionen von Ketamine wurde das chirurgische Toleranzstadium nach 20–30 sec erreicht und hielt 10–20 min an. Durch die zusätzliche Gabe eines Lachgas-Sauerstoffgemisches in einer Dosierung von 2:1 l/min konnten ohne Nachinjektion Operationen bis zu einer Dauer von 40 min durchgeführt werden. Andererseits mußte in einigen Fällen schon 5 min nach der Erstinjektion eine Nachinjektion erfolgen.

Bei intramuskulärer Verabfolgung von Ketamine wurde das Toleranzstadium nach 3–5 min erreicht und blieb 20–40 min erhalten. Durch zusätzliche Lachgas-Sauerstoff-Inhalation konnten Operationen an den Extremitäten bis zu 60 min Dauer vorgenommen werden.

Unter 107 Fällen mit intramuskulärer Ketamine-Anwendung trat ein Versager auf. Bei einem 2jährigen Kind konnte durch Injektion von 5 mg/kg Körpergewicht keine narkotische Wirkung erzielt werden. Ein später vorgenommener zweiter Narkoseversuch mit Ketamine hatte bei diesem Kind das gleiche negative Ergebnis.

Bei den mit Pethidin prämedizierten Kindern war das Toleranzstadium im allgemeinen gegenüber den Kindern ohne Prämedikation verlängert.

Die Pharynx- und Larynxreflexe blieben während der Narkose erhalten. Kurze intraorale Eingriffe konnten deshalb ohne Aspirationsgefahr unter Verzicht auf die sonst notwendige Intubation durchgeführt werden. Auch wenn bei hängendem Kopf operiert wurde, trat keine Atembehinderung ein. Das Einlegen eines Guedel-Tubus löste bei einigen Kindern Abwehrbewegungen aus, während der operative Eingriff toleriert wurde.

Das Erwachen aus der Narkose erfolgte bei intravenöser Applikation 30–45 min nach der letzten Injektion. Es geschah langsam, und erst nach einer 2–4stündigen Erholungsphase waren die Kinder wieder im Vollbesitz ihrer geistigen und körperlichen Kräfte.

Bei intramuskulärer Applikation erfolgte das Erwachen erst 1–2 Std nach der Injektion. Über weitere 2–3 Std bestand darüber hinaus noch ein starkes Nachschlafbedürfnis.

Blutdruck und Pulsfrequenz

Der bei Erwachsenen zu beobachtende Blutdruckanstieg nach Ketamine-Injektion ist bei Kindern in den meisten Fällen nicht so ausgeprägt. Dafür kommt es in den ersten Minuten nach der Injektion zu einem erheblichen Anstieg der Pulsfrequenz, besonders bei vorheriger Atropingabe. Wir haben Pulsfrequenzsteigerungen um 60% des Ausgangswertes beobachtet, bezogen auf die Frequenz vor Verabfolgung der Prämedikation (Abb. 1). Um die Auswirkung der Verstärkung des sympathicomimetischen Effektes des Ketamine durch die vagolytische Wirkung des Atropin auf die Pulsfrequenz zu vermeiden, haben wir in letzter Zeit auf eine Prämedikation bei der Ketamine-Mononarkose verzichtet.

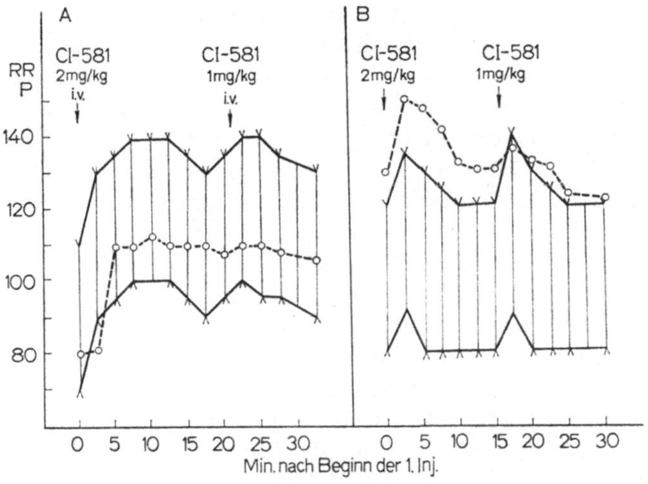

Abb. 1. Verhalten von Blutdruck und Puls während Ketamine-Narkosen
A ohne und B mit Prämedikation

Ketamine zur Einleitung einer Inhalationsnarkose

In 55 Fällen wurde Ketamine zur Einleitung einer Inhalationsnarkose mit Lachgas-Halothan unter gleichzeitiger Relaxation durch Succinylcholin angewendet. Bei der Mehrzahl der Kinder kam es 10–15 min nach

Beginn der Halothan-Inhalation in einer Konzentration von 0,3–1% zu einem Abfall des Blutdrucks auf die Ausgangswerte, bei 7 Patienten bis unter den Ausgangswert. Im Gegensatz dazu beobachteten wir bei 4 Kindern trotz der Halothan-Inhalation ein Anhalten der initialen Blutdruckerhöhung über eine Stunde. In diesen Fällen war bereits der Blutdruckanstieg nach der Ketamine-Injektion besonders ausgeprägt und erreichte Werte von 180 mmHg systolisch und 110 mmHg diastolisch (Abb. 2).

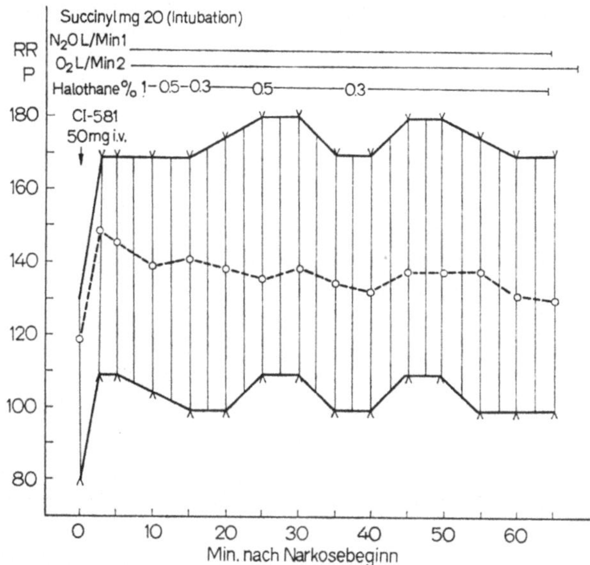

Abb. 2. Verhalten von Blutdruck und Pulsfrequenz bei einem 6jährigen Kind während einer Lippenplastik

Nebenwirkungen

Als Nebenwirkung (Tab. 2) trat besonders eine vermehrte Salivation in Erscheinung, die uns ungefährlich erscheint, da es durch die erhaltenen Schluck- und Hustenreflexe in keinem Fall zu einer Aspiration kam.

Eine in 3 Fällen beobachtete Muskelrigidität wurde als Zeichen einer zu oberflächlichen Narkose gewertet und konnte durch Nachinjektion beseitigt werden.

Bei einem zweijährigen Kind wurde durch Einlegen eines zu langen Guedel-Tubus ein Laryngospasmus ausgelöst. Das gleiche Ereignis trat bei einem 1¹/₂jährigen Kollegenkind beim Intubationsversuch durch das Berühren der Epiglottis ein. Die Intubation konnte erst nach Succinylcholingabe durchgeführt werden. Wir haben seitdem auf die Intubation in Ketamine-Mononarkose verzichtet und den Endotrachealtubus erst nach Vertiefung der Narkose durch Halothan oder in Relaxation mit Succinylcholin eingeführt.

Tabelle 2. *Beobachtete Nebenwirkungen bei 150 Ketamine-Narkosen*

| | Prämedikation | | |
	Keine (45 Pat.)	Atropin (50 Pat.)	Pethidin/Atropin (55 Pat.)
A. Während der Narkose			
Muskelrigidität	1	2	—
Hypersalivation	3	1	3
Bronchospasmus	—	1	—
Laryngospasmus	—	1	—
B. Postnarkotische Phase			
Brechreiz	—	—	1
Erbrechen	—	—	3
Schweißausbruch	—	—	2
Erregungszustände	1	1	—

Postoperative Übelkeit und Erbrechen haben wir nur bei Kindern beobachtet, die Pethidin in der Prämedikation erhielten. Wir möchten diese Nebenwirkung deshalb nicht dem Ketamine anlasten.

Bei 2 dreijährigen Kindern, wobei es sich in einem Falle wieder um ein Kollegenkind handelte, traten postnarkotisch schwere Erregungszustände auf, die trotz Psyquilgaben 2 Std anhielten. In beiden Fällen fielen durch eine unvorhergesehene Verzögerung der Operation die letzten Hautnähte und das Anlegen des Verbandes bereits in die Aufwachphase.

Ketamine hat sich besonders durch die Möglichkeit der intramuskulären Anwendung sowohl als Mononarkotikum als auch zur Einleitung einer Inhalationsnarkose in der Kinderchirurgie bewährt. Als besondere Indikationsgebiete haben sich für uns kurze Eingriffe im Gesicht und in der Mundhöhle, Frakturstellungen sowie in letzter Zeit urologische Untersuchungen bei stationären Kindern ergeben. Eine Anwendung bei ambulanten Patienten halten wir nur dann für gerechtfertigt, wenn die Möglichkeit einer mehrstündigen postnarkotischen klinischen Beobachtung besteht.

Summary

Ketamine was given in 150 children (age: 5 months to 12 years, weight: 3.5 to 61 kg) so well as an monoanaesthetic as or induction of combined anesthesia with nitrous oxide, oxygen, halothan and muscle relaxants.

The average doses were 5 mg/kg intramusculary and 2.3 mg/kg intravenously. If Ketamine will be used without any other anaesthetic, premedication is not necessary with respect to the undiminished protective reflexes. The recovery period is – sometimes – extended until 4 hours. This fact will be a restriction for the qualification of Ketamine in ambulatory patients.

Unsere klinischen Erfahrungen mit Ketamine in der Kinderchirurgie (100 Fälle)

Von **G. N. Gemperle, M. Gemperle** und **G. Szappanyos**

Aus der Anaesthesieabteilung der Universitätskliniken des Kantonsspitals Genf
(Direktor: Priv.-Doz. Dr. med. M. GEMPERLE)

Wir untersuchten CI-581 bei 100 Kindern im Alter von $1^1/_2$ Monate bis zu 16 Jahren. 36 Kinder waren jünger als vier Jahre, die übrigen hatten ein mittleres Alter von 8 Jahren. In der Hauptsache handelte es sich um Kinder in gutem Allgemeinzustand, die sich schmerzhaften Untersuchungen oder chirurgischen Kurzeingriffen zu unterziehen hatten: Gastroskopie, Luftencephalogramm, Phimoseoperationen, Repositionen von Frakturen, Verbindungen, etc.

Bei 76 Kindern handelte es sich um programmierte Operationen, 26 wurden notfallmäßig operiert.

Tabelle 1. *Programmoperationen und Notfalleingriffe*

n:	Programmoperationen	Notfalleingriffe	N.S.
103	76	26	1

I. Technik

Prämedikation. Die Kinder, die notfallmäßig operiert wurden, hatten keine Prämedikation; die übrigen erhielten 45 min vor Narkoseeinleitung Atropin allein, Atropin/Valium oder Atropin/Dehydrobenzperidol.

Anaesthesie. 49 Kindern wurde Ketamine in 5%iger Lösung intramuskulär, 50 Kindern in 1%iger Lösung intravenös verabreicht. In einem Fall kamen beide Applikationsarten zur Anwendung. Einzig bei Überschreiten der vorgesehenen Zeit wurde zusätzlich ein Gemisch von Lachgas/Sauerstoff mit Halothan gegeben. Bei ausschließlicher Applikation von Ketamine atmeten die Kinder spontan in Zimmerluft. Ausgewertet werden lediglich Kinder, die Ketamine als alleiniges Narkosemittel erhielten; die Verteilung ist folgendermaßen:

Tabelle 2. *Anwendung von CI-581 als alleiniges Anaesthetikum*

n:	Anwendungsart	1. Injektion	2. Injektion	3. Injektion	4. Injektion
48	i.v.	29	15	4	0
31	i.m.	31	0	0	0
1	i.m. und i.v.	0	0	0	1
80	total	60	15	4	1

Die benötigte Dosis (intramuskulär oder intravenös) ist im folgenden Schema zusammengestellt.

Tabelle 3. *Benötigte Dosis von CI-581 bei einmaliger Injektion*

n:	Ver-abreichung	mg/kg CI-581									
		—1	—2	—3	—4	—5	—6	—7	—8	—9	—10
33	i.v.	1	17	9	2	0	0	0	0	0	0
49	i.m.	2	1	0	0	2	5	23	14	1	1
82	total	3	18	9	2	2	5	23	14	1	1

Bei intravenöser Verabreichung beträgt die mittlere Dosis 2–3 mg pro Kilogramm Körpergewicht, bei intramuskulärer Applikation bewegt sie sich zwischen 7–8 mg pro Kilogramm.

II. Ergebnisse

1. Narkose. Der Schlafzustand wich stark vom klassischen Narkoseschlaf ab. Die Kinder hatten sehr oft weit geöffnete, tränende Augen mit lebhaften Lidreflexen. Der Narkoseschlaf hielt in der Regel länger an als die Analgesie. Im allgemeinen dauerte er nach intramuskulärer Verabreichung von Ketamine 45 min, nach intravenöser Injektion 15 min.

Tabelle 4. *Ansprechbarkeit nach ausschließlicher Anwendung von CI-581*

Anzahl der Injektionen	n:	Zeit bis zur Ansprechbarkeit (min)		
		Streubreite	Mittelwert	N.S.
1. (i.m.)	31	20–120	45	1
1. (i.v.)	29	8–25	14	1
2. (i.v.)	15	10–45	27	0
3. (i.v.)	4	12–25	15	0

Die Orientierung in Zeit und Raum war ungefähr nach 72 min möglich.

Tabelle 5. *Wiederherstellung der Orientierung nach CI-581*

Anzahl der Injektionen	n:	Zeit bis zur völligen Orientierung (min)		
		Streubreite	Mittelwert	N.S.
1. (i.m.)	31	30–180	72	4
1. (i.v.)	29	12– 60	30	1
2. (i.v.)	15	8– 60	33	1
3. (i.v.)	4	25– 30	25	0

Nach intravenöser Injektion waren die Kinder nach 30 min orientiert. Wurde in der Prämedikation Dehydrobenzperidol gegeben, so war der Narkoseschlaf verlängert.

2. Analgesie. Nach intramuskulärer Injektion wurde 2-5 min und nach intravenöser Verabreichung 30–90 sec später eine sehr gute Analgesie festgestellt.

Tabelle 6. *Eintritt der totalen Schmerzlosigkeit nach der Erstinjektion von CI-581*

Verabreichung	n:	Eintritt der totalen Schmerzlosigkeit (sec)							
		$\leq$50	51 bis 100	101 bis 150	151 bis 200	201 bis 300	301 bis 400	401 bis 500	501 bis 600
i.m.	31	1	3	8	4	8	0	2	5
i.v.	48	19	13	3	6	5	0	0	0

Tabelle 7. *Erste Schmerzreaktion nach der letzten Injektion von CI-581*

Anzahl der Injektionen	n:	Erste Schmerzreaktion nach Verabreichung von CI-581 (min)		
		Streubreite	Mittelwert	N.S.
1. (i.m.)	31	15–70	30	1
1. (i.v.)	29	7–20	11	2
2. (i.v.)	15	5–25	15	3
3. (i.v.)	4	10–20	13	0

Nach intramuskulärer Injektion hielt sie im Mittel 30 min, nach intravenöser Injektion jedoch nur 14 min an. Die Analgesie war genügend und erlaubte kurze chirurgische Eingriffe, jedoch ohne Muskelerschlaffung. Die zweite und dritte intravenöse Injektion war in der Regel in Abständen von je 6–9 min nötig.

3. Atmung. Klinisch konnte in keinem Fall eine Atemdepression festgestellt werden (keine Gasanalysen). Der Rhythmus war gestört und zeitweise durch tiefe Atemzüge unterbrochen. Die oberen Luftwege waren nie verlegt, die Larynx- und Pharynxreflexe waren immer vorhanden und verhinderten Aspiration und Regurgitation bei Notfällen mit vollem Magen. Der Tonus der Zungen- und Rachenmuskulatur blieben in jedem Fall erhalten, das Einführen eines Airways war unnötig.

4. Kardio-vasculäres System. Es wurde bei allen Fällen, die Ketamine allein erhielten, ein deutliches Ansteigen der Pulsfrequenz, sowie des diastolischen und systolischen Blutdruckes beobachtet.

Tabelle 8. *Pulsfrequenz nach aussschließlicher Anwendung von CI-581*

n:	Verabreichung	vor Anaesthesiebeginn	Pulsfrequenz während der Anaesthesie maximal	minimal
31	i.m.	110	144	120
48	i.v.	86	125	110

Tabelle 9. *Blutdruckmessungen nach ausschließlicher Injektion von CI-581*

n:	Ver-abreichung	vor Anaesthesiebeginn syst.	diast.	Blutdruck während der Anaesthesie syst. (max.)	diast. (max.)	syst. (min.)	diast. (min.)
31	i.m.	120	70	140	90	120	70
48	i.v.	120	80	140	95	125	80

Trotz Verabreichung von Dehydrobenzperidol in der Prämedikation konnten diese Veränderungen der Kreislaufverhältnisse nicht behoben werden.

5. Nebenwirkungen. Nach intramuskulärer Injektion von Ketamine beobachteten wir bei fast allen Patienten eine ausgesprochene Muskelstarre.

Tabelle 10. *Nebenwirkungen nach CI-581*

	Während der Anaesthesie	nach der Anaesthesie
Keine Nebenwirkungen	39	62
Hautrötung	9	1
Tachykardie	49	12
Hypertension	32	3
Speichelfluß	11	2
Erbrechen	2	6
Diplopie	0	11
Nystagmus	22	26
Angstzustände	0	3

Sie konnte von klonischen Zuckungen von Muskelgruppen der Extremitäten und von unkoordinierten Zungenbewegungen begleitet sein. Häufig waren vertikale oder horizontale Augenbewegungen. Diese Nebenwirkungen störten den chirurgischen Eingriff, verhinderten jedoch letzteren in keinem Fall. Selbst bei spastischen, encephalopathischen Kindern, bei welchen Ketamine verwendet wurde, kamen keine Konvulsionen zur Beobachtung.

Kinder über 4 Jahre klagten, nach dem sie befragt wurden, weder über unangenehme Träume, noch über Pseudo-Halluzinationen. Hingegen werden von größeren Kindern die Konvergenzstörungen mit Leseschwierigkeiten, die über mehrere Stunden andauern konnten, als sehr unangenehm empfunden.

III. Diskussion und Schlußfolgerung

Ketamine findet nach unserer Ansicht in der Kinderchirurgie ein gutes Anwendungsgebiet, da die oben erwähnten Nebenwirkungen, wie Puls- und Blutdruckerhöhungen und die psychomimetischen Effekte bei Kindern nicht störend sind. Sie ist besonders geeignet für Kurzeingriffe und schmerzhafte Untersuchungen, deren Dauer 20–30 min nicht überschreitet. Die Einfachheit der Technik ohne Intubation, der schnelle Analgesieeffekt, die verkürzte Wartezeit bei Kindern mit vollen Magen, die beim Chirurgen eine Begeisterung auslöst, soll den kritischen Anaesthesisten jedoch zu vorsichtiger Propagierung dieses neuen Narkoseverfahrens mahnen. Die Technik ist originell, weißt jedoch noch zu viele Nebenwirkungen auf; sie leistet aber vorzügliche Dienste in Notfallsituationen bei psychisch schlecht vorbereiteten Kindern. Für ambulante Eingriffe ist Ketamine nicht geeignet.

Summary

Ketamine was given in 100 children (age: 1.5 months to 16 years) for anesthesia in small orthopaedic and ENT-procedures.

The dosis was 7–8 mg/kg intramusculary or 2 mg/kg intravenously. Using repeated intravenous applications, the 2. injection contains 1 mg/kg and the 3. injection 0,5 mg/kg.

In case of extended duration of the procedure, anesthesia was maintained by nitrous oxide, oxygen and halothane. The respiratory system so well as the protective reflexes were not depressed. Systolic and diastolic blood-pressure and pulse-rate were increased. Premedication with droperidol could not avoid these changes of cardiovascular parameter. Avoiding atropine premedication strong selevation occurs. Occasionally muscle regidity was observed after intramusculary application of Ketamine.

Klinische Erfahrungen mit der intrasmuskulären Anwendung von Ketamine bei Kindern

Von **G. Westhues**

Aus der Anaesthesie-Abteilung (Leiterin: Dr. G. WESTHUES)
der Chirurgischen Abteilung der Kinderklinik der Universität München
(Direktor: Professer Dr. A. OBERNIEDERMAYR)

Als 1965 G. CORSSEN in Zürich erstmals in Europa über CI-581 berichtete, waren wir sehr bestrebt, dieses Mittel in unserer Klinik zu verwenden; besonders auch, weil es intramuskulär gegeben werden kann. Man ist ja dauernd auf der Suche nach einem Narkosemittel für die Ambulanz, das man den nur kurz vorbereiteten Kindern geben kann, das sie in eine für die chirurgischen Eingriffe genügende Narkosetiefe versetzt und sie bald wieder aufwachen läßt, damit sie das Haus verlassen können.

Für die Kinderchirurgie, bzw. Kinderanaesthesie, suchen wir natürlich besonders ein Mittel, das leicht zu applizieren ist und unsere kleinen Patienten möglichst wenig erschreckt.

Aus diesem Grunde faßten wir den Entschluß, CI-581 intramuskulär zu verwenden. Das Punktieren einer Vene zur intravenösen Anaesthesie ist bei kleinen Kindern oft sehr schwierig und zeitraubend, so daß wir in der Ambulanz und bei kleinen Eingriffen darauf gerne verzichten.

Tabelle 1. *Aufteilung des Beobachtungsmaterials*

Anzahl der Narkosen	100
Durchschnittsalter	4,57 Jahre
Durchschnittsgewicht	17,4 kg
Art des Eingriffs:	
Circumcisionen	74
Rectoscopien	3
Angiographien	3
Sphincterdehnungen	4
Cystoscopien	2
Rectumexcisionen	2
Tomogramme	2
Verschiedenes	10

Um die mit CI-581 narkotisierten Kinder auch nach dem Eingriff lange genug beobachten zu können, wählten wir aus unserem Krankengut 100 stationär liegende Kinder aus, bei denen kleinere Eingriffe durchgeführt werden sollten.

Die Kinder waren im Alter von 8 Monaten bis 13 Jahren (Tab. 1). Sie hatten ein Gewicht von 3–34 kg und waren in guter bis ausreichender gesundheitlicher Verfassung.

Tab. 1 zeigt die Verteilung unserer Patienten auf die verschiedenen Eingriffe.

Etwa 30 min vor Narkosebeginn wurden die Kinder mit Thalomonal und Bellafolin i.m. prämediziert. Die Wirkung der Prämedikation war in 83% der Fälle sehr gut, sonst ausreichend.

Alle Kinder – bis auf eines – bekamen zur Narkose eine einzige Dosis CI-581 intramuskulär. Ein Kind erhielt eine 2. Dosis nachinjiziert (Tab. 2). Wir begannen mit einer Dosis von 3 mg/kg. Erreichten aber damit in keinem Fall die benötigte Narkosetiefe und mußten bei mehr als der Hälfte der Fälle gleich zu Beginn (die genaue Anzahl der Fälle in Klammern auf der Tabelle), den anderen Kindern bald danach, Lachgas-Sauerstoff-Fluothane geben. Wir steigerten unsere Dosis auf 4 mg/kg. Aber auch damit trat keine genügende Narkose ein.

Tabelle 2. *Anzahl der Patienten mit verschiedenen Dosen von CI-581*

Art der Medikation	Anzahl der Patienten	Dosen von CI-581 in mg/kg					
		3	4	5	6	10	15
CI-581 als Monoanaesthetik	53	—	—	10	12	29	2
CI-581 mit Zusatzanaesthesie	46	5 (3)	2 (1)	12 (2)	20 (3)	7 (1)	—

Erst bei 5 mg/kg erreichten wir bei nicht ganz 50% eine ausreichende Narkose und die Zahl der Kinder, die gleich zu Beginn Fluothane brauchten, ging auf etwa 10% zurück. Ein ähnliches Bild bei 6 mg/kg.

Eine Dosis von 10 mg/kg jedoch ließ die Kinder in der überwiegenden Zahl tief und lange genug schlafen. Diese Dosis deckt sich mit Corssens 5 mg/Pfund.

Man muß also schon sehr hoch dosieren im Vergleich zu der üblichen i.v. Dosis von 1–2 mg/kg, um für die Chirurgie eine gute Narkose zu erreichen. Die Dosis von 15 mg/kg erzeugt einen sehr tiefen langen Schlaf und zeigt die große therapeutische Breite des Mittels.

Oft mußten wir Fluothane zusätzlich geben, weil der Eingriff länger dauerte als vorgesehen. Wir haben nicht nachgespritzt, um den Nachschlaf

nicht über Gebühr auszudehnen und um eine bestimmte Dosis beurteilen zu
können.

Die Injektion dauerte durchschnittlich 10 sec.

Das Mittel wird sehr schnell resorbiert (Tab. 3) und innerhalb weniger
Minuten liegt das Kind meistens in tiefem Schlaf. (Die Patienten, die von
Anfang an ein Zusatznarkotikum brauchten, sind in der Tabelle nicht
aufgeführt).

Tabelle 3. *Dauer bis zum Beginn der Operabilität in min*

Art der Medikation	Anzahl der Pat.	min					
		3 mg/kg	4 mg/kg	5 mg/kg	6 mg/kg	10 mg/kg	15 mg/kg
CI-581 als Mono-Anaesthetic	54	—	—	6,15	6,67	4,05	7,00
CI-581 mit Zusatz-Anaesthesie	36	7,00	11,00	10,60	6,33	4,416	0

Vom Beginn der Injektion bis zum Beginn der Operationsfähigkeit
dauerte es durchschnittlich 6–7 min. Die Patienten, die später ein Zusatz-
Narcotikum brauchten, schliefen schon langsamer ein (Tab. 4). Die nur
mit CI-581 narkotisierten Patienten reagierten nach 26–53 min wieder auf
Schmerzen. Bis zur Ansprechbarkeit dauerte es 60–124 min und bis zur
Reorientierung 128–180 min (Tab. 5, 6).

Tabelle 4. *Zeit bis zur ersten Schmerzreaktionen*

Art der Medikation	Anzahl der Pat.	Zeit in min					
		3 mg/kg	4 mg/kg	5 mg/kg	6 mg/kg	10 mg/kg	15 mg/kg
CI-581 als Mono-anaesthetic	53	—	—	26,20	28,41	37,86	52,50
CI-581 mit Zusatz-anaesthesie	46	22,67	37,50	31,11	23,76	34,16	—

Tabelle 5. *Zeit bis zur Wiederansprechbarkeit*

Art der Medikation	Anzahl der Pat.	Zeit in min					
		3 mg/kg	4 mg/kg	5 mg/kg	6 mg/kg	10 mg/kg	15 mg/kg
CI-581 als Mono-anaesthetic	53	—	—	59,10	64,41	94,10	123,00
CI-581 mit Zusatz-Anaesthesie	46	62,33	44,50	63,91	68,60	93,71	—

Tabelle 6. *Zeit bis zur völligen Reorientierung*

Art der Medikation	Anzahl der Pat.	Zeit in min					
		3 mg/kg	4 mg/kg	5 mg/kg	6 mg/kg	10 mg/kg	15 mg/kg
CI-581 als Mono-anaesthetic	53	—	—	128,60	120,08	152,10	181,50
CI-581 mit Zusatz-Anaesthesie		91,67	80,50	142,58	131,70	147,28	—

Der mit einer 2. Dosis behandelte Patient schlief ungleich länger (60, 140, 160 min.).

Der lange Nachschlaf der mit Fluothane unterstützten Patienten ist aber sicher auch auf CI-581 zurückzuführen.

Die Frequenz der Atmung änderte sich, bei einem Ausgangswert von 23/min, während 15 min bei 70% der Fälle nicht.

Fast alle Kinder bekamen aber eine initiale Bradypnoe mit geringer Atemdepression, 2 eine oberflächliche Atmung während der ganzen Narkose. 11 andere Kinder wechselten zwischen leichter Bradypnoe und einer geringen Unregelmäßigkeit der Atmung. Cyanose sahen wir in 2 Fällen, auf die noch einzugehen ist.

Bei 88 Patienten traten keine störenden Reflexe auf, bei 12 Kindern ein leichter Singultus am Anfang und während der Operation.

Die Pulsfrequenz stieg im Durchschnitt von 105/min auf 142/min und fiel am Ende der Anaesthesie auf 124/min ab. Wurde zum Ketamin ein anderes Narkosemittel gegeben (Fluothane), stieg der Puls ebenfalls von 105/min auf 141/min und fiel auch auf 125/min am Ende der Narkose. Der Blutdruck stieg im Durchschnitt um 20–30 mmHg und fiel am Ende auf den Ausgangswert. Es war auffallend, daß der Blutdruck durch zusätzliche Fluothanegabe keine anderen Werte ergab.

Zur Beurteilung muß man also sagen, daß eine Dosis von 10 mg/kg zu einem befriedigendem Ergebnis führt. Über 75% der Patienten schliefen lange und tief genug, um die notwendigen Eingriffe durchzuführen. Sie benötigten kein Zusatznarcotikum. Dazu muß man bemerken, daß alle Eingriffe äußerst schmerzhaft waren und eine sehr tiefe Narkose verlangten.

An Nebenerscheinungen fiel uns eine starke Muskelrigidität auf, die so weit ging, daß eine Intubation im Bedarfsfall ohne Relaxans in der Mehrzahl der Fälle nicht möglich gewesen wäre. Auf der anderen Seite erleichterte diese Rigidität die Narkose für unsere Zwecke und auch für die postoperative Pflege, weil der Kiefer nicht zurückfiel und damit der Atemweg frei blieb. Allerdings scheint das Mittel damit nicht zur Anlage von Gipsverbänden und dergleichen geeignet, wenn eine weitgehende Muskelentspannung notwendig ist.

Ein manchmal recht kräftiger Nystagmus trat häufig auf, auch wenn zusätzlich Lachgas-Fluothane gegeben wurde. Die Augen blieben während der Narkose meist offen. Die Chirurgen klagten häufig über starke Blutungsneigung, die sicher eine Folge des Blutdruckanstiegs ist.

Bei 50% der Fälle trat ein flüchtiges Exanthem auf, Lidflattern und leichte bis kräftige Streckkrämpfe, die aber bald vergingen. Einen nicht unerheblichen Opisthotonus haben wir bei 15 Kindern festgestellt.

Wir beobachteten 2 Zwischenfälle bei Anwendung von Ketamine:

1. Ein zweijähriges Kind mit einem Zungengrundtumor sollte bestrahlt werden. Nach der Injektion von 5 mg/kg bekam es einen Atemstillstand, der aber wohl auf die Lokalisation des Tumors und die dadurch bedingte Verlegung der Atemwege zurückzuführen ist. Das Kind wurde intubiert, beatmet und erholte sich gut.

2. Ein vierjähriger Junge kam nach der üblichen Prämedikation zu einer Zirkumcision auf den Tisch. Blutdruck 90/60. Nach der Injektion von 10 mg/kg stieg er auf 110/70 und fiel nach etwa 10 min auf 60 systolisch. Kurz danach war er nicht mehr meßbar. Das Kind wurde blaß, livide und feucht; die Atmung erst oberflächlich, dann hörte sie auf. Puls nicht tastbar, Herztöne leise. Nach Anlegen einer Infusion, Kreislaufmitteln und Sauerstoff-Beatmung kam der Druck langsam wieder und nach einer Stunde waren die Kreislaufverhältnisse stabil. RR 90/60. Wir konnten den Grund für diesen Vorfall nicht finden. Bei 98 Narkosen war der Verlauf komplikationslos.

Abschließend ist zu bemerken, daß CI-581 sicher *kein* „Kurzanaestheticum" ist, wie wir es in unserer Ambulanz brauchen. Wenigstens nicht bei der i.m. Applikation. Der Nachschlaf ist zu lange für unsere Verhältnisse. Auch für sehr schmerzhafte Eingriffe ist es nach unserer Ansicht nicht das Mittel der Wahl, da man eine hohe Dosis gebrauchen muß, um eine ausreichende Narkosetiefe zu erreichen. Eine große Bedeutung hat das Mittel zur Herbeiführung eines längeren Nachschlafes bei Kindern, wenn man diesen für diagnostische Eingriffe, Röntgenuntersuchungen, Angiographien und dergleichen haben will. Ein solch tiefer Schlaf ist bei Kindern sonst schwer zu erreichen. Bei Verwendung von 5 mg/kg dauert der tiefe Nachschlaf 60–90 min und das dürfte für solche nicht operativen Zwecke genügen. Das Kind kann dabei von einem Nicht-Anaesthesisten bewacht werden, was uns sehr günstig zu sein scheint.

Zusammenfassung

Es wird über 100 Narkosen an Kindern von 8 Monaten bis 13 Jahren berichtet, die mit CI-581 intramuskulär durchgeführt wurden.

Eine Dosis von unter 6 mg/kg stellte sich als ungenügend für chirurgische Eingriffe heraus. Mit einer Dosierung von 10 mg/kg schlafen über 75% der Kinder bis zu 53 min tief und können operiert werden.

Das Mittel flutet schnell an und hat eine große therapeutische Breite.

Die Patienten reagierten nach 26–53 min wieder auf Schmerzen. Bis zur Ansprechbarkeit dauerte es 60–124 min und bis zur Reorientierung 128–180 min.

Die Atmung war initial bei einigen verlangsamt oder oberflächlich, die Pulsfrequenz stieg an, ebenso der Blutdruck um 20–30 mmHg. Auch wenn zusätzlich Fluothane gegeben wurde.

An Nebenerscheinungen fiel eine starke Muskelrigidität auf, ein manchmal recht kräftiger Nystagmus, flüchtiges Exanthem, Lidflattern und vereinzelt leichte bis kräftige Streckkrämpfe zu Beginn der Narkose.

CI-581 ist kein Kurznarkoticum in unserem Sinn. Der lange, tiefe Nachschlaf läßt es aber günstig erscheinen, um Kinder für diagnostische und nicht schmerzhafte therapeutische Eingriffe ruhig zu stellen. Dabei können sie auch von Nicht-Anaesthesisten bewacht werden.

Summary

Ketamine was given intramusculary (10 mg/kg) in 100 children (8 months to 13 years). The recovery time was in respect to pain-response 23–26 minutes, to accessibility 60–124 minutes and to orientation as to time and place 128–180 minutes. In some children respiration was slow and flat. Pulse-rate and blood-pressure were increased. These changes were also observed, when halothane was given additionally. Side-effects like muscle-rigidity, nystagmus, transitory exanthema, flicker and light or strong convulsions during the inductive period. Because of the long lasting recovery period, Ketamine is not a so called short-acting anesthetic.

Erfahrungen mit Ketamine bei ophthalmologischen Eingriffen im Kindesalter

Von **I. Podlesch**

Aus der Abteilung für Anaesthesiologie der Universtität Düsseldorf
(Direktor: Prof. Dr. M. ZINDLER)

1965 berichteten FALLS, HOY und CORSSEN [3] über die Anwendung von Ketamine in der Ophthalmologie.

Wir haben Ketamine als Narkosemittel bei mehr als 300 Kindern im Alter von 2–15 Jahren bei ophthalmologischen diagnostischen und therapeutischen Maßnahmen benutzt. Die Beschränkung auf das Kindesalter erfolgte wegen der hypertensiven und psychomimetischen Wirkung dieser Substanz bei Erwachsenen [1, 4]. In der Mehrzahl der Fälle handelte es sich um *Operationen an den extraoculären Muskeln* zur Behebung eines Strabismus, die in Abhängigkeit von der Zahl der zu operierenden Muskeln 10–60 min dauerten.

Mit zunehmender Erfahrung hat sich folgende Narkosetechnik am besten bewährt:

Prämedikation

Vorabend: Keine.
40–60 min. präoperativ: 1 mg Promethazin (Atosil)/kg KG   i.m.
                1–2 mg Pethidin (Dolantin)/kg KG   i.m.
       0,01–0,02 mg Atropin/kg KG   i.m.
Anfangs wurden Atosil und Dolantin zeitlich getrennt injiziert.

Um den Kindern eine Injektion zu ersparen, haben wir später alle Substanzen zusammen in einer Mischspritze verabfolgt. Bei einigen Kindern mit heftiger Aversion gegen eine intramuskuläre Injektion wurden 20–40 mg Thiopental/kg KG rectal verabreicht.

Durchführung der Narkose

Einleitung: 1–2 mg Ketamine/kg KG i.v.
Fortsetzung: 0,5–1 mg Ketamine/kg KG i.v.
Die Einleitungsdosis wurde in 10–20 sec injiziert.

1–2 mg Ketamine/kg bewirkten Analgesie und Bewußtlosigkeit in 20–40 sec. Die gelegentlich auftretenden Augenbewegungen nach erfolgter

Narkoseeinleitung störten nicht, da vor der Augenmuskelpräparation eine
Fixierung des Augenbulbus vorgenommen wurde. Die Dauer der Analgesie
betrug nach einer Dosis von 1–2 mg/kg ca. 6 min. Das Flacherwerden der
Narkose kündigte sich durch Bewegungen der Extremitäten, tiefe Seufzer
oder Stöhnen an. Durch Nachinjektionen in der angegebenen Dosierung
war es möglich, die Narkose komplikationslos bis zum Operationsende
zu verlängern. Für eine Operationsdauer von 28 min wurden im Mittel
4,8 mg/kg Ketamine benötigt.

Bei 18 Kindern, die sehr ängstlich waren oder schwer auffindbare
Venen hatten, haben wir die Narkose über eine Maske mit N₂O/Halothan
eingeleitet und danach Ketamine i.v. appliziert. In 3 Fällen haben wir dabei
mit der üblichen Dosis eine starke Atemdepression erlebt. Wir empfehlen
deshalb eine Reduktion der Ketamine-Dosis.

Die meisten Kinder waren etwa 100 min nach Narkosebeginn wieder
ansprechbar. Da die vitalen Reflexe während dieser Zeit erhalten sind, sehen
wir in der verzögerten Wiedererlangung der verbalen Kontaktfähigkeit
keinen Nachteil. Zwischen Dosis und Zeitpunkt der Ansprechbarkeit
bestand eine lineare Beziehung (Abb. 1).

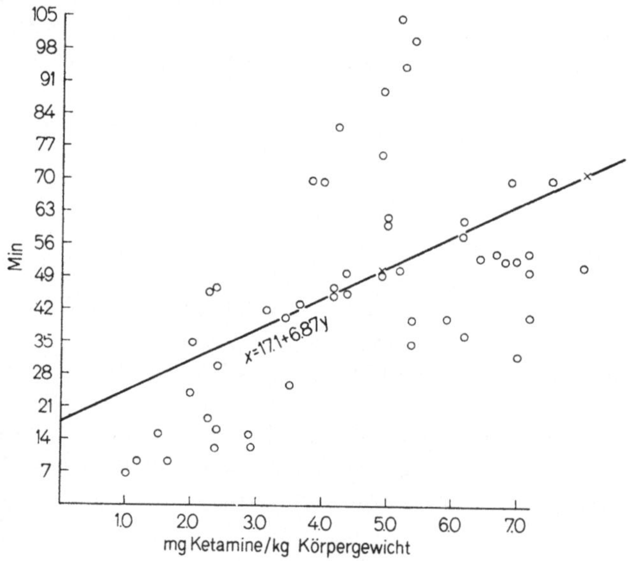

Abb. 1. Beziehung zwischen Ketamine-Dosis und Wiedererlangung
der Ansprechbarkeit

Nur wenigen Kindern haben wir Ketamine intramuskulär gegeben,
weil diese Applikationsform für ophthalmologische Operationen eine
Dosierung von mindestens 10 mg Ketamine/kg erforderte, und die damit
erzielte Narkose oft unzureichend war.

Nebenwirkungen auf Atmung und Kreislauf

Die Atmung wird nach Atropinbehandlung durch Ketamine bei Kindern weniger beeinflußt als bei Erwachsenen.

Arterielle Blutgasanalysen bei 22 Patienten ergaben, daß bei Atmung von Zimmerluft eine ausreichende Arterialisierung des Blutes erfolgt (Abb. 2). Nach Prämedikation mit Promethazin-Pethidin kann gelegentlich eine Atemdepression auftreten. Bei 2% unserer Patienten haben wir nach der Narkoseeinleitung mit Ketamine eine apnoische Phase beobachtet, die im äußersten Falle 4 min anhielt und künstliche Beatmung erforderte. Man sollte deshalb ein Beatmungsgerät bereitstellen. In diesen Fällen hat sich auch die intravenöse Gabe von 0,3–0,5 ml Micoren bewährt.

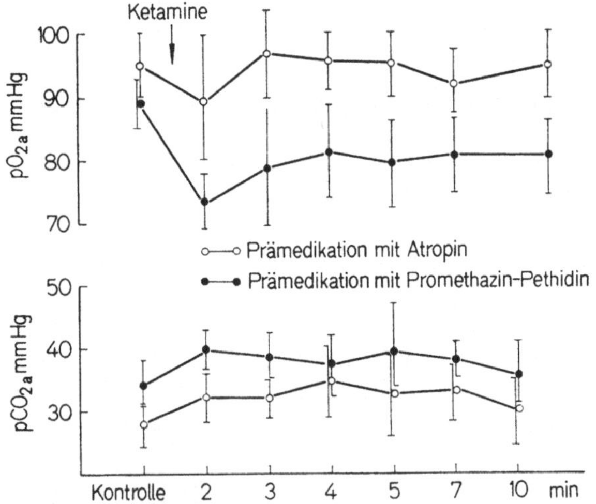

Abb. 2. Verhalten von Mittelwerten des arteriellen Sauerstoff- oder Kohlensäuredruckes nach intravenöser Gabe von 1–2 mg Ketamine/kg

Selten sahen wir uns veranlaßt, zur Freihaltung der Luftwege einen Guedel-Tubus einzulegen oder den Unterkiefer zu halten. In den meisten Fällen war ein ausreichender Tonus der Kiefermuskulatur vorhanden.

Ketamine bewirkte einen Anstieg des systolischen und diastolischen Blutdruckes sowie der Pulsfrequenz. Dieser Effekt überdauerte die analgetische Phase.

Blutdruck und Pulsfrequenz steigen nach Promethazin-Pethidin-Prämedikation geringer an als nach Atropin-Vorbereitung [5].

Sonstige Nebenwirkungen

Eine vermehrte Blutungsneigung machte sich intra operationem bei Kindern mit starkem Blutdruckanstieg störend bemerkbar. Schieloperationen verursachen meist einen Blutverlust unter 1,0 ccm, jedoch kann eine gesteigerte Blutungstendenz die Augenmuskelpräparation schwierig gestalten. Durch lokale subkonjunktivale oder intramuskuläre Injektionen einer Adrenalinlösung (1:6000 bis 1:100000) läßt sich diese Komplikation ausschalten. Oculocardiale Reflexe, die sich in 30–180 sec dauernden Pulsfrequenzverlangsamungen, Extrasystolien, Pulsus bigeminus oder seltener auch in Pulsbeschleunigung äußerten, traten in rund 70% der Fälle auf.

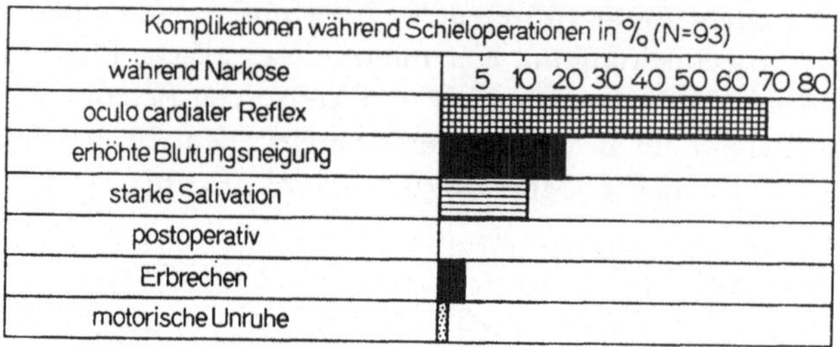

Abb. 3. Übersicht über Nebenwirkungen nach Ketamine

Da die Pulsfrequenz nie 60/min unterschritt und keine bedrohlichen Blutdrucksenkungen zustande kamen, halten wir dieses Ereignis für harmlos. In einer Vergleichsserie von Kindern, die in Hexobarbital-Lachgas-Halothan-Narkose operiert wurden, konnten oculocardiale Reflexe in 76% der Fälle festgestellt werden [6]. Übermäßige Speichelproduktion führen wir in den meisten Fällen auf nicht zeitgerecht verabfolgte Atropin-prämedikation zurück. Die mit Ketamine narkotisierten Kinder erbrachen innerhalb der ersten 24 Std post operationem kaum. Motorische Unruhe und psychomimetische Effekte traten selten und nahezu ausschließlich bei Kindern auf, denen nur eine Atropin-Prämedikation gegeben worden war.

Wirkung auf den Innendruck des normalen Auges

Nach Prämedikation mit Atropin (N = 5) oder Promethazin + Pethidin und Atropin (N = 8) haben wir in 3 Fällen mit dem Schiotz-Tonometer 5 min nach intravenöser Gabe von 1–2 mg Ketamine/kg einen Druckanstieg zwischen 2–4 mmHg gemessen. Von Corssen u. Hoy [2] wurden an 14 Kindern sofort und 3 min nach Injektion von 1 mg/lb Ketamine intraoculare Drucke bestimmt und in 5 Fällen Anstiege zwischen 2 und 7 mmHg gefunden. Systematische Untersuchungen an Glaukompatienten fehlen.

Gonioskopien, Goniotomien, Stardiscisionen, Wundversorgungen und Lidoperationen

Ketamine wurde mit Erfolg auch bei diesen Operationen angewandt. Die Narkosetechnik unterschied sich nicht von der bereits bei Schieloperationen beschriebenen. Trübungen der Hornhaut bei Kindern mit

Hydrophthalmus und Glaskörperverlust bei Verletzungen oder Star-operationen infolge akuten Augeninnendruckanstieges wurden unter Ketamine nicht beobachtet.

Für Untersuchungen oder Operationen an ambulanten Kindern halten wir Ketamine wegen seiner längeren Nachwirkung nicht indiziert.

Abschließend stellen wir fest, daß Ketamine nicht für jeden Patienten und jeden Eingriff zu empfehlen ist. Bei ophthalmologischen Operationen bei stationären Kindern halten wir es jedoch gegenwärtig für die Methode der Wahl.

1. Auf eine Intubation, die im Kindesalter nicht selten zu Laryngo-spasmus und Glottisödem führt, kann verzichtet werden.

2. Eine Kreislaufdepression fehlt.

3. Postoperatives Erbrechen tritt selten auf.

4. Die postoperative Phase verläuft ruhig, was die Pflege der Kinder, denen postoperativ beide Augen verbunden werden, erleichtert.

Summary

In 300 children (2–15 years) Ketamine was given as a monoanaesthetic for anaesthesia in strabotomies.

After premedication with Atropine or a mixture of Atropine, promethazine and pethidine anaesthesia was started by intravenous injection of 1–2 mg/kg Ketamine. Repeated doses of 0.5–1 mg/kg were given if required. After premedication with Promethazine, Pethidine and Atropine the required amount of Ketamine was smaller than after premedication with Atropine alone. Cough and swallowing reflexes were not influenced during this kind of anaesthesia.

In average 42 minutes after start of anaesthesia the children were conscious. After premedication with Promethazine, Pethidine and Atropine this time was prolonged up to 104 minutes.

Sufficient spontaneous respiration under anaesthesia with Ketamine is one particular advantage in strabotomy, because endotracheal intubation can be avoided.

Literatur

1. Corssen, G., and E. F. Domino: Anesth. Analg. **45**, 29 (1966).
2. —, and J. E. Hoy: J. Ped. Ophthalm. **20** (1967).
3. Falls, H. F., E. J. Hoy, and G. Corssen: Amer. J. Ophthal. **61**, 1093 (1966).
4. Langrehr, D., P. Alai, J. Andjelković u. I. Kluge: Anaesthesist **16**, 308 (1967).
5. Podlesch, I., u. M. Zindler: Anaesthesist **16**, 299 (1967).
6. —, H. Görtz u. K. Quint: Klin. Mbl. Augenheilk. **152**, 405 (1968).

Ketamine in der pädiatrischen Chirurgie

Von **P. Dangel**

Aus der Anaesthesieabteilung des Kinderspitals Zürich, Leiter Dr. P. Dangel

Im Kinderspital Zürich wurden bisher 100 Anaesthesien mit dem Anaestheticum CI-581 durchgeführt. Aus Tab. 1 ist die Altersverteilung unserer Patienten ersichtlich. Der jüngste Patient war nur knapp 4 Wochen alt, die Anaesthesie wurde zur Vornahme eines Pneumoencephalogrammes durchgeführt.

Tabelle 1. *Altersverteilung*

0–1 Monat	2
1–6 Monate	5
6–12 Monate	6
1–2 Jahre	16
2–3 Jahre	3
3–4 Jahre	10
4–6 Jahre	13
6–8 Jahre	15
8–10 Jahre	13
ältere	17
	100

Aus Tab. 2 ist die Art der Eingriffe, welche unter Anaesthesie nur mit CI-581 durchgeführt wurden, ersichtlich.

Als Prämedikation haben wir in den meisten Fällen nur Atropin verwendet. Es ist uns nicht gelungen, zur Prämedikation eine Medikamentenkombination zu finden, welche die Dosis von CI-581 möglichst klein halten und den ziemlich langen Nachschlaf etwas abkürzen würde. Schließlich schien uns am besten eine Kombination von Atropin (Dosierung je nach Alter) und Diazepam (Valium, Dosierung 2 mg/5 kg) zu sein.

In 79 Fällen haben wir gute Resultate erzielt, die Kinder haben ruhig geschlafen, die Atemwege wurden spontan frei gehalten, auch in sitzender Stellung, wie z. B. für die Durchführung der Luftencephalographie. Es traten keine Abwehrreaktionen auf, so daß auch die Operateure mit der Methode zufrieden waren.

Tabelle 2. *Art der Eingriffe*

Pneumoencephalographien	36
Urologische Eingriffe	14
(Cystoskopien,	
Circumcisionen,	
Hypospadie,	
Kath. Wechsel)	
Frakturrepositionen	13
Verbrennungen	10
Wundversorgungen	8
(Excisionen,	
Incisionen)	
Orchidopexien	8
Mundplastik nach elektrischer Verbrennung	6
Leistenhernien	2
Analfistel, Rectoskopie	2
Nabelhernien	1
	100

Tabelle 3. *Prämedikation*

Keine	9
Atropin	45
Atropin + Valium	21
Taractan	11
Atropin, Pethidin + Inapsin	4
Taractan + Valium	1
	100

Tabelle 4. *Resultate*

Ruhiger Patient, ungestörte Operation	79
Unterdosierung	5
Überdosierung	1
Konvulsionen	1
Erbrechen während Operation	2
Störende motorische Unruhe bei guter Analgesie	11
Bradykardie, Hypotension	1
	100

Bei 5 Fällen haben wir eindeutig unterdosiert und deshalb starke Abwehrreaktionen oder eine störende Muskelspannung, z. B. bei der Reposition von Frakturen, nicht genügend verhütet. Immer konnte aber die Operation ohne weitere Maßnahmen zu Ende geführt werden. Einmal ist unabsichtlich eine starke Überdosierung aufgetreten:

Ein 1¹/₂jähriges Kind mit Microcephalie, nach Vorbereitung mit Atropin 0,3 mg i.m., wurde mit 40 mg/kg CI-581 i.m. zur Luftencephalographie anaesthesiert. Die Operation dauerte 24 min. Blutdruck, Puls und Respiration waren völlig normal. Das Kind war ziemlich blaß, sonst war aber nichts Pathologisches festzustellen. Die ersten Schmerzreaktionen traten nach 67 min auf, das Kind war nach 1 Std 25 min ansprechbar und nach 4 Std 32 min wieder völlig wach. Nach 3 Std 17 min konnte es bereits wieder selbst sitzen. Der postoperative Verlauf war, abgesehen von mehrmaligem Erbrechen nach der Anaesthesie, ohne Besonderheiten. Die therapeutische Breite von CI-581 scheint eine vierfache Überdosierung noch zuzulassen.

Einmal sahen wir Konvulsionen bei einem Kind, welches an einer bereits bekannten Epilepsie litt und zur Durchführung einer Luftencephalographie eine Narkose mit CI-581 erhielt:

Der Patient war 9²/₁₂jährig, in gutem Allgemeinzustand. Vorbeitetung mit Atropin 0,4 mg, Narkoseeinleitung mit CI-581 10 mg/kg i.m. Nach vorher unauffälligem Verlauf treten in der 13. min während der Luftfüllung in sitzender Stellung des Patienten, tonisch-klonische Zuckungen des Gesichtes und aller Extremitäten auf, welche erst auf die Injektion von Diazepam 2×5 mg i.v. wieder verschwanden. Gleichzeitig Hypertension von 170/120 mmHg und sehr starke Salivation. Der weitere Verlauf war ohne Besonderheiten, allerdings ist das Kind erst 4 Std 5 min nach der Injektion von CI-581 wieder voll orientiert gewesen. Wir glauben, daß bei diesem Patienten mit einer Krampfanamnese die Indikation zur Anaesthesierung mit CI-581 falsch gestellt worden ist und daß solche Kinder mit anderen Mitteln narkotisiert werden sollten.

Zweimal kam es zu Erbrechen während der Anaesthesie:

Bei einem 5jährigen Patienten wurde zur Versorgung eines Gaumenrisses nach Vorbereitung mit Atropin 0,3 mg die Anaesthesie mit CI-581, 2 mg/kg i.v., eingeleitet. Beim Versuch, den Riß am weichen Gaumen zu nähen, kommt es zur Auslösung von Würgreflexen, eines Laryngospasmus und zu massivem Erbrechen. Das Kind hat aber nicht aspiriert, da alle Schutzreflexe vorhanden waren. Postoperativ komplikationsloser Verlauf. Auch hier folgerten wir eine falsche Indikationsstellung. Operationen im Rachengebiet können wegen der unter CI-581 allein immer noch vorhandenen Abwehrreflexe nicht durchgeführt werden.

Bei einem 6¹/₂jährigen Patienten, Vorbereitung mit Atropin und Diazepam, Narkose mit 10 mg/kg CI-581 i.m., kam es nach vollendeter Luftfüllung und 17 min nach einer 2. Injektion von 5 mg/kg CI-581 bei der Umlagerung auf den Bauch zur Vornahme der Röntgenaufnahmen zu Erbrechen. Auch hier keine Aspiration und komplikationsloser postoperativer Verlauf.

Andererseits konnten wir mehrere Kinder, welche kurz vor der notfallmäßigen Anaesthesie mit CI-581 noch gegessen hatten, behandeln, ohne daß es zu Erbrechen gekommen wäre.

Bei 11 Fällen war die Operation wegen einer anhaltenden motorischen Unruhe trotz guter Analgesie stark gestört. Besonders bei spastischen Patienten (Fälle von Pneumoencephalographie) traten atethotische Ruderbewegungen mit allen Extremitäten auf, so daß in einem Fall sogar der Versuch abgebrochen und das Kind mit Halothan weiter anaesthesiert werden mußte. CI-581 scheint in der üblichen Dosierung bei motorisch zentral gestörten Patienten solche Bewegungen nicht zu unterdrücken, im Gegenteil sogar eher zu stimulieren.

Einmal kam es bei einem 11–12jährigen Kind mit Hydrocephalus und Entwicklungsrückstand während der Anaesthesie unter CI-581 (6 mg/kg) zu einer vorübergehenden Hypotonie und Bradykardie mit ausgeprägter Blässe bei erhaltener Spontanatmung. Sofortige Besserung des Zustandes auf Atropin i.v. und nachher komplikationsloser Verlauf.

Der längste unter reiner CI-581-Anaesthesie durchgeführte Eingriff, eine Verbrennungsbehandlung bei einem 4jährigen Patienten mit 40%iger drittgradiger Verbrennung dauerte 1 Std 39 min. Es wurden dazu lediglich 2 × 6 mg/kg CI-581 i.m. benötigt. Das Kind war mit Taractan per os, 2 mg/kg prämediziert. Eine Blutgasanalyse in der 48. min ergab völlig normale Verhältnisse. Der Patient zeigte keinerlei Nebenerscheinungen, die Spontanatmung war immer suffizient, die Schmerzreaktion trat 49 min nach der 2. Injektion auf, der postoperative Verlauf war ohne Befund. Nach 1 Std 9 min war das Kind ansprechbar, es erwachte allerdings erst voll nach $4^1/_2$ Std.

Verschiedene Eingriffe dauerten zwischen 50 und 60 min, wobei wir nie besondere Schwierigkeiten bei der Aufrechterhaltung der Anaesthesie mit CI-581 i.m. oder i.v. sahen.

Zusammenfassung

Ketamine ist auch bei der Anwendung an pädiatrischen Patienten nicht ein kurzwirkendes Mittel. Die Aufwachphase, besonders bei mit intramuskulärer Anwendung anaesthesierten Patienten dauert immer länger als nach einer Inhalationsnarkose mit Halothan.

Kenntnisse in der Atmungsreanimation sind unerläßlich. Es ist zu hoffen, daß die scheinbare Leichtigkeit, mit welcher in fast allen Fällen die Spontanatmung aufrecht erhalten werden kann, nicht zur fahrlässigen Verwendung dieses Narkosemittels durch unausgebildete Ärzte führt.

Unangenehme Wahrnehmungen in der Aufwachphase scheinen im Kindesalter selten zu sein. Nur zweimal erzählten Kinder von als subjektiv angenehm empfundenen Träumen.

Krampfanamnesen scheinen uns eine Kontraindikation gegen die Verwendung von Ketamine zu sein. Wir glauben zwar nicht, daß das Ketamine als Ursache für die bei einem Fall aufgetretenen Konvulsionen anzusehen ist. Immerhin müssen wir aber von einem Narkosemittel verlangen können, daß es mit Sicherheit das Auftreten von Konvulsionen während eines chirurgischen Eingriffes unterdrückt.

Eingriffe im Rachenraum können nicht unter CI-581 allein durchgeführt werden, da die immer vorhandenen natürlichen Schutzreflexe kein

ruhiges Arbeiten gestatten und da Erbrechen und Laryngospasmus ausgelöst werden können.

Besonders günstig scheint die Anwendung dieses neuen Anaesthesie-
mittels bei Eingriffen im Gesicht zu sein, wo der Zugang zu den Atem-
wegen durch die Operation erschwert ist, wie z. B. bei plastischen Operationen im Gesicht oder bei der Behandlung von im Gesicht verbrannten Kindern. Bei anderen Indikationen scheint uns Ketamin weniger deutlich den
üblichen Narkoseverfahren, z. B. der Inhalationsnarkose mit Halothan,
überlegen zu sein. Nach unserer Erfahrung ziehen die Kinder das Einschlafen mit einem Inhalationsmittel fast in jedem Fall der Narkoseeinleitung mit der Spritze vor. Dies wird besonders deutlich bei Patienten, welche
wiederholt anaesthesiert werden müssen.

Diskussion

Corssen: Wir sind natürlich mit den heutigen Vorträgen sehr zufrieden und können feststellen, daß besonders die Herren, die uns in Ann Arbor besucht haben (Herr ZINDLER und Herr HORATZ) uns Ergebnisse präsentiert haben, die sich sehr mit unseren eigenen decken. Ganz besonders erfreut war ich natürlich zu hören, daß Herr MUNDELEER dieselben Erfahrungen wie wir gemacht hat an einer Serie von Patienten mit Verbrennungen. Es könnte doch sehr wichtig sein, noch einmal die Frage der Aufwachphase zu diskutieren. Wir haben in den letzten 14 Tagen, bevor ich aus Ann Arbor abflog, noch einmal in unserer Zahnklinik 11 Patienten behandelt, um zu beweisen, daß wir doch berechtigt sind, von einem kurzwirkenden Anaestheticum zu sprechen.

Wir verglichen 2 Patienten mit 1 mg/Pfund, 2 Patienten mit $^2/_3$ mg/Pfund 3 Patienten mit $^1/_2$ mg/Pfund, 2 Patienten mit $^1/_2$ mg/Pfund und schließlich 2 Patienten mit $^1/_4$ mg/Pfund Ketamine intravenös. Es wurden Zahnextraktionen bis zu 12 Zähnen in einer Sitzung durchgeführt. Mit 1 mg/Pfund wurde eine Analgesie von ungefähr 12 min Dauer erreicht. Bei den Patienten mit $^2/_3$ und $^1/_3$ mg/Pfund wurde jeweils eine Analgesise von ungefähr $9^1/_2$ min erreicht. Die Patienten mit $^1/_4$ mg/Pfund hatten eine Analgesiedauer von 6–7 min. Die Dauer des chirurgischen Eingriffes in dieser Gruppe war erheblich kürzer, so daß es berechtigt erscheint, für Eingriffe von 5–8 min Dauer (also z. B. Zahnextraktionen) die Dosis erheblich herabzusetzen. Wir kämen mit $^1/_4$ mg/Pfund aus. Der chirurgische Eingriff dauert ungefähr so lange, wie die Analgesie anhält. Die Aufwachzeiten waren bei allen untersuchten Patienten immer sehr kurz, und alle Patienten konnten eine halbe Stunde später aus der Klinik entlassen werden. Was ich hiermit zeigen möchte ist, daß man die Dosis für diese sehr kurzen Eingriffe niedriger als 1 mg/Pfund ansetzen kann und dann in der Lage ist, innerhalb einer halben Stunde den Patienten nach Hause zu schicken. Wie Herr Dr. DILLON noch im Laufe des heutigen Vormittags bestätigen wird, ist das eine Zeit, die für amerikanische Verhältnisse ausreichend ist. Wir wollen die Patienten nicht 10 min nach einer Anaesthesie nach Hause schicken, weil wir glauben, daß das absolut unvernünftig wäre. Wenn wir in der Lage sind, Patienten nach der genannten Dosierung innerhalb einer halben Stunde nach Hause zu schicken, dann glauben wir, daß wir es mit einem kurzwirkenden Anaestheticum zu tun haben; mit einem Anaestheticum also, das durchaus geeignet ist, im Rahmen der Ambulanzanaesthesie einen Platz einzunehmen. Wir verfahren in dieser Weise an jedem Tag bei 2–5 Patienten. Wir haben bisher noch keinen Patienten in der Klinik behalten müssen, weil seine Aufwachphase verlängert war. Allerdings vermeiden wir die intramuskuläre Injektion, denn wir glauben, daß diese Applikationsart für poliklinische Eingriffe ungeeignet ist.

Kreuscher: Herr CORSSEN, ich glaube, wir müssen uns zunächst darüber einigen, was wir unter Wirkungsdauer verstehen wollen. Wir meinen, daß wir unter Wirkungsdauer die tatsächlich nachweisbare Zeit pharmakologischer Wirkungen eines Arzneimittels verstehen sollten. Und diese Zeit bezieht sich im Hinblick auf ambulante Patienten ganz besonders auf die Beeinträchtigung ihrer Eigenverantwortlichkeit bzw. auf die Notwendigkeit ihrer Versorgung durch andere Personen.

Corssen: Aber was wollen Sie bei einem 2jährigen Kind von Verantwortlichkeit reden?

Kreuscher: Es handelt sich hierbei nicht nur um Kinder, sondern auch um Erwachsene! Wenn wir von einem kurzwirkenden oder sogar ultrakurzwirkenden Mittel sprechen, dann laufen wir immer Gefahr, daß dieses Mittel für ambulante Narkosen angewandt wird. Denken Sie bitte an die Erfahrungen mit den Thiobarbituraten!

Ich möchte aber im Hinblick auf zwei sehr traurige Arzneimittelkatastrophen, die hinter uns liegen, noch den Pharmakologen zwei grundsätzliche Fragen stellen: Sind Untersuchungen über eine mögliche teratogene Wirkung von CI-581 gemacht worden? Weiterhin möchte ich fragen, ob Untersuchungen über die Verträglichkeit oder Unverträglichkeit einer versehentlichen intraarteriellen Injektion gemacht wurden? Denken Sie bitte an die Katastrophen, die wir mit Estil erlebten!

Zindler: Ich kann Ihnen nur sagen, daß die arterielle Verträglichkeit geprüft wurde und dabei keine Unverträglichkeiten oder besondere Reaktionen gesehen wurden.

Kaump: We have studied in dogs, rabbits and rats quite extensively with no exaggerated fact beyond that which we saw with other animals.

In dogs we gave the compound intramusculary 25 mg/kg, in rats 10–20 mg/kg intramusculary and in rabbits 10 mg/kg intravenously and 20 mg/kg intramusculary respectively. A group of mated dogs were treated: 1 group during the first trimester, 1 group during the second trimester, 1 group during the third trimester of pregnancy, twicely for 6 doses in each group with no undesirable effects on pregnancy.

Lassner: Ich möchte jetzt noch die Frage stellen, ob jemand der Anwesenden eine intraarterielle Injektion mit Ketamine erlebt hat und welche Folgen sie gehabt hat.

Langrehr: Eine intraarterielle Injektion haben wir bei Menschen nicht erlebt. Wir haben aber bei drei Katzen zur Untersuchung der direkten Gefäßwirkung eine 5%ige Lösung intraarteriell injiziert und keinen Effekt an der Arterie gesehen. Auch konnten wir keine Gewebsveränderungen beobachten.

Corssen: Wir haben bei unseren insgesamt 1600 Fällen, von denen wir nur 1500 hier präsentierten, nicht eine einzige Venenirritation oder Thrombophlebitis beobachtet, obwohl wir regelmäßig danach geschaut haben. Auch bei unseren über 200 intramuskulären Injektionen wurde nicht eine einzige Gewebsunverträglichkeit festgestellt. Ich glaube, daß die Gewebsverträglichkeit ungewöhnlich gut ist.

Szappanyos: There is one more indication for the use of Ketamine, as an analgetic. We use it for acute pancreatitis, where the patient requires 100 mg Pethidine and more every hour. We changed to CI-581 using a continuous i.v.-drip. We gave 1 mg/kg for half an hour, that would be a little more than 3.000 mg Ketamine/die. From that technique we've found a satisfactory analgetic effect and no effect on the respiration, and we did not see any tachycardia or increased blood-pressure. I think it would be quite useful to try this method much more in such cases.

Peters: Aufgrund meiner Erfahrungen an der Ophthalmologischen Universitätsklinik in Amsterdam kam ich zu der Überzeugung, daß CI-581 das einzige uns bekannte Narkosemittel ist, bei dem der Ophthalmologe imstande ist, den Augendruck so zu messen, daß er klinisch brauchbare Werte erhält. Ich glaube, Frau PODLESCH sagte, daß sie bei einem ihrer Fälle ein leichtes Ansteigen des Augendruckes beobachtete. Die Früherkennung eines Glaukoms durch Augendruckmessung ist aber nicht möglich, wenn der Augendruck durch die Narkose gesenkt wird. Ich möchte diese Eigenschaft des Ketamine als einen besonderen Vorteil bezeichnen.

Allgemeine Erfahrungen mit Ketamine bei Risikopatienten

Von **H. Kassel**

Aus der Allgemeinen Anaesthesieabteilung (Chefarzt Dr. H. Kassel)
des Oldenburgischen Landeskrankenhauses Sanderbusch i. O.

Nach zunehmender Kenntnis und Beschäftigung mit dem Phencyclidinderivat CI-581 haben wir das Präparat bei der klinischen Prüfung in den letzten 2 Jahren u. a. bei sogenannten *Risikopatienten* eingesetzt, bei denen wegen der Begleitkrankheiten die Anwendung von Ketaminen nach den bisherigen Richtlinien kontraindiziert war oder der schlechte Allgemeinzustand ein erhebliches Operationsrisiko beinhaltete.

Es handelte sich um 22 Patienten, vorwiegend des höheren Lebensalters. Das Durchschnittsalter betrug 65 Jahre, die älteste Patientin war 81 Jahre.

Als *Prämedikation* gaben wir 0,5 mg Atropin und 1–2 ml Thalamonal je nach Alter und Körpergewicht.

Wir verwendeten Ketamine bei risikoreichen Operationen aus verschiedenen Fachgebieten (Tab. 1).

Tabelle 1

Fachgebiet	*Anzahl*
Allgemeine Chirurgie	
Eingriffe im Abdomen	10
Amputationen	2
Urologie	7
Gynäkologie	2
Kieferchirurgie	1
	22

CI-581 wurde in üblicher Dosierung bei 14 Fällen als intravenöses Mononarkoticum verwendet. 5 Patienten erhielten zusätzlich ein Sauerstoff-Lachgas-Halothan-Gemisch bei erhaltener Spontanatmung. 2 Patienten wurden endotracheal intubiert und unter Wechseldruck mit Sauerstoff-Lachgas beatmet. Bei 1 Patienten wurde zusätzlich eine Lokalanaesthesie gegeben.

Das erhöhte Anaesthesierisiko wurde durch Begleitkrankheiten wie Schock, Volumenmangel, Herzinsuffizienz, Hochdruck, Zustand nach Herzinfarkt, Emphysem, Intoxikation, Inanition bei metastasierender Carcinose bedingt (Tab. 2).

Tabelle 2

Risiko	*Anzahl*
Schock, Volumenmangel, Gefäßsklerose	4
Hochdruck und Myokardschaden	7
Zustand nach Herzinfarkt	2
Dekompensierte Herzinsuffizienz, Hochdruck, absolute Arrhythmie	2
Intoxikation, Inanition, Carcinose	7
	22

Bei 3 Patienten bestand zusätzlich ein manifester Diabetes mellitus, bei 2 Patienten eine Lebercirrhose, bei 1 Patient ein Asthma bronchiale.

Im Vergleich zu den bisher gebräuchlichen Narkosemitteln stellt CI-581 eine Substanz dar, die bei alleiniger Anwendung neben einer flüchtigen Atemdepression eine Zunahme von Blutdruck und Pulsfrequenz bewirkt. Dieser blutdrucksteigernde Effekt schien uns bei Schockzuständen und Intoxikationen wünschenswert. Wir beobachteten in mehreren Fällen die erstrebte Blutdrucksteigerung, bei ausgeprägtem Volumenmangel jedoch einen Blutdruckabfall. Erst nach Volumenersatz kam es nach der Zweitinjektion zu der üblichen Anhebung des Blutdrucks.

Kasuistik

1. Bei einem 68jährigen Mann wurde nach früherer suprasymphysärer Teilexstirpation der Prostata die Prostatektomie nach FREYER durchgeführt. Histologisch handelte es sich um ein Prostata-Carcinom. 5 Std nach der Operation kam es plötzlich zu einer starken Blutung aus dem Prostatabett mit Blasentamponade. Die Re-Operation mußte sofort vorgenommen werden. Der Patient befand sich im hämorrhagischen Schock. Der Anaesthesieverlauf ist in Abb. 1 dargestellt.

2. Ein 47jähriger Patient mit seit Jahren bestehendem Hochdruck (um 180/110 mmHg), arteriellen Durchblutungsstörungen und Zustand nach lumbaler Grenzstrangresektion erlitt 8 Tage vor der jetzigen Operation ein Aortengabelsyndrom mit arteriellem Durchblutungsstop beider Beine. Es wurde eine Thrombektomie nach Eröffnung der Aorta und der Aa. iliacae vorgenommen. Danach bot sich zunächst ein glatter Operationsverlauf mit Besserung der Durchblutungsverhältnisse. Nach 6 Tagen trat ein Dünn-

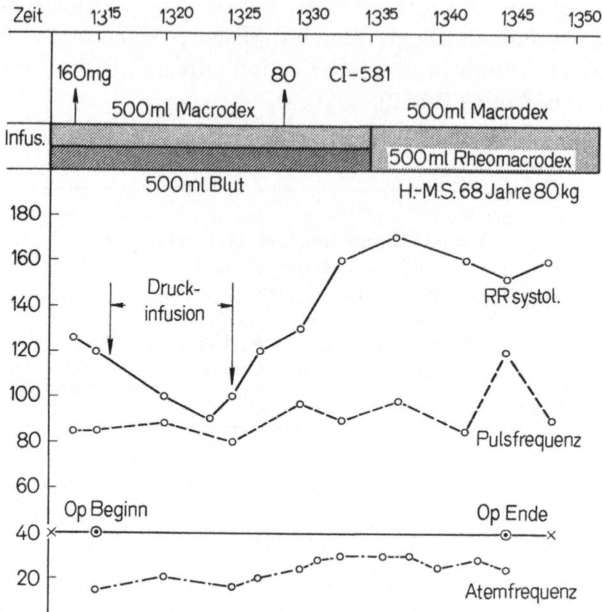

Abb. 1. Ketamine-Anaesthesie bei hämorrhagischem Schock

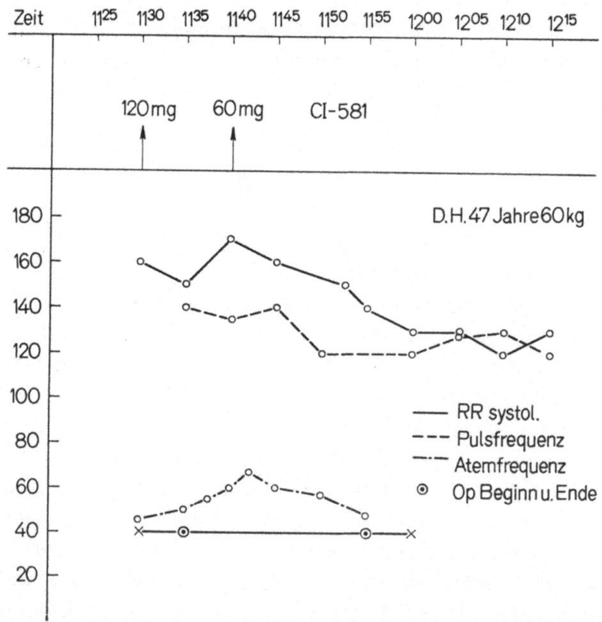

Abb. 2. Ketamine-Anaesthesie bei schwerer Intoxikation

darmileus auf. Ein Adhäsionsstrang im Operationsgebiet der Aorta mußte operativ beseitigt werden. Nach weiteren 24 Std kam es erneut zu einer massiven arteriellen Embolie des rechten Beines, die Thrombektomie im Femoralisbereich zeigte keinen Erfolg, so daß die Amputation, 24 Std später, bei schlechtem Allgemeinzustand wegen Ileusintoxikation und ausgedehnter arterieller Embolie nicht zu umgehen war (Abb. 2).

Der Patient überstand den Eingriff gut, zeigte in den nächsten Stunden zunehmende Besserung, kam jedoch 24 Std später unter den Zeichen erneuter massiver Embolien, vorwiegend des linken Beines, durch akutes Kreislaufversagen ad exitum.

3. 67jährige adipöse Frau (157 cm; 88,5 kg). Seit 10 Jahren mittelschwerer Diabetes mellitus und seit 12 Jahren Herzinsuffizienz bei Hochdruck. Zur Vorgeschichte wurden außerdem eine Lungenembolie und ein durchgemachter Herzinfarkt angegeben. Die Patientin wurde uns wegen einer beginnenden feuchten Gangrän des linken Armes von einer anderen Klinik überwiesen. Angeblich bestanden seit einer Woche wechselnde arterielle und venöse Durchblutungsstörungen. Konservative Behandlungsmaßnahmen brachten nur vorübergehenden Erfolg.

Die Blutdruckwerte lagen zwischen 220/110 und 145/110. Klinisch fanden sich die Zeichen einer dekompensierten Herzinsuffizienz mit Lippencyanose, Dyspnoe, Leberstauung und Unterschenkelödemen. Im EKG war ein Linkstyp mit Coronarinsuffizienz bei wechselnder Extrasystolie und vorübergehender absoluter Arrhythmie nachweisbar.

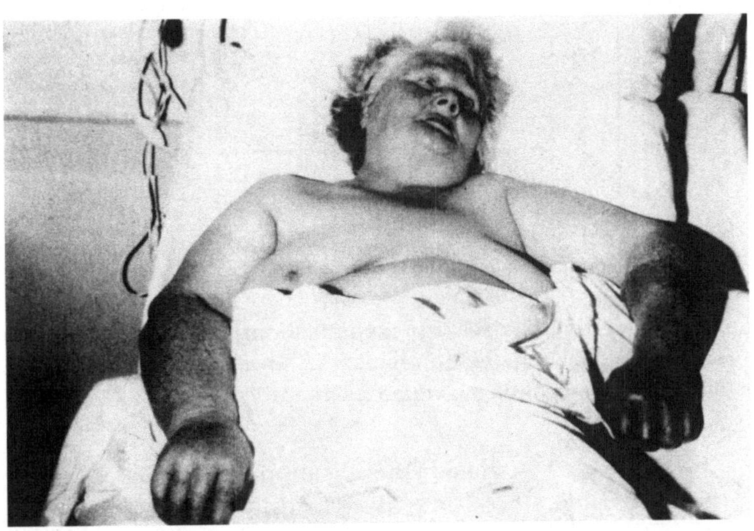

Abb. 3. T. M., 67 J., feuchte Gangrän des linken Unterarmes
bei dekompensierter Herzinsuffizienz, Hochdruck und Diabetes mellitus

Während der 1 wöchigen internen Vorbehandlung war es nicht gelungen, die Herzinsuffizienz zu kompensieren. Die zunehmend feuchte Gangrän des linken Armes verlangte eine baldige Amputation (Abb. 3).

Vor Beginn der Anaesthesie wurde über die Vena femoralis ein Cava-Katheter gelegt, da eine periphere Venenpunktion infolge ausgedehnter Thrombosierung nicht möglich war.

Während der Anaesthesie sahen wir oscillographisch im EKG keine Besonderheiten, der zentrale Venendruck schwankte prä- und postoperativ zwischen $+1$ und $+5$ cm H_2O. Dabei war der Oberkörper leicht erhöht gelagert.

Der Anaesthesieverlauf ist in Abb. 4 dargestellt.

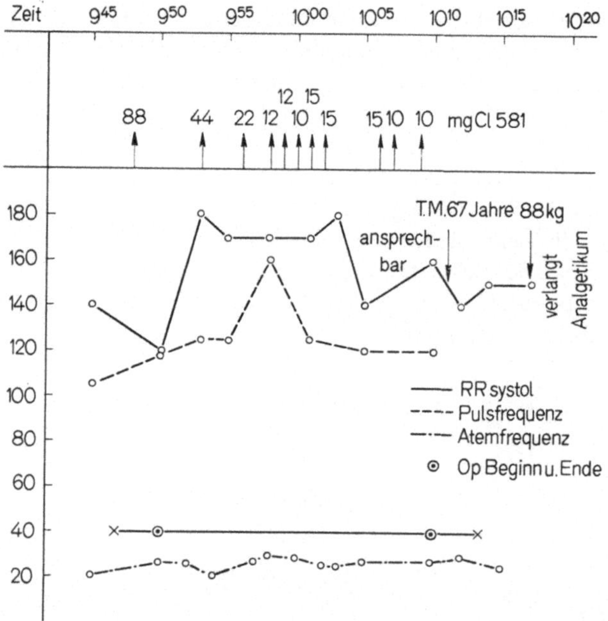

Abb. 4. Ketamine-Anaesthesie bei dekompensierter Herzinsuffizienz

Der postoperative Verlauf war komplikationslos, die Patientin erholte sich gut, die Herzdekompensation bildete sich nach Tagen zurück, wesentliche Blutzuckerschwankungen traten nicht auf.

Zusammenfassung

Das Phencyclidinderivat CI-581 hat sich bei der klinischen Prüfung in unserer Abteilung bei Risiko-Anaesthesien sehr gut bewährt. Insgesamt kamen 22 Patienten zur Operation, bei denen neben dem höheren Lebensalter wegen wesentlicher Begleitkrankheiten ein erhöhtes Operationsrisiko bestand.

Von diesen 22 Patienten erlagen 9 nach 1–11 Tagen ihrem Grundleiden. Ein ursächlicher Zusammenhang mit der Anaesthesie war in keinem Fall gegeben.

Bedrohliche Zwischenfälle während der Anaesthesie wurden nicht beobachtet.

Mit anderen Autoren sind wir der Meinung, daß CI-581 neben der geringen Toxicität eine große therapeutische Breite besitzt und eine Bereicherung unserer Anaesthesiemethoden, insbesondere auch bei Risikopatienten, darstellt.

Summary

In 22 poor risk patients (mean age 64 years) Ketamine was given intravenously for surgical, urological, gynaecological and maxillodental procedures.

The high risks consist of hypovolaemia, intoxication, cardiac insufficiency and arterial sclerosis.

No casualties, caused by Ketamine, occur.

The new anaesthetic seems to be suitable for anaesthesia in high risk patients.

Literatur

1. DOMINO, E. F., P. CHODOFF and G. CORSSEN: Clinical Pharmacology and Therapeutics 3, 279 (1965).
2. KREUSCHER, H. u. H. GAUCH: Anaesthesist 8, 229 (1967).
3. — u. J. GROTE: Anaesthesist 10, 304 (1967).
4. LANGREHR, D., P. ALAI, J. ANDJELKOVIC u. I. KLUGE: Anaesthesist 10, 308 (1967).
5. PODLESCH, J. u. M. ZINDLER: Anaesthesist 10, 299 (1967).

Klinische Erfahrungen mit Ketamine bei Eingriffen im Zahn-, Mund- und Kieferbereich

Von **L. Stöcker**

Anaesthesieabteilung des Klinikum Essen der Ruhr-Universität
(Leiter: Dr. L. Stöcker)

Krankengut

Von bisher 126 insgesamt mit CI-581 intravenös durchgeführten Mono-
anaesthesien entfielen 84 auf Kurz-Eingriffe in der Zahn- und Kieferklinik.
Das Alter der Patienten lag zwischen 6 und 68 Jahren. Das durchschnittliche
Lebensalter betrug 29 Jahre.

Die weitere Aufschlüsselung der unter Ketamine ausgeführten kieferchirurgischen Eingriffe zeigt ein selektives Überwiegen von Incisionen
perimandibulär und mundbodenwärts gelegener Abscesse mit nachfolgen-
der Drainage.

Tabelle 1. *Kieferchirurgische Eingriffe unter CI-581-Anaesthesie*

Abszeß-Spaltung, perimandibulär	68
Mundbodenphlegmone, Incision, Drainage	6
Kieferfrakturen, Reposition und Fixation	2
Sequesterotomie, Mandibula	1
Summe	84

Die Narkoseführung muß als mögliche Komplikation eine Abszeß-
Perforation in die Mundhöhle während der Incision von außen in Rechnung
stellen und Vorsorge gegen eine endobronchiale Aspiration treffen. Eine
endotracheale Intubation als Methode der Wahl zur Aspirationsprophylaxe
muß häufig blind und nasal durchgeführt werden, weil die begleitende
entzündliche Kiefersperre den oralen Zugang zum Kehlkopf blockiert. In
vier Fällen konnte ein in- und exspiratorischer Stridor als Hinweis auf ein
entzündliches Ödem im Bereich des Kehlkopfeinganges gelten. In dieser
Situation sind per inhalationem wie intravenös eingeleitete Allgemein-
narkosen nur *nach* vorangegangener Tracheotomie oder zumindest in
Tracheotomie-Bereitschaft gefahrlos durchzuführen.

Alle Patienten waren stationär aufgenommen. Als Prämedikation wurde in 58 Fällen ausschließlich Atropin 5 min vor der Ketamine-Injektion i.v. verabfolgt (Erwachsene: 0,5 mg; Kinder: 0,01 mg/kg). Die restlichen 26 Patienten erhielten 30–45 min vor dem Eingriff die zur Halothan-Lachgas-Anaesthesie bei uns übliche Prämedikation intramuskulär (Dolantin: 1 mg/kg; Atosil: 0,5–1,0 mg/kg und Atropin).

Dosis-Wirkungsrelation

Auf Grund der Voruntersuchungen von DOMINO, CHODOFF, CORSSEN, LANGREHR u. Mitarb. [2, 3, 10] und der eigenen Erfahrungen [16] lassen sich für die Dosierung von Ketamine bei intravenöser Applikation für Kurzeingriffe folgende Richtwerte angeben:

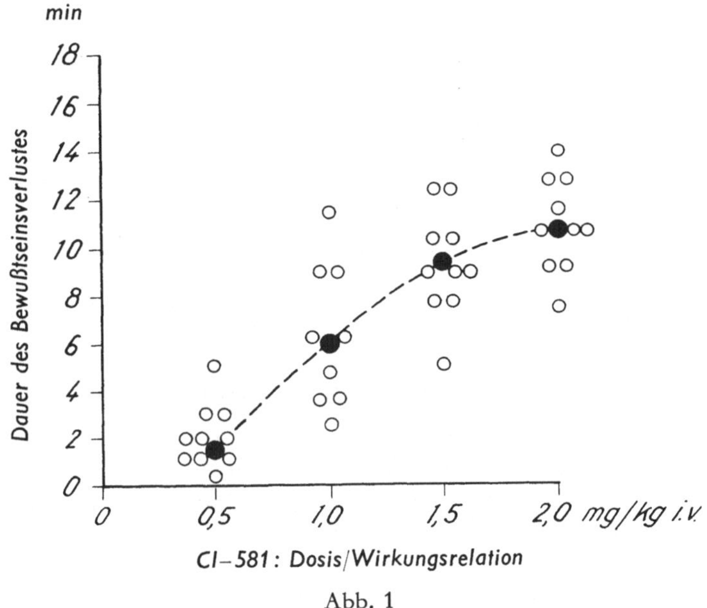

Abb. 1

Bei einer i.v.-Gabe von 0,5 mg/kg, verteilt über eine Injektionsdauer von jeweils 30 sec, wird nur in der Hälfte der Fälle Bewußtlosigkeit erreicht; die operativ nutzbare Zeit beträgt etwa 1 min. Die andere Hälfte der Patienten verbleibt ansprechbar, weist jedoch Zeichen hochgradiger Analgesie für einen Zeitraum von etwa 5 min auf.

Bei einer Dosierung von 1 mg/kg i.v. beträgt die Operationstoleranz zwischen 3 und 12 min, im Mittel 6 min. Alle Patienten zeigten eine in Frequenz und Tiefe unbeeinflußte Atmung. Die Corneal-, Husten- und Schluckreflexe blieben erhalten. Die Lidspalte des Auges wird häufig nicht geschlossen, in einigen Fällen wurde ein grobschlächtiger horizontaler Nystagmus beobachtet.

Bei generell erhöhtem Skeletmuskel-Tonus und gesteigert auslösbaren Sehnenreflexen erübrigten sich alle Maßnahmen zur Freihaltung der oberen Luftwege wie die Einlage eines Guedel-Mundtubus oder auch nur die Überstreckung des Kopfes. Ohne ausreichende Atropin-Prämedikation kam regelmäßig eine starke, dünnflüssige Salivation in die Mundhöhle zur Beobachtung. Der Speichel wurde von den Patienten intermittierend verschluckt, ohne Dysphagien auszulösen.

Bei einer Dosierung von 1,5 mg/kg i.v. beträgt die nutzbare Operationszeit im Mittel 10 min bei Schwankungen zwischen 6 und 14 min. Eine weitere Steigerung der Dosis auf 2 mg/kg i.v. führte nur zu einer geringen Zunahme der Dauer der Operationstoleranz auf einen Mittelwert von 12 min. Bei gleichzeitiger Dolantin-Prämedikation (1 mg/kg) sank das Ventilationsvolumen der ersten 3 min merklich ab, weil bei gesteigerter Frequenz die Atemtiefe abflacht und kurzfristige Apnoe-Intervalle von 15–20 sec Dauer, gefolgt von tieferen Atemzügen, auftreten. Bei einem mit 2 mg/kg Dolantin i.m. prämedizierten 42jährigen Patienten dieser Gruppe trat 3 min nach der Injektion von 2 mg/kg Ketamine i.v. unter Luftatmung eine mäßige Hautcyanose auf, die eine assistierte Beatmung mit Sauerstoff über etwa 5 min erforderte.

Klinischer Narkoseverlauf

In Abhängigkeit von der Kreislaufzeit tritt 1–1,5 min nach der über 30 sec verteilten i.v.-Injektion die Medikamentwirkung schlagartig ein. Diese bietet für den mit der intravenösen Barbiturat- oder Propanididnarkose (Epontol) vertrauten Anaesthesisten ein befremdendes Bild:

Die Unterhaltung mit dem Patienten verstummt, der Gesichtsausdruck wird eigentümlich leer, verliert seine Mimik, erscheint „mineralisiert". Bei in der Regel erhaltenem Conjunctival- und Cornealreflex öffnen sich die Lidspalten. In 30% kommt ein horizontaler Nystagmus zur Beobachtung, der bis in die Aufwachphase anhält.

Bis zu einer Dosierung von 2 mg/kg i.v. sind die Schluck- und Hustenreflexe sicher und vollständig erhalten. Der ungestörte Skeletmuskeltonus garantiert die selbständige Freihaltung der oberen Luftwege ohne „Halten des Unterkiefers" (Essmarch'scher Handgriff) oder Einlegen eines Guedel-Mundtubus.

Für Operationen im Bereich der Zahnreihen ist ein Kiefersperrer erforderlich. Operationen in Höhe des weichen Gaumens und des Rachenringes (Tonsillektomie) werden durch den erhaltenen Schluck- und Hustenreflex gestört.

Die Rückkehr des Bewußtseins kündigt sich durch Schließen der bisher weit geöffneten Augenlider und durch unwillkürliche Bewegungen an. Die Analgesie überdauert die Phase der Amnesie um etwa 10–20 min. Während der Übergangsphase ist die Sprache anfänglich verwaschen. Es finden sich Echolalie und Wort-Formulierungsstörungen.

Trotz anschließender schneller Reorientierung über Raum und Zeit vermag es der Patient offensichtlich nur mit großer Mühe, wieder eine Beziehung zu sich und seinem Körper aufzunehmen.

Das Vermögen, sich aus der Horizontalen selbständig zum Sitzen aufzurichten, ist selbst bei der niedrigen Dosierung von 1 mg/kg Ketamine i.v. über 15–20 min gestört. Läßt man später – also nach 30–45 min –, den Patienten mit Unterstützung durch eine Begleitperson gehen, so erweisen sich die orthostatischen Kreislaufregulationen als stabil. Der Gang aber ist unsicher, schwankend und läßt eine ausgesprochene Ataxie erkennen.

Bei einer Dosierung von 1 mg/kg Ketamine i.v. sind nach 1 Std alle durch das Mittel hervorgerufenen und klinisch faßbaren Veränderungen einschließlich der Ataxie abgeklungen. Bei einer Dosierung von 1,5 mg/kg i.v. war das Verhalten nach 90–120 min unauffällig. Die Prämedikation mit Opiaten (Dolantin 1 mg/kg; 30 min vor Anaesthesie-Beginn i.m.) verlängerte die Wirkungsdauer der jeweiligen Ketaminedosen um durchschnittlich 30–50%.

Herz- und Kreislaufeffekte unter Ketamine

Wie in den Tierversuchen an Kaninchen, Hunden und Affen [9], so führt auch beim Menschen die intravenöse Injektion von CI-581 zu einem regelmäßig zu beobachtenden Pulsanstieg um 20–30 Schläge/min, der in der 3. min nach der Injektion sein Maximum erreicht und über 5–12 min anhält. Eine maximale Frequenzsteigerung wird bereits bei einer Dosierung von 0,5 mg/kg Körpergewicht erreicht; eine Erhöhung der Dosis führt zu keiner weiteren Steigerung.

Synchron mit der Herzfrequenzsteigerung – diese aber zeitlich überdauernd –, verläuft ein Anstieg des systolischen und des diastolischen Blutdrucks, dessen Ausmaß dosisabhängig ist.

Der bemerkenswerte Anstieg des diastolischen Blutdrucks weist auf eine sympathikotone Wirkung des Ketamine hin. Von KREUSCHER u. Mitarb. [9] wurden nach 1,5 mg/kg CI-581 i.v. eine Steigerung des Herzschlagvolumens um 25–28%, eine Vergrößerung des Herzminutenvolumens um 75% ermittelt.

Orthostatische Belastungen lassen sich in einem zahnärztlichen Behandlungsstuhl nicht ganz umgehen. Sie wurden vom Kreislauf unserer Patienten gut toleriert, weil Ketamine eine Erhöhung des Venendrucks, des elastischen Widerstandes und eine frequenzabhängige Vermehrung des Herzzeitvolumens bedingt.

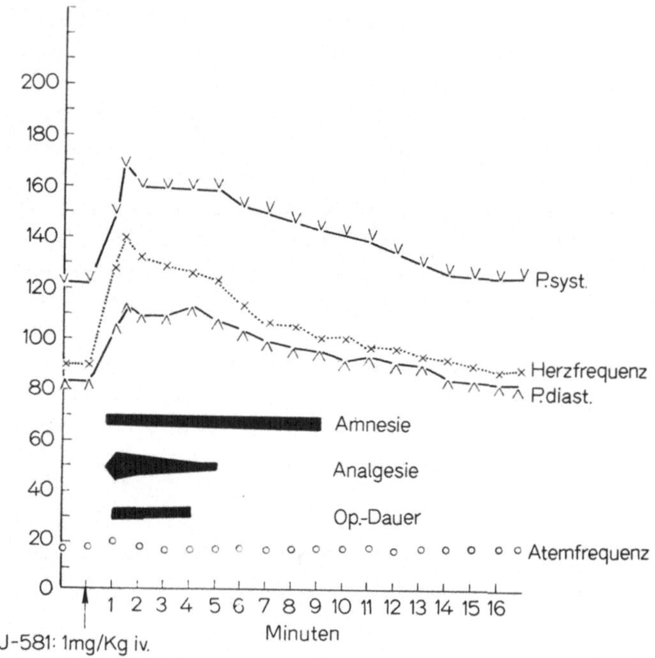

Abb. 2. Mittelwerte von 3 Patienten unter i.v. Narkose mit 1 mg/kg Ketamine. Verhalten von Puls, Blutdruck und Atmung

Die stimulierende Wirkung von Ketamine auf Herz und Kreislauf legen seine Anwendung bei Hypotonikern, orthostatisch belastenden Lagerungen (HNO- und zahnärztliche Praxis) und bei kardiodepressiven diagnostischen Untersuchungen (Serien-Angiographie, Pneumencephalographie) nahe. Sinngemäß gelten als relative Kontraindikationen fixierte Hypertonien mit einem systolischen Blutdruck über 180 mmHg.

Atmung

Plethysmographische Untersuchungen [3] und Messungen des Atemminutenvolumens an Patienten, die zuvor in Lokalanaesthesie intubiert wurden, haben ergeben, daß Ketamine nur eine sehr kurzfristige, dosisabhängige Ventilationsminderung geringen Ausmaßes bedingt, die 2–3 min nach der i.v. Injektion ihr Maximum erreicht und bis zu 20% des Ausgangswertes beträgt. Durch blutgasanalytische Untersuchungen konnte die Entstehung einer respiratorischen Acidose unter CI-581 ausgeschlossen werden [3, 10, 14). Eine Prämedikation mit Opiaten (Dolantin 1–2 mg/kg i.m.) kann die Atemdepression manifest werden lassen.

Zentralnervensystem, Reflexverhalten, Psyche

Während oder nach mit Ketamine durchgeführten Allgemeinanaesthesien kamen keine Krampfanfälle zur Beobachtung. Der Muskeltonus ist mäßig erhöht, die Sehnenreflexe sind leicht gesteigert.

Unmittelbar mit Einsetzen der komatösen Phase kommt es unter der Einwirkung von CI-581 zu der für Phencyclidin-Derivate charakteristischen Veränderung des EEG:

An Stelle des Ruhe-EEG mit alpha-Rhythmus tritt über beiden Hemisphären eine generalisierte theta-Aktivität zu Tage (b), die bei Rückkehr der Ansprechbarkeit mit beta-Wellen durchsetzt ist (c).

Der präanaesthesiologische alpha-Rhythmus kommt ungestört erst wieder zur Beobachtung, wenn der klinische Eindruck längst unauffällig geworden ist. Bei einer Dosierung von 1 mg/kg i.v. ist dies nach 60–90 min, bei einer Dosierung von 1,5 mg/kg i.v. nach 90–120 min der Fall.

Krampfpotentiale wurden nicht registriert.

Bei 19 Patienten wurde ein grober horizontaler Nystagmus beobachtet. Die Augenlidspalte blieb in 60% der Fälle während der Anaesthesie offen. Spontane Bewegungen und Schließen der Augenlider kündigen das Aufwachen des Patienten an. Bei läppischem Gesichtsausdruck erscheint der Patient ansprechbar, bevor nach weiteren 3–5 min das Kommunikations- und Erinnerungsvermögen einsetzt.

Eigenversuche haben gezeigt, daß während der Aufwachphase die Minderung der Tiefensensibilität und der Berührungsempfindlichkeit sich subjektiv störend auswirkten. Trotz schneller Rückkehr des Orientierungsvermögens kann der Patient offensichtlich nur mit Mühe wieder eine Beziehung zu sich und seinem Körper finden.

Obwohl der Bewußtseinsverlust objektiv unter der Ketamine-Injektion schlagartig einsetzt, fehlt subjektiv bei einer Mononarkose mit CI-581 die für Barbiturat- oder Propanidid-Anaesthesie typische Bewußtseinslücke.

Vielmehr wurden von 13% spontan und von 19% zusätzlich auf Anfrage „Narkose-Träume" angegeben, die bei intellektuellen Patienten vorwiegend als interessant und angenehm, bei naiven Patienten als beängstigend und unangenehm empfunden wurden.

Ursächlich für die Traumerlebnisse dürfte der Ausfall sensorischer Afferenzen (Berührungs- und Schmerzempfindung, Tiefensensibilität) wäh-

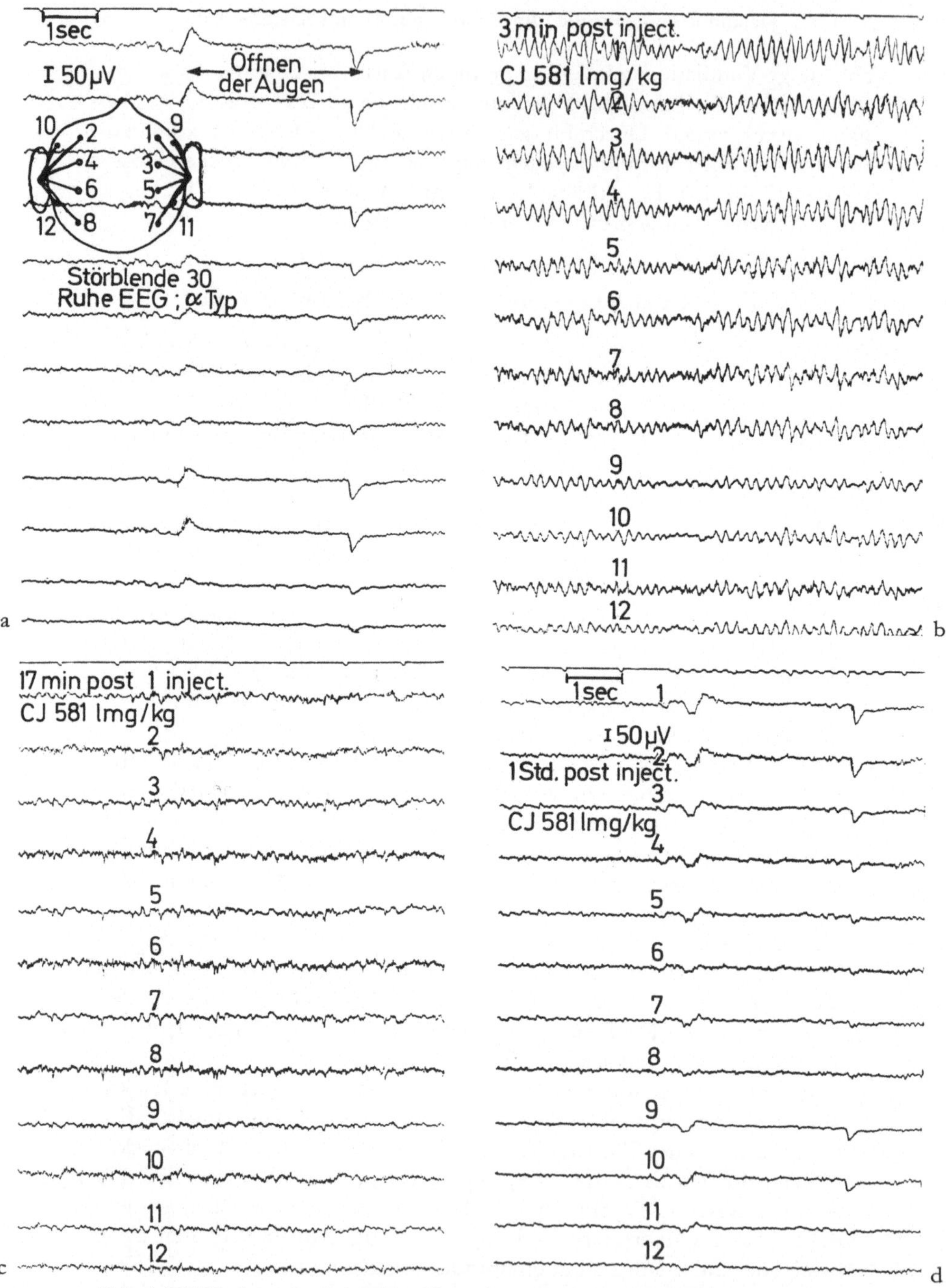

Abb. 3. EEG; a) vor der Injektion, b) 3 min nach 1 mg/kg Ketamine i.v., c) 17 min nach 1 mg/kg Ketamine i.v., d) 60 min nach 1 mg/kg Ketamine i.v.

rend der Aufwachphase anzuschuldigen sein, der mit optischen Störungen wie Doppeltsehen, Nystagmus und Astigmatisus häufig gekoppelt ist.

Äußerungen wie „ich war im Weltraum" oder „ich bin mit einer Mondrakete gefahren" oder „ich war tot und im Himmel" werden so verständlich. In 4 Fällen war der Charakter der Traumerlebnisse ausgesprochen beängstigend und unangenehm. Eine 12jährige Schülerin äußerte das Empfinden „von einer riesigen Dampfwalze platt gedrückt zu werden"; eine 63jährige Patientin gab an „wie von warmen Sand lebendig begraben worden zu sein."

Die Beobachtungen von LANGREHR, KREUSCHER und anderen [9, 10], daß eine nachfolgende Inhalationsnarkose diese Traumerlebnisse auslöscht, bzw. diese gar nicht erst entstehen läßt, kann als weiterer Hinweis für die zeitliche Genese dieser Wachträume während des Abklingens der Ketamine-Einwirkung gewertet werden.

Tabelle 2. *Psychotomimetische Nebenwirkungen unter CI-581*

„Narkoseträume" spontan	16; auf Nachfrage	25 = 41
subjektiv angenehm	28	
subjektiv unangenehm	4	
subjektiv indifferent	52	
Erregungszustände in der unmittelbaren Aufwachphase		2
Erregungszustände 10–30 min nach Rückkehr des Bewußtseins anhaltend (chronischer, agressiver Alkoholist)		1

Psychische Veränderungen traten in der weiteren postoperativen Phase nicht auf. Nur bei einem wegen chronischem Alkoholismus entmündigten Landstreicher wurde ein etwa 40 min anhaltender Unruhezustand beobachtet, der mit Äußerungen der Selbstanklage Gott gegenüber, mit Singen von Kirchenliedern und Zeichen allgemeinen Katzenjammers einherging.

Entscheidend für die Wahl des Ketamine zur Durchführung kieferchirurgischer Kurzeingriffe war die Beobachtung, daß bei erhaltenem Tonus der Schlund- und Mundbodenmuskulatur und bei ungestörten Schluck- und Hustenreflexen schmerzfrei operiert werden konnte. Auch bei den vier Fällen mit in- und exspiratorischem Stridor und Kehlkopfeingangsödem konnte ohne Beeinträchtigung der Atmung ein Mundbodenabsceß incidiert werden. Speichel oder in die Mundhöhle durchgebrochener Absceßeiter wurde entweder reaktionslos verschluckt oder lief bei Kopftieflagerung nach außen ab.

Da nach bisherigen Erfahrungen durch Ketamine kein Erbrechen ausgelöst wird und subjektives Übelkeitsgefühl auch nach Applikation des

CI-581 auf vollen Magen 30 min nach dem Mittagessen vermißt wird (Eigenversuche), läßt sich unseres Erachtens die Intubation der Trachea zur Aspirationsprophylaxe umgehen, ohne die Sicherheit des Patienten zu beeinträchtigen.

Bei der entzündlich bedingten Kiefersperre müßte die endotracheale Intubation nasal und blind durchgeführt werden; eine weitere Traumatisierung würde der Ausbildung eines Kehlkopfeingangsödems Vorschub leisten.

Laboruntersuchungen

Bei 10 Patienten, die zur Anaesthesie 1,0–1,5 mg/kg Ketamine i.v. und zur Prämedikation ausschließlich 0,5 mg Atropin i.v. erhalten hatten, erfolgte die Kontrolle der Leber- und Nierenfunktion an Hand der Bestimmungen von SGOT, SGPT, LDH, Harnstoffstickstoff und Kreatinin im Serum

    a) vor dem Eingriff,

    b) 24 Std nach der Narkose und

    c) 3 Tage nach der Ketamine-Anaesthesie.

Wie Einzel- und Mittelwerte zeigen, war eine Veränderung über die physiologische Variationsbreite hinaus nicht festzustellen [Tab. 3. Mittelwerte von 10 Patienten unter Ketamine-Anaesthesie a) vor, b) 24 Std nach und c) 3 Tage nach der Applikation.].

Einen blutzuckersteigernden Effekt konnten wir durch Serienbestimmung des Blutzuckers 1, 2 und 3 Std nach Injektion von CI-581 nicht nachweisen. Die hämatologischen Veränderungen waren uncharakteristisch; eine vermehrte Leukocytose ist durch die Auswahl des operativen Krankengutes (perimandibuläre Abscesse und Mundbodenphlegmonen) hinreichend geklärt.

Summary

Ketamine for oral surgery

The report deals with 126 cases of short-lasting Ketamine-Anaesthesia, introduced by intravenous injection of CI-581 in patients from 6 to 68 years of age. Dose range: 0.5–2.0 mg./kg. body weight. 84 cases were done in oral surgery.

The characteristics of Ketamine-Anaesthesia are marked analgesia, slightly increased mucsle tone and lack of respiratory depression, if no premedication with opiates is given. The eyelids remain open, horizontal nystagmus frequently is observed. Corneal, pharyngeal and laryngeal reflexes are well preserved. There were no convulsions.

Tabelle 3. *Bestimmungen von SGOT, SGPT, LDH, Harnstoffstickstoff und Kreatinin im Serum vor und 24 bzw. 72 Std nach der Injektion von CI-581 (70 Patienten)*

Nr.	SGOT	SGPT	LDH	Harnstoff-N.	Kreatinin
1 a)	13,5	11,2	76	22,5	0,7 (vor Ketamine)
b)	*13,5*	*9,0*	*114*	*28,0*	*0,9 (nach 24 Std)*
c)	*11,2*	*11,2*	*102*	*18,0*	*0,4 (nach 3 Tagen)*
2 a)	36,0	13,5	210	15,0	0,9
b)	*20,2*	*18,0*	*124*	*18,0*	*1,0*
c)	*20,2*	*7,5*	*114*	*19,0*	*1,0*
3 a)	13,5	18,0	306	22,5	1,4
b)	*11,2*	*6,7*	*238*	*21*	*0,9*
c)	*11,2*	*7,7*	*306*	*18*	*0,9*
4 a)	4,5	6,7	76	18	0,55
b)	*11,2*	*6,7*	*114*	*23*	*0,8*
c)	*7,2*	*11,2*	*76*	*20,5*	*0,9*
5 a)	11,2	7,2	124	22,5	1,4
b)	*13,5*	*7,7*	*114*	*11,0*	*0,5*
c)	*7,5*	*11,2*	*210*	*15,0*	*0,8*
6 a)	36	13,5	238	18	1,1
b)	*20,2*	*11,2*	*114*	*19*	*1,2*
c)	*13,5*	*7,7*	*210*	*20,5*	*1,0*
7 a)	4,5	6,7	124	18,5	0,8
b)	*7,2*	*11,2*	*210*	*15,0*	*0,65*
c)	*11,2*	*9,0*	*114*	*18,0*	*0,7*
8 a)	20,5	4,5	95	18,5	0,9
b)	*20,2*	*7,7*	*102*	*22,5*	*1,1*
c)	*4,5*	*6,7*	*76*	*20,5*	*1,4*
9 a)	4,5	7,7	322	18	1,1
b)	*7,5*	*11,2*	*238*	*20,0*	*1,4*
c)	*11,2*	*9,0*	*124*	*12*	*0,9*
10 a)	36	13,5	76	20,5	1,5
b)	*20,5*	*11,2*	*114*	*18,0*	*1,1*
c)	*13,5*	*7,5*	*114*	*18,0*	*1,2*
Mittelwerte:					
a)	17,7	10,3	165	17,9	1,0
b)	14,5	10,0	148	19,6	0,95
c)	11,3	8,9	145	18,9	0,95

The average time in which operative procedures following intravenous injection of Ketamine were well tolerated, are 6 min at a dose of 1 mg./kg., 10 min at a dose of 1.5 mg./kg. and 12 min if 2 mg./kg. body weight are given.

Atropin is recommended for premedication to prevent the induced salivation. Pethidin, 1–2 mg./kg. 30 min prior to induction i.m., not only increases the duration of anaesthesia for about 30–50%, but also lengthens the awakening period and depresses ventilation. Its use seems to be superflous in a potent analgesic agent as Ketamine.

The use of CI-581 in short-lasting oral surgery is advantageous for the following reasons:

1. The maintenance of vital reflexes obviates the need for endotracheal intubation, even in the presence of locked mandibular joint or in- and exspiratory stridorous breathing. If during the procedure blood or purulent material enters the oral cavity, it is either swallowed or runs out of the mouth.

2. Complete lack of emetic properties allows the procedure to be done also in patients whose stomach is not empty.

3. Sympathicomimetic stimulation of the cardiovascular system counteracts the effects of the semi-sitting position which frequently is maintained in dentistry.

However, a fixed hypertension of more than 180 mmHg systolic should be considered as a contraindication for the use of CI-581.

Psychomimetic side-effects showed up only during the awakening period and were manifested in 32% of the cases by vivid, but rather amorphous and unreasonable dreams which in 4 Patients (3%) had a very unpleasant contents that led to anxiety.

Further complaints of this period were double vision, nystagmus, astigmatism and "numbness" of the total body.

Observations of other investigators were confirmed, that additional inhalation anaesthesia, extending beyond the period of Ketamine-action, will abolish these undesirable side-effects.

Intravenous as well as intramuscular Ketamine-Anaesthesia in the adult should *not* be called short-acting, since it takes at least 2–3 h following the i.v. injection of 2 mg./kg. CI-581, before the clinical and EEG findings return to normal.

Children however, given the same dose, may be left without medical observation after 30–60 min, if the horizontal position is maintained and transportation cared for.

Under these preliminaries the drug can be used as i.v.-anaesthetic for outpatient care.

Literatur

1. Chen, G., C. Ensor, D. Russel, and B. Bohner: J. Pharmacol. exp. Ther. **127**, 241–250 (1956).
2. Corssen, G., and E. F. Domino: Anesth. Analg. **45**, 29 (1966).

3. Domino, E. F.: Int. Rev. Neurobiol. 6, 303 (1964).
4. —, P. Chodoff, and G. C. Corssen: Clin. Pharmacol. Ther., Vol. 6, No 3, 279–291 (1965).
5. Greifenstein, F. E., M. de Vault, J. Yoshitake, and J. E. Gajewpki: Anesth. Analg. 7, 283–294 (1958).
6. Gött, U.: Anaesthesist 9, 261–264 (1960).
7. Johnstone, M.: Anaesthesist 9, 114–115 (1960).
8. —, V. Evans, and S. Baigel: Brit. J. Anaesth. 31, 433 (1959).
9. Kreuscher, H., u. H. Gauch: Anaesthesist 16, Heft 8: 229–233 (1967).
10. Langrehr, D., Palai I. Andjelkovic, u. J. Kluge: Anaesthesist 16, Heft 10: 308–318 (1967).
11. Lear, E., R. Suntay, I. M. Pallin, and A. E. Chiron: Anesthesiology 20, 330 (1959).
12. McCarthy, D. A., and C. M. Chen: Fed. Proc. 24, 268 (1965).
13. — —, D. H. Kaump, and C. Ensor: J. New Drugs, Vol. 5, No. 1 (1965).
14. Podlesch, I., u. M. Zindler: Anaesthesist 16, Heft 10, 229–303 (1967).
15. Scholler, K. L., H. Thies, u. K. Wiemers: Anaesthesist 9, 163–169 (1960).
16. Stöcker, L.: Dtsch. zahnärztl. Z., 21. Jahrgang, Heft 10, 1241–1243 (1966).

Clinical Experience
with Ketamine (CI-581) in Surgical Interventions
of Short Duration

By **A. Soetens**

Department of Anesthesia – Civilian Hospital –
Hoboken-Antwerp (Belgium)

CI-581 was tested in 7 cases, 3 of which were males. The age of the patients ranged from 19 to 60 years. Weight ranged from 60 to 100 kg. In five instances the surgical intervention was of very short duration: from 3 to 5 min. The other two cases lasted 17 and 45 min.

The drug was injected intravenously without any premedication. Analgesia was sufficient after 2 min allowing the surgeon to start his intervention. In all but two cases a second dose was injected 2 or 3 min after the beginning of the operation.

The total amount of drug injected ranged from 1.4 to 2.6 mg. per kg. bodyweight, the average dose being 1.95 mg. per kg. bodyweight.

In all cases analgesia was very satisfactory and the surgical intervention was very well accepted. No respiratory depression occurred.

But when side effects are considered, satisfaction is not so complete. First of all, already during the anaesthetic period, we noticed sometimes an important muscular rigidity. In one case we even experienced a sort of catatonia: the upper and lower limbs remained as they were positioned.

In the post-operative course, during the awakening period, in 3 cases out of 7 trials, some untoward psychic effects were noticed in the form of hallucinations, strange feeling and in one case frightful dreams made the patient scream, disturbing her neighbours in the ward. In this particular case it has to be outlined that the patient was allowed to awake in a quiet sorrounding and that no question was asked until she was fully awake in order not to "evoke" dreams.

These psychic troubles were noticed exclusively in women. We had no trouble whatsoever with none of the 3 men. Maybe this is ascribable to the greater psychic lability of women.

However we feel that these untoward psychic effects in adults constitute a definite contraindication to the use of CI-581.

Zusammenfassung

Ketamine wurde bei 7 Patienten im Alter von 19–60 Jahren ohne vorherige Prämedikation intravenös appliziert. Die bei einer Dosierung von 1,9 mg/kg erreichte Narkosedauer betrug 3–5 min. In allen Fällen wurde eine zufriedenstellende Analgesie erreicht und in keinem Fall Atemdepression beobachtet. Bei einigen Patienten wurde eine vermehrte Muskelrigidität festgestellt. Bei 3 Patienten traten in der Aufwachphase unerwünschte psychische Nebeneffekte wie Halluzinationen, furchterregende Träume und allgemeine Unruhe auf. Diese psychischen Störungen wurden ausschließlich bei Frauen beobachtet und schränken die Anwendbarkeit des Mittels bei Erwachsenen ein.

Erfahrungen mit Ketamine im Selbstversuch

Von **J. Lassner**

Die Berichte über psychische Störungen nach Ketamin haben mich veranlaßt, Selbstversuche mit dieser Substanz durchzuführen. Die Dosierung war in dem 1. Versuch 0,3 mg/ml im intravenösen Dauertropf bis zu einer Gesamtdosis von 0,5 mg/kg, im 2. Versuch bis zu einer Gesamtdosis von 1 mg/kg und im 3. Versuch eine Schnellinjektion mit einer Dosis von 3 mg/kg. Im 1. Versuch wurde eine Prämedikation mit 0,5 mg Atropin gegeben. Die beiden anderen Versuche erfolgten ohne Prämedikation. Der Versuchsablauf wurde in der üblichen Weise registriert und von meinen Mitarbeitern überwacht. Meine Äußerungen wurden mittels Tonband aufgezeichnet. Bei den ersten beiden Versuchen bemühte ich mich besonders, meine Eindrücke und persönlichen Erlebnisse so gut wie möglich zu verbalisieren und gleichzeitig von den Beobachtern ihre Bemerkungen synchron notieren zu lassen, um dann später beide konfrontieren zu können. Ich glaube, daß der Zeitpunkt nach dem Vortrag von Herrn SOETENS aus Antwerpen besonders günstig ist, um diese Selbstbeobachtungen kurz zu rekapitulieren. Vielleicht können wir auf diese Weise die klinischen Beobachtungen besser verstehen.

Beim Eintropfen der Lösung kam es schon nach 3 mg (ich wiege 80 kg) zu leichter Sehstörung, zur Schwierigkeit zu fixieren, bald zu Schwierigkeiten beim Artikulieren der Worte. Um den Mund herum ein Gefühl von „Dicke", so wie nach einer Injektion von einem Lokalanaestheticum durch den Zahnarzt. Dann eine Umwölkung und Umnachtung des Bewußtseins, obwohl die Verbalisierung weiterhin, wenn auch mit Schwierigkeiten, durchzuführen war. Ein gradueller Verfall des Körperbewußtseins und Unmöglichkeit bestimmte Gegenden, die Körperinseln, wie sie SCHMIDT genannt hat, zu lokalisieren. Das Selbstgefühl, das Ich-Gefühl, zog sich gewissermaßen mehr und mehr in die craniale Gegend zurück, bis schließlich das Selbstbewußtsein in eine Gegend um Stirn und Augen beschränkt war. Trotzdem war weiterhin eine Verbalisierung möglich, wenn auch mit erheblichen Schwierigkeiten beim Aussprechen: Stottern, Echolalie und ähnliche Erscheinungen. Zugleich kam es, vielleicht aus dem experimentellen Zusammenhang heraus, zu einer eigenartigen Schwierigkeit, gleichzeitig Beobachter und Beobachteter zu sein. Dieser Versuch, festzustellen, was erlebt wird, führte zu einer Entzweiung des Beobachteten und des

Beobachters selbst, und zwar stärker bei der höheren Dosierung als der niedrigeren, zugleich mit einem merkwürdigen Wiederholungsphänomen. Es war so, wie wenn man, zwischen 2 Spiegeln sitzend, das Spiegelbild und das gespiegelte Spiegelbild immer schwieriger voneinander unterscheiden kann.

Im 2. Versuch führte diese Aufgabe, weiter zu beobachten und gleichzeitig Beobachteter zu sein, zu einer äußerst beängstigenden Störung der Zusammenhänge, so daß einen Moment der Gedanke auftrat, es würde nie mehr möglich sein, herauszubekommen, was eigentlich Wirklichkeit wäre und was Beobachtung. Nun war das schon beim 1. Versuch passiert und die Angstäußerungen von den Umstehenden so verstanden worden, daß sie tatsächlich den intravenösen Tropf für einen Moment angehalten hatten. Weil ich gleich wieder zu Bewußtsein gekommen war, hatte ich den Auftrag gegeben, in keinem Fall diese Äußerungen irgendwie Einfluß auf den Fortgang des Versuchs nehmen zu lassen, sondern den Versuch weiterzuführen. Dadurch kam es dann kurz nach dieser Verwirrung mit Realitäts- und Selbstbewußtseinsverlust zu einem Unbewußtsein aber gleich wieder, nach Verlangsamung der intravenösen Zufuhr, zum Wiederauftreten derselben Schwierigkeit.

Wenn die Dosierung höher war und der tatsächliche Bewußtseinsverlust zustandegekommen war, traten beim Aufwachen oder beim Wiedereintreten des Beobachtungsvermögens verschiedene interessante Phänomene auf: Das wesentlichste dabei war das Wiederkehren des Sprechvermögens zu einem Zeitpunkt, wo sowohl die Innenbeobachtung wie die optische Beobachtung durch das Sehen des Körpers zu erheblichen Störungen führte. Das interessanteste war dabei, daß die vorhergesehenen Schmerzreize durch Einstechen von Nadeln in verschiedene Körperpartien (Beine, Arme, Wangen und Nacken) in allen Zustandsmomenten als normal schmerzhaft empfunden wurden, aber in keiner Weise mit dem Körper in Zusammenhang zu bringen waren. Ketamine ist kein Analgeticum im üblichen Sinn. Der Schmerzreiz wird als solcher durchaus erfahren, aber nicht sensu strictiore einverleibt. So wurde z. B. in einem dieser Versuche auf den Arm geklebtes Heftpflaster langsam abgezogen. Dabei wurde an den bei mir sehr zahlreichen Haaren gezogen. Das ist eigentlich eine geringe Unannehmlichkeit, war aber der Ausdehnung des Hautreizes wegen interessanter als das bloße Einstechen von Nadeln. Dieser Reiz war deutlich verstärkt, fühlbar wie eine Verbrennung, aber nicht am Arm, sondern etwa 25–30 cm seitwärts vom Arm, d. h. an einer Stelle, wo sich der physische Arm nicht befand.

Zur gleichen Zeit wurde der Körper als gewichtslos empfunden. Bewegung der Glieder überraschte dadurch, daß sich die Arme und Beine spontan bewegten, – schwerelos und mühelos, so wie bei den Astronauten im Weltraum. In diese schwerelos empfundenen Gegenden können

Schmerzreize gesetzt werden, die aber nicht als im Körperteil sich ereignend zum Bewußtsein kommen.

Die Schwierigkeit zu sehen ist von einer besonderen Art. Die Gegenstände und Personen erscheinen so wie in Zerrspiegeln. Das Seherlebnis erfolgt, als ob die Spiegel verschieden angeordnet wären. Das Störendste ist, daß die Fluchtlinien des Raumes nicht in der normalen perspektivischen Anordnung zusammenlaufen. Die Wände sind nicht mehr gerade; die Personen und die Abstände sind nicht mehr durch das Sehen zu erfahren. Die Größenverhältnisse der Gegenstände sind zueinander ohne verstehbaren Zusammenhang.

Die Störungen der Koordination und des Konzentrationsvermögens halten lange an. Persönlich habe ich mit Prüfungen, die wir durchgeführt haben, nach der 1 mg/kg-Dosis 3 Std lang deutlich Schwierigkeiten gehabt. Nach der 3 mg/kg-Dosis für über 4 Std. Das Gehen nach der Dosis von 0,5 mg/kg wurde 30 min später so wie sich Bewegen auf einem Schiff bei Sturm empfunden.

Diskussion

Langrehr: Herr Lassner, wie lange dauerte diese Tropfinfusion, d. h. in welcher Gesamtzeit wurden die 0,5 mg/kg und 3 mg/kg appliziert?

Lassner: Die 0,5 mg/kg-Dosis dauerte etwa 2 min, die 1 mg/kg-Dosis 3 min und die 3 mg/kg-Dosis wurde schnell injiziert.

Corssen: Ich möchte eine Bemerkung zu Herrn Lassners Behauptung machen, daß wir es nicht mit einem Analgeticum zu tun haben. Es ist sehr schwer, den Begriff der Analgesie zu definieren. Wenn der Patient auf einen schmerzvollen Stimulus nicht reagiert, wenn er später, nach dem Erwachen, sich an diesen schmerzvollen Stimulus nicht mehr erinnern kann, dann würden wir das als eine Analgesie bezeichnen. Der Patient ist nicht in der Lage, den Stimulus, der im Assoziationszentrum ankommt, als schmerzvollen Stimulus zu interpretieren. Und da er später nicht in der Lage ist, sich daran zu erinnern, würde ich aus praktischen Gründen sagen, daß es sich um ein Analgeticum handelt. Stimmen Sie mir zu, Herr Lassner?

Lassner: I would not!

Corssen: There is a possibility that you felt the painful stimulus but you said you did interpretate this as a painful stimulus which is outside of the body. Now, then the pain-threshold was not high enough and the dosage apparently was not the one we have recommended for producing analgesia. We have, for example, in our volunteers in the prison done exactly the same. We have used an intravenous infusion and produced a similar conciousness and then subjected the volunteers to painful stimuli. The volunteers were not able to interpret this as a painful stimulus, when we later interviewed the volunteers and had forgotten, as a matter of fact, after the intravenous infusion was discontinued.

So, I am just objecting to your claim, that we do not deal with an analgetic compound with this drug.

Langrehr: Wir stimmen mit den Eigenerfahrungen von Herrn Lassner in allen Punkten überein, nur wurde bei mir Ketamine rasch gespritzt, wobei die Aufwachphase der protrahierten Einschlafphase entspricht. In bezug auf die Analgesie muß ich aber eine andere Erfahrung mitteilen. Die Empfindung des Schmerzreizes außerhalb des Körpers mag an dem geschwollenen, außerordentlich starken lokalanaesthetischen Gefühl der Extremitäten liegen. Selbst stärkste Schmerzreize werden bei schon wiedererlangtem Bewußtsein nur ganz undeutlich und „weit entfernt" empfunden. Man könnte mit einem Messer in die Extremitäten hineinschneiden, man empfindet das nicht. Ich würde doch meinen, daß diese Substanz eine außerordentlich starke analgetische Wirkung hat.

Lassner: Die Frage, was man eine Analgesie nennen soll und was nicht, ist so schwierig, daß ich glaube, wir sollten sie hier nicht anschneiden. Denken Sie doch zum Beispiel daran, daß wir immer wieder sagen, wir verwenden Analgetika in der Anaesthesie, was an und für sich schon ein rechter Unfug ist. Daß jemand, der nicht fühlt, noch zusätzlich keinen Schmerz mehr fühlen könne, hat ja kaum eine wirkliche Bedeutung. Daß ein Bewußtloser ein Analgeticum bekommen kann oder daß ein Mittel bei einem Bewußtlosen Analgesie hervorrufen soll, beinhaltet widersprüchliche Termini. Ich bin daher mit Herrn CORSSEN darin einverstanden, daß wir tatsächlich hauptsächlich vor einem Problem stehen. Ob ein Patient, der eine Operation durchmacht, ohne sich darüber zu beschweren, ein Analgeticum bekommen hat oder nicht, das ist an und für sich eine nebensächliche Angelegenheit. Das Mittel gestattet, schmerzfrei zu operieren, und das ist das Wesentliche. Ob wir es als Analgeticum klassifizieren sollen, ist eine Frage, die mehr die Pharmakologie oder Psychologie angeht. Ich kann nur sagen, daß ich im Selbstversuch in der Lage war, Schmerzreize deutlich als solche zu identifizieren, und zwar bei der Dosierung, bei der ich noch bei Bewußtsein war. Sobald man nicht mehr bei Bewußtsein ist, wird es schwer sein zu sagen, was man empfindet.

Zindler: Wir sehen doch, daß bei Erwachsenen in der Regel diese psychischen Effekte auftreten. Warum sind sie bei Kindern nicht vorhanden? Empfinden vielleicht Kinder Erscheinungen als nicht abnorm, die wir Erwachsenen so empfinden würden? Oder kommt es daher, daß Kinder diese unangenehmen Empfindungen zwar haben, sich aber verbal nicht ausdrücken können? Gibt es darüber Beobachtungen oder Ansichten?

Corssen: Dies ist natürlich eine Frage, die uns seit Beginn unserer Versuche beschäftigt. Wenn wir Ketamine bei ein und demselben Kind bis zu 18mal geben, sollte man doch annehmen, daß diese Kinder ihren Unwillen äußern, wenn der Anaesthesist wieder mit seiner Spritze kommt, um diese Art von Anaesthesie zu verabreichen. Wir haben das aber bei keinem unserer 10 oder 12 Fälle, bei denen wir bei den gleichen Patienten häufig Ketamine geben mußten, erlebt. Unter unseren Kindern waren auch ältere, d. h. 12–14jährige, von denen man annehmen muß, daß sie schon zu einer gewissen kritischen Äußerung in der Lage sind. Wir haben bei unseren Kindern niemals einen Anhalt dafür gehabt, daß psychogenetische Effekte empfunden wurden, so daß eine weitere Wiederholung dieser Anaesthesieform abgelehnt wurde.

Lassner: Es gibt eine Menge Untersuchungen psychologischer Natur über das Krankheitserlebnis bei Kindern. Ich stimme darin überein, daß je nach dem Lebensalter gewisse Erscheinungen, die der Erwachsene oder das Kind nach der Pubertät als krankhaft empfindet, insbesondere z. B. die

Herzkrankheit, von dem jüngeren Kind nicht als solche identifiziert wird; wohl erlebt, aber nicht als krankhaft empfunden wird. Es ist durchaus denkbar, daß die bei Erwachsenen beobachteten Seh-, Geh- oder Sprechstörungen auch beim Kind auftreten, aber von ihm nicht als beunruhigend oder störend interpretiert werden. Das Fehlen dieser Erscheinungen beim Kind kann ich mir schwer vorstellen.

Kreuscher: Wir haben nun gehört, daß diese Substanz eine ganze Reihe nicht erwünschter Nebenwirkungen hat, und wir suchen nach günstigen Indikationen. Bei der Anwendung für kieferchirurgische bzw. zahnärztliche Eingriffe scheint mir noch eine kleine Diskrepanz vorzuliegen, die ich gerne klären möchte. Herr STÖCKEL sagte, daß kieferchirurgische, zahnärztliche Eingriffe eine sehr gute Indikation für Ketamine seien, weil die Schutzreflexe erhalten bleiben. Herr DANGEL aber warnt davor, obwohl er, wenn ich ihn richtig verstanden habe, sogar einen Zwischenfall erlebte, der dank der erhaltenen Schutzreflexe günstig abgelaufen ist. Vielleicht sollte man diese Frage noch einmal diskutieren.

Dangel: Ich glaube, daß Herr STÖCKER und ich uns insofern nicht widersprochen haben, als er nur Eingriffe im Zahn-, Kiefer- und vestibulären Bereich des Mundes unter Ketamine-Anaesthesie durchgeführt hat. Ich habe nur von Eingriffen im Rachen und tieferen Bezirken gewarnt. Ich glaube, daß die Grenze dort liegt, wo Würg-, Brech- und Schluckreflexe ausgelöst werden.

Clinical Experience with Repeated Ketamine Administration for Procedures Requiring Anesthesia

By J. B. Dillon

University of California, Medical Center, School of Medicin, Department of Surgery, Division of Anesthesiology, Los Angeles, California, USA

We have given Ketamine repeatedly to eight patients, ages 15 years and less. The frequency of administration of the anesthetic has varied from a daily basis to a schedule of 2 or 3 injections per week. The period of treatment has ranged from 13 to 40 days. Seven of the patients, ranging in age from 2 months to 4 years, were being treated for primary or metastatic neoplastic disease of the eyes. Four of them had retinoblastomas; two had metastatic neuroblastomas, and one a sarcoma. They were anesthetized to facilitate keeping them in proper position for radiation therapy of the eye. No further manipulation was needed.

An older child with 50% body burns, and under care currently for the acute phase of this injury, has also received Ketamine for 10 times in 14 days so that painful dressings can be changed in a Hubbard tank.

The intramuscular route of administration has been employed in all patients because of difficulty in finding suitable veins. The 5% solution was used for most of the injections; but when the 10% solution became available, it was found preferable in most instances. Usually one injection sufficed.

Inasmuch as the effects after a single injection of the drug are brief and since neither the anesthetic or the procedure was associated with the gastro-intestinal disturbances, the routine feeding schedule of the small patients was not interrupted to any significant extent. These patients continued to gain weight.

Those patients that were ill from their disease, the radiation treatment or intercurrent infection were not made worse by the anesthetic.

No adverse effects on blood or marrow were noted in the patients who had these examinations in conjunction with the treatments.

No behavior problems arose in relation to the need for repeated treatments and injections.

Slight random movement and occasional nystagmus presented no real problem.

No tissue reaction was noted at the site of injection.

Tachyphylaxis did not occur.

The anesthesia was evaluated as satisfactory by the surgeon or radiologist.

The 10% solution available for IM use now appears especially valuable. Onset of anesthesia and analgesia is quicker than with the 5% preparation. The convenience of the smaller volume that can be used makes it very useful.

No tissue reaction has been noted with this concentration.

Zusammenfassung

Bei Kindern bis zum Alter von 15 Jahren wurden wiederholt Ketamine-Anaesthesien durchgeführt. Die Frequenz der Ketamine-Injektionen lag zwischen der täglichen Applikation bis zu 2 oder 3mal wöchentlich. Die Behandlungsdauer reichte von 13–49 Tage. Es wurde stets die intramuskuläre Injektion angewendet. Als Vorteil wurde hervorgehoben, daß die Kinder trotz der häufigen Anaesthesien keine Unterbrechung ihres Ernährungsplanes erfahren mußten, denn weder die Anaesthesie noch die erforderlichen Eingriffe waren mit gastrointestinalen Störungen verbunden. Alle Kinder nahmen kontinuierlich an Gewicht zu. Es wurden keine Gewebereaktionen an der Applikationsstelle beobachtet. Tachyphylaxien traten nicht auf.

Allgemeine klinische Erfahrungen und Indikationen für Ketamine bei mehr als 1600 Fällen

Von **D. Langrehr**

Aus der Anaesthesieabteilung des Zentralkrankenhauses Bremen-Nord, Städt. Krankenanstalten, Bremen (Direktor: O.-Med.-Rat Dr. D. Langrehr)

Die statistische Darbietung der von uns durchgeführten Ketamine-Anaesthesien möchte ich Ihnen ersparen. Ich will aus der Gruppe der Nebenwirkungen herausgreifen, daß man auch bei Ketamine mit einer Atemdepression rechnen muß. Eine Ketamine-Anaesthesie ist daher – wie jede andere Anaesthesie – von einem Anaesthesisten zu überwachen.

Einige Schwierigkeiten kann die Adaptation des Patienten in der Aufwachphase bereiten. Wir haben den Eindruck, daß man bei Berücksichtigung der verschiedenen Möglichkeiten des Zustandekommens der psychischen Phänomene diese richtig handhaben kann. Wir fürchten sie daher nicht; vielmehr sehen wir sie auch bei Erwachsenen immer seltener und geringer ausgeprägt. Die Befunde zur Elektrophysiologie der Reticulärformation erklären die Wirkung einer offensichtlich dort aktiven Substanz. Wir fanden auf Grund unserer Erfahrungen folgende Indikationen für Ketamine, die sich im wesentlichen mit den Mitteilungen anderer Untersucher in Einklang befinden:

1. Die kleine Chirurgie vor allem des Kindesalters, bei alten Menschen und bei Patienten in sehr schlechtem Allgemeinzustand.
2. ophthalmologische und otorhinologische Eingriffe
3. chirurgische Eingriffe im Gesichts- und Halsbereich
4. konservierende Zahnbehandlung, Zahnextraktionen
5. septische Chirurgie besonders bei Diabetikern
6. Frakturbehandlung und Wundversorgung
7. dringliche Erstversorgung im Schock
8. Tracheotomie
9. Radiumeinlagen
10. Bülau-Drainagen
11. schmerzhafte Verbandswechsel besonders bei Verbrennungen und Hauttransplantationen
12. endoskopische und diagnostische Eingriffe wie Bronchoskopien (zusammen mit Relaxantien), Bronchographien, Oesophagogastroskopien,

Cystoskopien, Pneumoencephalographien, Carotis-Angiographien, Myelographien, Laparoskopien.

Besonders geeignet ist Ketamine für die Narkoseeinleitung in der großen Risikochirurgie und bei geburtshilflichen Eingriffen.

Wir sind der Auffassung, daß Ketamine eine echte Bereicherung unseres anaesthesiologischen Arzneimittelschatzes darstellen könnte.

Erschienene Bände (Fortsetzung) :

28 Die Wiederbelebung der Atmung. Von H. Nolte. DM 8,—

29 Kontrolle der Ventilation in der Neugeborenen- und Säuglingsanaesthesie. Von U. Henneberg. DM 19,80

30 Hypoxie. Herausgegeben von R. Frey, K. Lang, M. Halmágyi und G. Thews. DM 48,—

31 Kohlenhydrate in der dringlichen Infusionstherapie. Herausgegeben von K. Lang, R. Frey und M. Halmágyi. DM 18,—

32 Örtliche Betäubung: Abdominal-Chirurgie. Von Sir Robert R. Macintosh und R. Bryce-Smith. DM 38,—

33 Planung, Organisation und Einrichtung von Intensivbehandlungseinheiten am Krankenhaus. Herausgegeben von H. W. Opderbecke. DM 34,—

34 Venendruckmessung. Herausgegeben von M. Allgöwer, R. Frey und M. Halmágyi. DM 24,—

35 Die Störungen des Säure-Basen-Haushaltes. Herausgegeben von V. Feurstein. DM 38,—

36 Anaesthesie und Nierenfunktion. Herausgegeben von V. Feurstein. DM 36,—

37 Anaesthesie und Kohlenhydratstoffwechsel. Herausgegeben von V. Feurstein. DM 24,—

38 Respiratorbeatmung und Oberflächenspannung in der Lunge. Von H. Benzer. DM 16,—

39 Die nasotracheale Intubation. Von M. Körner. DM 28,—

40 Ketamine. Herausgegeben von H. Kreuscher. DM 36,—

41 Über das Verhalten von Ventilation, Gasaustausch und Kreislauf bei Patienten mit normalem und gestörtem Gasaustausch unter künstlicher Totraumvergrößerung. Von O. Giebel. DM 18,—

42 Der Narkoseapparat. Von P. Schreiber. DM 19,80

In Vorbereitung :

43 Die Klinik des Wundstarrkrampfes im Lichte neuzeitlicher Behandlungsmethoden. Von K. Eyrich

44 Der primäre Volumenersatz mit Ringerlaktat. Von A. O. Tetzlaff

45 Vergiftungen: Erkennung, Verhütung und Behandlung. Herausgegeben von R. Frey, M. Halmágyi, K. Lang und P. Oettel